Future Perspectives in Primary Care Research

This book explores the current developments and future directions of primary care research, emphasising innovative approaches, methodologies and technologies that are shaping the field. The content examines the scope of primary care research in various contexts, including emerging trends in primary care research and recent innovations such as digitalisation, providing practical insights into the application of advanced research methods in primary care for both new and experienced researchers.

Structured to provide step-by-step guidance on various research techniques, addressing the economic evaluations of interventions and identifying areas for innovation in primary care research, readers will acquire a robust understanding of modern primary care research methods, enabling them to contribute significantly to the academic and practical aspects of the discipline.

Key Features:

- Describes the current state of primary care research and makes projections of its future trajectory
- Delves into the unique and specific nature of primary care research, discussing its ontological, epistemological and methodological foundations
- Explores cutting-edge research theories and methods, including pragmatic trials, complexity research and the implementation of innovative study designs
- Highlights the importance of the incorporation of digital tools and artificial intelligence in primary care research, addressing both their practical applications and ethical considerations

As a comprehensive guide for researchers, practitioners and policymakers, highlighting emerging trends and providing practical insights into the application of advanced research methods in primary care, this book is particularly valuable for academics and researchers at universities and institutions around the world, empowering them to conduct impactful research and develop evidence-based practices. It will be an essential tool for those looking to enhance their research skills, foster interdisciplinary collaborations and contribute to the global advancement of primary care.

WONCA Family Medicine

About the Series

The WONCA Family Medicine series is a collection of books written by world-wide experts and practitioners of family medicine, in collaboration with The World Organization of Family Doctors (WONCA). WONCA is a not-for-profit organization and was founded in 1972 by member organizations in 18 countries. It now has 118 Member Organizations in 131 countries and territories with membership of about 500,000 family doctors and more than 90 per cent of the world's population.

Migrant Health: A Primary Care Perspective
Bernadette N. Kumar and Esperanza Diaz

Global Primary Mental Health Care: Practical Guidance for Family Doctors
Christopher Dowrick

How To Do Primary Care Educational Research: A Practical Guide
Mehmet Akman, Valerie Wass and Felicity Goodyear-Smith

ICPC-3 International Classification of Primary Care: User Manual and Classification
Kees van Boven and Huib Ten Napel

Family Medicine in the Undergraduate Curriculum: Preparing medical students to work in evolving health care systems
Valerie Wass and Victor Ng

Anxiety and Depression in Primary Care: International Perspectives
Sherina Mohd-Sidik and Felicity Goodyear-Smith

Core Values in Family Medicine
Anna Stavdal, Johann Agust Sigurdsson and Felicity Goodyear-Smith

Digital Health for Primary Care
Ana Luisa Neves and Lilliana Laranjo

Challenges in Primary Mental Health Care
Christos Lionis and Christopher Dowrick

Working with Adolescents and Young Adults: A Guide for Family Physicians
Pierre-Paul Tellier, Muna Chowdhury and Maria Veronica Svetaz

Future Perspectives in Primary Care Research
Mehmet Akman, Bob Mash and Felicity Goodyear-Smith

For more information about this series please visit: https://www.crcpress.com/WONCA-Family-Medicine/book-series/WONCA

Future Perspectives in Primary Care Research

Edited by

Mehmet Akman, Bob Mash and
Felicity Goodyear-Smith

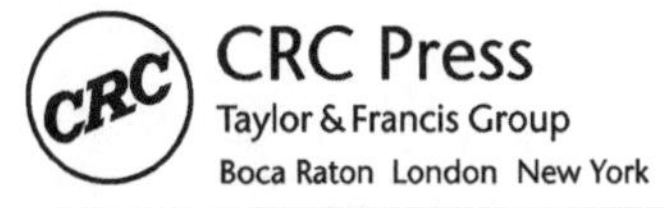

CRC Press is an imprint of the
Taylor & Francis Group, an **informa** business

Designed cover image: Getty Images

First edition published 2026
by CRC Press
2385 NW Executive Center Drive, Suite 320, Boca Raton FL 33431

and by CRC Press
4 Park Square, Milton Park, Abingdon, Oxon, OX14 4RN

CRC Press is an imprint of Taylor & Francis Group, LLC

ISBN: 978-1-041-09851-5 (hbk)
ISBN: 978-1-041-09850-8 (pbk)
ISBN: 978-1-003-65210-6 (ebk)

DOI: 10.1201/9781003652106

Typeset in Minion
by Apex CoVantage, LLC

Contents

Foreword

Strong and sustainable primary care forms the bedrock of effective health systems across the world. The World Health Organization has identified five core functions of primary care: (1) first contact accessibility ensures timely equitable access; (2) continuity builds trusted relationships; (3) coordination supports the integration of services; (4) comprehensiveness ensures access to a full range of services; and (5) people-centeredness empowers people to take an active role in their health.[1] These essential building blocks form the foundation for effective health provision that manages acute illness and chronic disease and provides health promotion and preventative care whilst considering the wider population health needs of the communities we work in.

Primary care needs to be underpinned with robust research that is appropriate to the setting where services are delivered. Too often, decisions made by clinicians and policymakers are based on evidence generated in secondary care, focusing on patient populations that simply do not represent the type of patients managed in the community. It is time for clinicians, policymakers, patients and grant funders to prioritise primary care research. Yet the complexity of research in this setting is often under-appreciated. The infrastructure to support high-quality research is often lacking and, where it does exist, it can be difficult to access. Engaging with the pubic and policymakers is difficult and can be resource intensive. Clinical training, at both undergraduate and postgraduate levels, frequently does not prepare health and care professionals to be research active, and funding for formal research training (at masters and doctoral levels) is hard to obtain and often too expensive or time consuming to be a realistic option.[2]

Primary care is diverse, and as such the approach taken to generating evidence in this setting needs to be carefully tailored. Strong methodological approaches underpin robust findings, and it is important that clinicians and academics are fully aware of innovation in this area. Furthermore, to be relevant, research must be inclusive, proactively working with communities not traditionally involved in research to ensure findings are truly representative. Clinicians and researchers need an ever-growing skill set, with a heightened awareness of the most appropriate methodological approach needed to address the issues raised.

The COVID-19 pandemic rapidly changed the way in which we work and highlighted the need to embrace technology. Digital technologies have the potential to revolutionise the approach we take for research.[3] Electronic medical records can provide unique data at both the local and national levels, providing large databases to inform training, health planning and service provision. Routine consultation data, if rigorously collected, is a valuable resource that is even richer when practices work together, providing a more comprehensive resource. Technology-enabled research, including clinical trials, can reach remote and rural communities, allowing people previously excluded from research to participate. Not only does this enhance the richness of the evidence generated, but it is an important educational outlet for patients and clinicians. On-line focus groups, surveys completed through an email link, text message and WhatsApp responses to questions are all increasingly used and can help reduce costs. However, inclusivity needs to be at the heart of all our approaches, taking care not to reinforce digital exclusion and marginalised socioeconomically deprived communities.

The importance of patient and public involvement and community engagement are well established, yet this critical component is too frequently missing or tokenistic. This fails to recognise the key role patients play in co-designing research and risks disengagement, lack of study uptake and problems in study delivery when missing. Only through building trusted partnerships with patients, families and community leaders can research be designed and delivered that addresses unmet needs and generates wider impact. Meaningful engagement can be challenging and resource intensive, but the process can build a highly productive and long-lasting legacy that empowers communities, supports researchers and generates relevant research that best addresses the needs of local populations. This approach needs to be embedded from the earliest stages of research, with patients treated as equal partners, removing traditional hierarchy and through promoting mutual respect for the skills each team member brings.[4]

One of the strengths of primary care is our commitment to multi-disciplinary working. This approach reinforces the holistic nature and person-centredness associated with primary care that improves outcomes for patients. High-quality research should also be multi-disciplinary, drawing in talent from a broad range of professional backgrounds. By transcending traditional barriers, complex and challenging questions can be addressed from a diverse range of perspectives, providing new insight that benefits patients, clinicians and policymakers. Moving beyond the biomedical model of disease, to actively include the psychosocial components of health and well-being, gives us a more comprehensive understanding and provides evidence that is hugely beneficial to end users.

The research journey should not end with publication. Those conducting research have an ethical responsibility to mobilise the evidence, helping clinicians and policymakers to access and implement findings that help patients. This process is often more difficult than conducting the original study and needs to start at study conception. Getting evidence into practice is an active process that needs strong networks, community engagement to appreciate the local context, and an understanding of behaviour change.

This new book, edited by Akman, Mash and Goodyear-Smith, is an essential addition to the family medicine toolkit and should be core reading for the multidisciplinary primary healthcare team and established academics alike. Written by international leaders in primary care research with strong track records in the design and delivery of clinical studies, *Future Perspectives in Primary Care Research* builds on the fundamentals of study design and provides new insight into a rapidly evolving field. To address the contemporary health issues we face, we need to innovate, embracing new ways of working and using diverse methodological approaches. Primary care is facing an epidemic of obesity, the growing burden of long-term conditions and a rapidly aging population. To tackle these issues head-on and generate the evidence we urgently need, we have to start to think differently and adopt new approaches to research. Only then can we provide the care our patients deserve.

Professor Christian Mallen
Professor of General Practice and Public Health
Executive Dean, Keele University
Director, NIHR School for Primary Care Research

References

1. Integrated primary care for UHC. World Health Organization. [Available from: https://www.who.int/teams/integrated-health-services/clinical-services-and-systems/primary-care]
2. Bonfim D, Belotti L, Yamawaka de Almeida L, Eshriqui I, Velasco S, Monteiro C, Jantsch A. Challenges and strategies for conducting research in primary health care practice: An integrative review. *BMC Health Serv Res.* 2023 Dec 8;23(1):1380. https://doi.org/10.1186/s12913-023-10382-1
3. Rosa C, Marsch LA, Winstanley EL, Brunner M, Campbell ANC. Using digital technologies in clinical trials: Current and future applications. *Contemp Clin Trials.* 2021 Jan;100:106219. https://doi.org/10.1016/j.cct.2020.106219
4. Arumugam A, Phillips LR, Moore A, Kumaran SD, Sampath KK, Migliorini F, Maffulli N, Ranganadhababu BN, Hegazy F, Botto-van Bemden A. Patient and public involvement in research: Review of practical resources for young investigators. *BMC Rheumatol.* 2023 Mar 9;7(1):2. https://doi.org/10.1186/s41927-023-00327-w

Editors

Mehmet Akman, MD, MPH, is a general practitioner and professor of family medicine at the Faculty of Medicine and Health Sciences, Karabakh University, and Chief of the family health center at Karabakh University Clinic, Khankendi, Azerbaijan. He is also Emeritus Professor at Marmara University School of Medicine, Istanbul, Türkiye. Dr Akman is the immediate past Chair of the WONCA Working Party on Research and co-editor of the WONCA series book *How to Do Primary Care Educational Research.* He is Co-Editor-in-Chief of *Primary Health Care Research & Development* and an executive board member of the European Forum for Primary Care. He has published over 100 peer-reviewed papers. His research focuses on chronic disease management, primary care organisation and health systems strengthening.

Bob Mash, MBChB, PhD, FRCP, is a family physician and professor at the Division of Family Medicine and Primary Care, Stellenbosch University, South Africa. He is the Editor-in-Chief of the *African Journal of Primary Health Care and Family Medicine* and has published over 300 peer-reviewed papers. He is an international member of the National Academy of Medicine in the US and currently the President of the WONCA Africa Region. He has co-edited two previous WONCA books on primary care research.

Felicity Goodyear-Smith, MBChB, MGP, MD, FRNZCGP (Dist), is a general practitioner and professor of general practice and primary healthcare at the University of Auckland, New Zealand. She has a long involvement with WONCA, including past Chair of its Working Party on Research. She has previously co-edited five books in the WONCA Family Medicine series and has also contributed chapters to three other books in this series. Dr Goodyear-Smith was the founding editor-in-chief of the *Journal of Primary Health Care*, which she has now co-edits. She has published over 360 peer-reviewed papers as well as a number of books and book chapters.

Contributors

Monica Aggarwal, PhD
Assistant Professor
Dalla Lana School of Public Health and Department of Family and Community Medicine
University of Toronto
Toronto, Canada

Max O Bachmann, MBChB, bDOH, MSc, PhD, FFCH
Professor of Health Services Research
Norwich Medical School, University of East Anglia
Norwich, England

Erica Barbazza, MSc, PhD
Public and Occupational Health
University of Amsterdam
Meibergdreef 9 and Amsterdam Public Health Research Institute, Quality of Care
Amsterdam, The Netherlands

Duygu Ayhan Başer
Department of Family Medicine
Hacettepe University
Ankara, Türkiye

Shona Bates, BSc, MSc, PhD
International Centre for Future Health Systems
University of New South Wales
Sydney, Australia

Peter Brown, BIT, PhD
International Centre for Future Health Systems
University of New South Wales
Sydney, Australia

Amber Wheatley Buckell, BSc, MBMCh
Primary Care Registrar
British Virgin Islands Health Service Authority
British Virgin Islands

Christopher C Butler, BA, MBChB, DCH, CCH, MD, FRCGP, (Hon) FFPH, FMedSci
Professor of Primary Care
Nuffield Department of Primary Care Health Sciences
University of Oxford
Oxford, England

Plaxcedes Chiwire, PhD
Department of Health Services Research, CAPHRI Care and Public Health Research Institute
Maastricht University
Maastricht, The Netherlands

Rafal Chomik, BCom, MSc, PhD
International Centre for Future Health Systems
University of New South Wales
Sydney, Australia

Margarida Gil Conde, MD, FMS, PhD
Specialist in Family Medicine
University Clinic of Family Medicine
Faculdade de Medicina da Universidade de Lisboa
Lisbon, Portugal

Benjamin F Crabtree, PhD
Distinguished Professor
Rutgers Robert Wood Johnson Medical School
New Brunswick, New Jersey, United States

Lynden Crowshoe, MD
Associate Professor
Department of Family Medicine
Cuming School of Medicine, University of Calgary
Alberta, Canada

Anna Dania, PhD
Family Medicine
Faculty of Health, Medicine and Life Sciences
Maastricht University
Maastricht, The Netherlands

Patricia Mary Davidson, BNurs, MSc, PhD
Foundation Co-Director
International Centre for Future Health Systems
University of New South Wales
Sydney, Australia

Enrique Falceto de Barros
Professor
Universidade Feevale
Novo Hamburgo, Brazil

Chris Dietz, LLB, MA criminology, PhD
International Centre for Future Health Systems
University of New South Wales
Sydney, Australia

Kyle Eggleton, MBChB, MMedSci, MPH, PhD, FRNZCGP (Dist)
Associate Dean Rural, Associate Professor and General Practitioner
Department of General Practice and Primary Health Care
University of Auckland
Auckland, New Zealand

Enrique Falceto de Barros, MD, PhD Professor
Saúde Planetária Brasil
São Paulo, Brazil

Óscar Brito Fernandes, MSc, PhD
Public and Occupational Health
University of Amsterdam, Meibergdreef 9 and Amsterdam
Public Health Research Institute, Quality of Care
Amsterdam, The Netherlands

Thomas Frese
Professor and Head of Department
Institute of General Practice and Family Medicine
Martin-Luther-University
Halle-Wittenberg, Germany

Özden Gökdemir, MD, PhD
Associate Professor
Faculty of Medicine
Izmir University of Economics
İzmir, Türkiye

Trisha Greenhalgh, OBE, BM Bch, MD, FRCP, FRCGP, MedSci
Professor of Primary Health Care and General Practitioner
Nuffield Department of Primary Care Health Sciences
University of Oxford
Oxford, England

Robert J Havey, MD
Clinical Professor of Medicine and Deputy Director
Institute for Global Health, Feinberg School of Medicine
Northwestern University
Chicago, Illinois, United States

Lisa R Hirschhorn, MD, MPH
Professor, Medical Social Sciences
Department of Medical Social Sciences
Feinberg School of Medicine
Director, Ryan Family Center on Global Primary Care
Havey Institute for Global Health
Northwestern University
Chicago, Illinois, United States

Kiran Jobanputra, MBChB, BSc(Hons), MPH, MRCGP
Climate Action Accelerator
Geneva, Switzerland

Alan Katz, MBChB, MSc, CCFP
Professor in Family Medicine
Max Rady College of Medicine
University of Manitoba
Winnipeg, Manitoba, Canada

Martina Kelly, MB Bch, BAO, MA, PhD, FRCGP, CCFP
Professor and Family Physician
Department of Family Medicine and Community Health Sciences
Cumming School of Medicine, University of Calgary
Alberta, Canada

Candan Kendir
Directorate for Employment, Labour and Social Affairs
Organisation for Economic Co-Operation and Development (OECD)
Paris, France
Public and Occupational Health,
University of Amsterdam,
Meibergdreef 9 and Amsterdam, The Netherlands

Michael Kidd, AO, MBBS, MD, FAHMS
Professor and Foundation Director
International Centre for Future Health Systems
University of New South Wales
Sydney, Australia

Buğu Usanma Koban, MD, PhD
Family Medicine Department
Marmara University
Istanbul, Türkiye

Dilge Kocabaş, MD
Hakan Joint Occupational Health and Safety Unit
İzmir, Türkiye

Dionne Kringos, MSc, PhD
Public and Occupational Health
University of Amsterdam
Meibergdreef 9 and Amsterdam
Public Health Research Institute, Quality of Care
Amsterdam, The Netherlands

Jialing Lin, BMed, MMed, PhD
International Centre for Future Health Systems
University of New South Wales
Sydney, Australia

Akim Tafadzwa Lukwa, PhD
Health Economics Unit, School of Public Health and Family Medicine
University of Cape Town
Cape Town, South Africa

William L Miller, MD, MA
Chair Emeritus
Lehigh Valley Health Network
Allentown, Pennsylvania, United States

Stephanie Montesanti, MA, PhD
Professor and Canada Research Chair (Tier 2) in Health System Integration
University of Alberta
Edmonton, Alberta, Canada

Paulo Jorge Nicola, MD, FMS, MSc (Clin Res)
Specialist in Family Medicine
Epidemiology Unit, Instituto de Medicina Preventiva e Saúde Pública
Faculdade de Medicina da Universidade de Lisboa
Lisbon, Portugal

Samuela Ofanoa, MPH, PhD
Research Fellow
Pacific Health, School of Population Health
University of Auckland
Auckland, New Zealand

William R Phillips, MD, MPH, FAAFP
Professor Emeritus of Family Medicine
University of Washington
Seattle, Washington, United States

Sankha Randenikumara, MBBS, MCGP
Chief Family Physician
The Family Health Clinic
Colombo, Sri Lanka
Chair of WONCA Working Party on Planetary Health

Joseph B Ross, BA, MPA
Associate Director
Ariadne Labs, Harvard School of Public Health
Brigham and Women's Hospital
Boston, Massachusetts, United States

Ginetta Salvalaggio, MSc, MD, CCFP(AM)
Professor
Department of Family Medicine
University of Alberta
Edmonton, Alberta, Canada

Patricia Nayna Schwerdtle, BN, BAppSc(HealthProm), MIntHlth, Dr sc hum
Faculty of Medicine
Heidelberg Institute of Global Health (HIGH)
University Hospital, Heidelberg University
Heidelberg, Germany
The Climate Action Accelerator
Geneva, Switzerland

Florian O Stummer, MPH, MBA, PhD
Institute of General Practice and Family Medicine
Martin-Luther-University
Halle-Wittenberg, Germany

Elizabeth Sturgiss, BMed, PhD, FRACGP, MPH, MForensMed, FHEA
Professor
Faculty of Health Sciences and Medicine
Bond University
Queensland, Australia

Tokuharu Tanaka, MD, PhD
Assistant Professor
Department of Emergency and Family Medicine
University of Fukui Hospital
Fukui City, Japan

Patricia Thille, BSc (PT), MA, PhD
Associate Professor
Department of Physical Therapy, College of Rehabilitation Sciences
University of Manitoba
Winnipeg, Canada

Siobhan Tu'akoi, BHSc (hon), PhD
Senior Research Fellow
Pacific Health, School of Population Health
University of Auckland
Auckland, New Zealand

Karen Tu, MD, MSc
Professor
Department of Family and Community Medicine
University of Toronto
Toronto, ON, Canada

Ülkü Sur Ünal, MD
Assistant Professor
Marmara University School of Medicine
Department of Family Medicine
Istanbul, Türkiye

Jose M Valderas
Department of Family Medicine
National University Health System
Singapore, Singapore

Braulio Mark Valencia, MD, MSc, PhD
International Centre for Future Health Systems
University of New South Wales
Sydney, Australia

Maria van den Muijsenbergh, MD, PhD
Emeritus Professor of Health Disparities
Primary Care and General Practitioner
Radboud University Medical Center
Nijmegen, Netherlands

Nathaly Karina Velásquez Ipanaqué, MD, PhD
Specialist in Family and Community Medicine and Head
Villa Campoy Community Mental Health Center
Lima, Peru
Young Doctors' Liaison
WONCA Working Party on Planetary Health

Marc R Wilkins, BSc (hons), PhD, DSc.
International Centre for Future Health Systems
University of New South Wales
Sydney, Australia

Sabrina T Wong, RN, PhD, FCAHS, FAAN
Professor
School of Nursing and Centre for Health Services and Policy Research
University of British Columbia
Vancouver, Canada

SECTION

1

Introduction

CHAPTER

1 Purpose and Scope of This Book

Mehmet Akman, Bob Mash and Felicity Goodyear-Smith

This book, *Future Perspectives in Primary Care Research*, is a timely contribution to the CRC Press WONCA Family Medicine series, following three previous volumes: *International Perspectives on Primary Care Research*,[1] *How To Do Primary Care Research*,[2] and *How To Do Primary Care Educational Research*.[3] While these earlier books offered foundational knowledge and practical guidance for conducting and teaching research in primary care, this volume looks purposefully to the future. It focuses on emerging paradigms, expanding boundaries and innovative methodologies that are reshaping how primary care research is conceptualised, conducted and used. It explores current developments and future directions of primary care research, emphasising approaches that are both scientifically rigorous and contextually sound. As primary care evolves in response to global health challenges—rising multimorbidity, digitalisation, climate change and shifting population needs—researchers are called to develop new methods and frameworks that capture this complexity. The book aims to serve as a comprehensive guide for researchers, educators and policymakers, offering critical insights into how research in primary care can remain responsive, inclusive and impactful.

Rather than viewing research through a narrow biomedical lens, this book recognises the unique nature of knowledge and reality as experienced within primary care. It acknowledges that the discipline demands methodologies reflecting the relational, continuous, person- and community-centred nature of care. Accordingly, the chapters explore themes such as complexity thinking, reflexivity, ethical considerations in digital and artificial intelligence (AI) research and the creative integration of arts in health inquiry. These approaches, while diverse, are unified by a shared commitment to capturing the lived experience of health and illness within the real-world context of primary care.

Technological innovation is one of the central axes of this book. Several chapters examine how big data, digital tools and AI are increasingly being incorporated into

DOI: 10.1201/9781003652106-2

primary care research, offering opportunities to enhance data-driven insight while raising important ethical and methodological questions. The volume addresses the governance of digital data, the ethics of AI deployment and the importance of protecting patient autonomy and trust in the digital age. These explorations are grounded in the recognition that technology must serve—not overshadow—the human dimensions of care.

The book widens the research lens of primary care, addressing topics that reflect the field's growing complexity and societal relevance. Chapters discuss the research implications of genomic and personalised care, the value of linking individual and community health perspectives, and the role of planetary health in reshaping healthcare priorities. These thematic expansions invite primary care researchers to adopt a transdisciplinary lens, forging connections between clinical care, public health and ecological sustainability.

As primary care research expands in breadth and complexity, its methodological approaches must evolve accordingly. The book includes discussions on new clinical trial designs tailored to primary care realities, the use of scoping reviews and mapping exercises, implementation research for closing the evidence–practice gap and participatory methods that engage patients and communities in co-producing knowledge. Special attention is given to qualitative rigour through chapters on reflexive analysis, coding strategies and the use of theoretical and analytical frameworks appropriate to the complexity of primary care systems. The closing section reflects on what lies ahead—emphasising the need to build and sustain research capacity, to strengthen institutional foundations and to ensure that research becomes an embedded, routine aspect of clinical care. These chapters envision a future where researcher development is prioritised—especially in underserved regions—and where academic settings fully embrace research that bridges local impact with international insight.

This book is intended for an international audience of primary care researchers, educators, clinicians and policymakers. It is particularly relevant to faculty and postgraduate students working in departments of family medicine, general practice, nursing and allied health sciences, as well as to professionals engaged in community health, public health and health services research. The book also provides valuable perspectives for early-career researchers and those working in resource-constrained settings. The vision and values that shape this book are closely aligned with the goals of the World Organization of Family Doctors (WONCA), and the volume is developed through the active contributions of the WONCA Working Party on Research.

By the end of this book, readers will have acquired not only a deeper understanding of future-focused research approaches but also a renewed sense of purpose in advancing the discipline of primary care. The chapters collectively demonstrate that primary care research is not only methodologically diverse and intellectually rich—it is also essential to achieving better health outcomes, more responsive health systems and greater social accountability. As the editors, we believe that this book will be both a map and a mandate for researchers who are determined to shape the future of healthcare through the lens of primary care.

References

1. Goodyear-Smith F, Mash B, editors. International perspectives on primary care research. Boca Raton: CRC Press; 2016.
2. Goodyear-Smith F, Mash B, editors. How to do primary care research. Boca Raton: CRC Press; 2018.
3. Akman M, Wass V, Goodyear-Smith F, editors. How to do primary care educational research. Boca Raton: CRC Press; 2021.

CHAPTER

2

The Need for Future-Oriented Primary Care Research

Alan Katz

2.1 Introduction

Primary care stands at a critical juncture in healthcare evolution. As the foundation of high-functioning health systems worldwide, it faces unprecedented challenges, while being presented with transformative opportunities that could reshape how we understand, deliver and research healthcare. The traditional paradigms of primary care research, rooted in a biomedical and descriptive/observational paradigm, while remaining valuable, are proving insufficient to address the complex, interconnected challenges of 21st-century healthcare delivery.

The landscape of primary care is rapidly evolving, driven by technological advancement, demographic transitions, climate change, recognition of the importance of the social determinants of health and the growing recognition that health extends far beyond clinical encounters. This evolution demands a fundamental reimagining of how we conduct primary care research, one that embraces complexity, anticipates future challenges and develops innovative methodologies capable of generating actionable insights for an uncertain future.

Future-oriented primary care research represents a paradigm shift from reactive to proactive inquiry, from siloed disciplines to interdisciplinary collaboration, and from standardised interventions to personalised, context-sensitive approaches. This chapter explores the imperative for this transformation, examining the trends and challenges that necessitate new research approaches while outlining the innovative methodologies that will shape the future of primary care research.

2.2 The Evolving Landscape of Primary Care

2.2.1 Demographic and Epidemiological Transitions

The global burden of disease has undergone dramatic transformation over the past several decades. The epidemiological transition from acute infectious diseases,

DOI: 10.1201/9781003652106-3

prevalent in low- and middle-income countries, to chronic non-communicable diseases, has fundamentally altered the primary care landscape, mirroring the challenges of high-income countries.[1] Today's primary care providers increasingly manage complex patients with multiple comorbidities, requiring sophisticated care coordination and long-term management strategies, which traditional biomedical models struggle to effectively address.

Simultaneously, population aging presents unprecedented challenges for primary care systems. By 2050, the global population aged 60 and older is projected to reach 2.1 billion, with many countries experiencing rapid increases in their elderly populations.[2] This demographic shift necessitates research approaches that can inform age-friendly primary care delivery, understand the complex interplay of biological aging with social determinants, and develop sustainable models of care for aging populations.

2.2.2 Technological Disruption and Digital Health

The digital revolution has fundamentally transformed healthcare delivery and opened new frontiers for primary care research. Electronic health records, telemedicine, mobile health applications and wearable devices generate vast amounts of real-world data that offer unprecedented opportunities for understanding health patterns, predicting disease progression and personalising interventions.[3] The COVID-19 pandemic precipitated a new acceptance of virtual primary care delivery, with many unanswered questions about safety and efficacy.[4] Chapter 6 looks at how digital tools can empower primary care research.

Artificial intelligence and machine learning applications in primary care are moving from tools facilitating practice efficiency such as ambient voice scribes, to clinical tools offering diagnostic support, risk stratification and treatment optimisation. However, these technological advances also raise critical questions about algorithm bias, data privacy, clinical decision-making autonomy and the digital divide that future-oriented research must address.[5]

2.2.3 Climate Change and Planetary Health

Climate change represents one of the most significant threats to human health in the 21st century, with primary care positioned as the frontline for addressing climate-related health impacts. From heat-related illness and vector-borne diseases to mental health impacts of climate anxiety and displacement, primary care providers increasingly encounter the health consequences of environmental degradation.[6,7] In addition, primary care delivery currently contributes to the problem. Research into ways to mitigate this contribution through clinic functioning to prescribing patterns is essential to reduce the impact of service delivery.

This reality demands research approaches that can understand the complex pathways through which environmental factors influence health, develop climate-resilient primary care systems and explore the role of primary care in promoting both human and planetary health. The concept of planetary health research represents a new frontier that integrates environmental sustainability with human health outcomes.[8] Chapter 16 further explores planetary health research.

2.2.4 Social Determinants and Health Equity

The recognition that health outcomes are primarily determined by social, economic and environmental factors rather than clinical interventions has profound implications for primary care research. Social determinants of health, including income, education, housing, food security and social supports, account for an estimated 80% of health outcomes, yet traditional clinical research often fails to adequately address these factors.[9]

This understanding demands research approaches that can capture the complexity of social determinants, understand their mechanisms of action and develop interventions that address root causes of health inequity. Community-based participatory research, implementation science and complex systems approaches are increasingly recognised as essential methodologies for addressing these challenges.[10,11]

2.3 Emerging Challenges in Primary Care Research

2.3.1 Research Infrastructure

Primary care delivery is predominantly community-based. This places a unique challenge on primary care disciplines to advance research outside of the framework of academic centres, in addition to developing academic clinician-researchers. This includes ensuring that trainees have a positive research attitude to lobby for primary care research funding. Practitioners who wish to do research in their own practices can be sustained through practice-based research networks to study important questions (see Chapter 10).

2.3.2 Complexity and Multimorbidity

Traditional research methodologies, particularly randomised controlled trials, are poorly suited to address the complexity of modern primary care practice. Most clinical trials exclude patients with multiple conditions, yet multimorbidity is the norm rather than the exception in primary care settings. Research approaches must evolve to address the complexity of real-world primary care, where patients present with multiple interacting conditions, treatments may have competing effects, and outcomes are influenced by a multitude of factors beyond the intervention under study.[12] Trish Greenhalgh's Chapter 3 explores complexity thinking in depth.

Complex adaptive systems thinking offers promising approaches for understanding primary care as a dynamic system characterised by non-linear relationships and unpredictable behaviours. This perspective suggests that research methodologies must be capable of capturing complexity rather than controlling for it.[13]

2.3.3 Personalisation and Precision Medicine

The promise of precision medicine delivering the right treatment to the right patient at the right time presents both opportunities and challenges for primary care research. Genomic medicine, biomarker development and algorithmic risk prediction offer unprecedented possibilities for personalising primary care interventions. However, implementing precision medicine in primary care requires research approaches that can address questions of clinical utility, cost-effectiveness, implementation feasibility and equity.[14] Chapter 11 discusses the research implications of genomics in personalised primary care.

The integration of genomics into primary care represents a particular challenge, requiring research that can bridge the gap between genomic discoveries and clinical application, while addressing issues of genetic literacy, counselling capacity and equitable access to genomic technologies. How to add these complexities to already unrealistic expectations, which have led to dramatic increases in the burnout of primary care providers, will require local context-based research.[15]

2.3.4 Implementation and Translation

The persistent gap between research evidence and clinical practice represents a fundamental challenge for primary care research. Traditional efficacy studies, conducted under controlled conditions, often fail to translate to real-world effectiveness when implemented in diverse primary care settings. Implementation science has emerged as a critical discipline for understanding how evidence-based interventions can be successfully adopted, adapted and sustained in primary care practice (see Chapter 19).[16]

Future-oriented primary care research must integrate implementation considerations from the outset, employing effectiveness-implementation hybrid designs that simultaneously test intervention effectiveness and implementation strategies.[17] This approach recognises that understanding 'what works' is inseparable from understanding 'how to make it work' in real-world primary care settings. The inclusion of the end users of research findings, which may include policymakers, health system managers, clinicians and patients, is a fundamental requirement of knowledge translation.[18]

2.3.5 Global Health Disparities

Primary care research has historically been dominated by studies conducted in high-income countries, with limited generalisability to LMICs, where the majority of the world's population live. LMICs face unique challenges, including resource constraints, evolving disease burdens, varying healthcare delivery models and distinct social and cultural contexts, that require locally relevant research approaches.[19]

The need for indigenous research capacity, culturally appropriate methodologies and locally relevant interventions represents a critical priority for future-oriented primary care research. This includes understanding how global health innovations can be adapted to LMIC contexts while avoiding the pitfalls of medical colonialism and ensuring that research benefits the communities where it is conducted—'nothing about us without us' and addressing systemic racism in healthcare.[20]

2.4 Innovative Research Methodologies for Future Primary Care

2.4.1 Master Protocol Clinical Trials

Traditional clinical trial methodology, with its emphasis on testing single interventions in homogeneous populations, is increasingly recognised as inadequate for addressing the complexity of primary care practice. Master protocol clinical trials such as 'platform trials' represent an innovative approach that allows multiple interventions to be tested simultaneously within a single trial infrastructure, with the ability to add or remove interventions based on accumulating evidence (see also Chapter 17).[21]

In primary care, master protocol trials offer the potential to efficiently test multiple interventions for common conditions, compare different implementation strategies and adapt trial designs based on real-world performance. This approach is particularly valuable for chronic disease management, where multiple therapeutic options exist, and personalised treatment selection is critical for optimal outcomes.

2.4.2 Big Data and Observational Studies

The proliferation of electronic health records, claims databases and digital health technologies has created unprecedented opportunities for generating real-world evidence about primary care interventions and outcomes. Big data approaches allow researchers to study large, diverse populations, examine long-term outcomes and identify rare but important adverse events that may not be detected in traditional primary data collection.[22] However, big data research also presents significant challenges, including data quality issues, indigenous data sovereignty, inability to address causation rather than association and the need for sophisticated analytical methods to extract meaningful insights from complex datasets. This is covered in full in Chapter 4.

2.4.3 Artificial Intelligence (AI) and Machine Learning

AI and machine learning techniques offer huge potential to transform primary care research and practice, with predictive modelling and clinical decision support and the automation of clinical workflows. Natural language processing can extract valuable information from unstructured clinical notes, while deep learning algorithms can identify subtle patterns in physiological signals that may not be apparent to human observers.[23]

In primary care research, AI applications include developing and testing clinical prediction rules, potentially identifying patients at risk for adverse outcomes or optimising treatment selection. However, the implementation of AI in all clinical research requires careful attention to algorithm transparency and bias mitigation. The lack of algorithm transparency is a major challenge in primary care where patient-provider trust is so fundamental. See Chapter 5 for further details on the use of AI in primary care research.

2.4.4 Transdisciplinary Research Approaches

The complex challenges facing primary care cannot be adequately addressed by any single discipline or sector. Transdisciplinary research, which works across disciplines and sectors so that interdisciplinary knowledge may breach the boundary between science and society, offers a promising approach for addressing complex primary care challenges (see also Chapter 13).[24]

Transdisciplinary primary care research might integrate biomedical sciences with social sciences, engineering, environmental sciences, humanities and communities to develop a comprehensive understanding of health and illness. This approach is particularly valuable for addressing complex challenges such as climate change and health, social determinants of health and the development of complex interventions that operate at multiple levels of the healthcare system. This paradigm of research is complex, involving larger teams from different sectors with different funding structures and cultures. Two examples of transdisciplinary research are presented.[25]

2.4.5 Creative Arts and Innovative Methodologies

The integration of creative arts into primary care research represents an emerging frontier that offers new possibilities for understanding and improving healthcare delivery. Arts-based research methods, including narrative inquiry, photovoice and creative expression, can provide rich insights into patient experiences, healthcare provider perspectives and the social contexts of health and illness.[26]

Creative arts approaches are particularly valuable for engaging marginalised communities, exploring sensitive topics and generating new forms of knowledge that complement traditional quantitative and qualitative research methods. These approaches can inform the development of culturally appropriate interventions and provide deeper understanding of the human experience of health and illness. This topic is covered in depth in Chapter 7.

2.4.6 Reflexivity and Participatory Research

Future-oriented primary care research must embrace reflexivity, the practice of critically examining one's own assumptions, biases and positionality in the research process. Reflexive research approaches recognise that researchers are not neutral observers but active participants who shape the research process and outcomes.[27] Miller and Crabtree expand on reflexivity in primary care research in Chapter 8 and Thille and Kelly on reflexive approaches to qualitative thematic analysis in Chapter 22.

Participatory research methodologies, including community-based participatory research and patient and public involvement in research, represent important approaches for ensuring that research is relevant, appropriate and beneficial to the communities it aims to serve. These approaches challenge traditional power dynamics in research and recognise community members as co-researchers rather than as research subjects.[28] See Chapter 21 for a full account of community engagement and co-design by and with disadvantaged populations.

2.5 Primary Care Research in Low- and Middle-Income Countries

2.5.1 Unique Challenges and Opportunities

Primary care research in LMICs faces distinct challenges that require innovative approaches and methodologies. Resource constraints, limited research infrastructure, and competing health priorities create a complex environment for conducting high-quality research. However, LMICs also offer unique opportunities for innovation, including the potential to leapfrog 'western' healthcare delivery models, implement novel providers to the primary care team and create technologies without legacy system constraints.[19]

The burden of disease in LMICs often differs significantly from that in high-income countries, with persistent challenges from infectious diseases alongside the growing burden of non-communicable diseases. This epidemiological transition requires research approaches that can address the dual burden of disease while considering resource constraints and healthcare system limitations in rapidly evolving societal structures.

2.5.2 Task-Shifting and Human Resources

Many LMICs face severe shortages of healthcare professionals, leading to innovative approaches such as task-shifting, where certain clinical responsibilities are transferred to less specialised healthcare workers. Research on task-shifting in primary care requires methodologies that can evaluate both clinical outcomes and implementation feasibility, while considering issues of training, supervision and quality assurance.[29]

The development of human resources for health research in LMICs represents a critical priority, requiring approaches that build local research capacity while avoiding brain drain and ensuring that research benefits remain within the communities where research is conducted.

2.5.3 Technology and Innovation

LMICs have demonstrated remarkable innovation in leveraging technology for healthcare delivery, including mobile health interventions, telemedicine and point-of-care diagnostics. Research on these innovations requires methodologies that can evaluate effectiveness in resource-constrained settings while considering issues of scalability, sustainability and equity.[30]

The digital divide within and between countries presents both challenges and opportunities for primary care research. Although some populations may lack access to basic digital technologies and connectivity, others may have access to advanced mobile technologies that enable innovative research approaches.

2.6 Building Resilience for Future Challenges

2.6.1 Climate Resilience and Adaptive Capacity

Climate change presents unprecedented challenges for primary care systems, requiring research approaches that can understand vulnerabilities, develop adaptive strategies and build resilience (see Chapter 15). Climate-resilient primary care research must consider both acute climate events, such as extreme weather, and chronic environmental changes, such as rising temperatures and changing disease patterns.[31]

Building adaptive capacity in primary care systems requires research that can identify early warning systems, develop flexible care delivery models and understand the social and economic factors that influence climate vulnerability. This research must be inherently transdisciplinary, integrating climate science, public health, social sciences and healthcare delivery research with the lived experience of local communities.

2.6.2 System Transformation and Innovation

The future of primary care will likely require fundamental transformation of current healthcare delivery models. Research approaches must be capable of studying system-level changes, understanding the dynamics of transformation and identifying factors that promote or hinder innovation adoption. Complex systems approaches, implementation science and organisational behaviour research offer valuable perspectives for understanding healthcare system transformation.[32]

Innovation in primary care may come from unexpected sources, including patient-driven innovations, community-based solutions and cross-sector collaborations. Transdisciplinary research methodologies provide flexibility and inclusion to capture and evaluate these diverse forms of innovation.

2.7 Methodological Considerations for Future-Oriented Research

2.7.1 Mixed-Methods Research

The complexity of future primary care challenges requires methodological approaches that can integrate quantitative and qualitative methods while drawing on diverse epistemological traditions. Mixed-methods research, while not new to primary care research, offers a framework for combining different methodological approaches to address complex research questions that cannot be adequately answered by any single method.[33]

2.7.2 Longitudinal and Life Course Approaches

Understanding health and illness in primary care requires longitudinal perspectives that can capture the dynamic nature of health status, the long-term effects of interventions and the complex trajectories of health and disease over the life course. Life course epidemiology offers a framework for understanding how early life experiences influence later health outcomes and how health trajectories can be modified through primary care interventions.[34] Life course epidemiology has the potential to influence our understanding of the development of chronic diseases and interventions to prevent their development.

Longitudinal research in primary care faces significant challenges, including participant retention, changing healthcare systems and the long time-horizons required to observe meaningful outcomes. However, advances in digital health technologies and linkage of electronic health records offer new opportunities for conducting large-scale, long-term studies of primary care interventions.

2.7.3 Ethics and Responsible Innovation

Future-oriented primary care research must grapple with complex ethical challenges related to emerging technologies, data privacy, equity and responsible innovation. The rapid pace of technological change often outpaces traditional ethical review processes, requiring new approaches to ethical oversight that can balance innovation with protection of research participants and communities.[35]

Responsible innovation frameworks offer approaches for ensuring that research and development processes consider ethical, social and environmental implications from the outset rather than as an afterthought. This approach is particularly important for primary care research, where interventions directly impact vulnerable populations and have the potential for widespread implementation. Transdisciplinary research teams are ideally suited to ensuring compliance with these values.

2.8 Conclusion

The future of primary care research lies in embracing complexity, uncertainty and innovation while maintaining rigorous scientific standards and ethical principles. The challenges facing primary care from climate change and technological disruption to health equity and global health disparities require research approaches that are adaptive, inclusive and capable of generating actionable insights for an uncertain future.

Future-oriented primary care research must be inherently transdisciplinary, drawing on diverse fields of knowledge while developing new methodological approaches that can address complex, real-world challenges. This research must be conducted in partnership with communities, patients and healthcare providers, ensuring that research priorities and methods are aligned with the needs and values of those who will be affected by research outcomes.

The transformation of primary care research will require significant investment in research infrastructure, training and capacity building, particularly in LMICs, where the need for locally relevant research is greatest. It will also require new forms of collaboration among researchers, healthcare providers, policymakers and communities that transcend traditional boundaries and power structures.

As primary care continues to evolve in response to changing population needs and technological capabilities, research must evolve in parallel, developing new methodologies and approaches that can guide this transformation. The future of primary care depends on our ability to conduct research that is not only scientifically rigorous but also relevant, applicable and responsive to the complex challenges of 21st-century healthcare.

The chapters that follow in this volume explore specific aspects of this future-oriented approach to primary care research, from platform clinical trials and genomics to creative arts and climate resilience. Together, they provide a roadmap for transforming primary care research to meet the challenges and opportunities of an uncertain but promising future.

Acknowledgements

The first draft of this chapter was generated by Claude Sonnet 4. That draft underwent significant editing and rewriting, including the deletion of some sections and the addition of new sections. The initial 28 references required significant updating. Thanks to Gillian Fransoo for your invaluable assistance.

References

1. Bollyky TJ, Templin T, Cohen M, et al. Lower-income countries that face the most rapid shift in noncommunicable disease burden are also the least prepared. *Health Aff.* 2017 Nov;36(11):1866–75.
2. United Nations. United Nations, department of economic and social affairs, population division. World Population Ageing 2019: Highlights. New York; 2019.
3. Topol EJ. High-performance medicine: The convergence of human and artificial intelligence. *Nat Med.* 2019 Jan 7;25(1):44–56.
4. Agarwal P, Fletcher GG, Ramamoorthi K, et al. Uses of virtual care in primary care: Scoping review. *J Med Internet Res.* 2025 Feb 14;27:e55007.
5. Rajkomar A, Dean J, Kohane I. Machine learning in medicine. *N Engl J Med.* 2019 Apr 4;380(14):1347–58.
6. Watts N, Amann M, Arnell N, et al. The 2020 report of The Lancet Countdown on health and climate change: Responding to converging crises. *Lancet.* 2021 Jan;397(10269):129–70.
7. Dzau VJ, Laitner MH, Balatbat CA, et al. Climate change and human health: A research agenda for action. *N Engl J Med.* 2025 Jul 3;393(1):88–92.
8. Whitmee S, Haines A, Beyrer C, et al. Safeguarding human health in the Anthropocene epoch: Report of the Rockefeller Foundation–Lancet Commission on planetary health. *Lancet.* 2015 Nov;386(10007):1973–2028.
9. Marmot M, Wilkinson R, editors. Social determinants of health. Oxford: Oxford University Press; 2006.
10. Riccardi MT, Pettinicchio V, Di Pumpo M, et al. Community-based participatory research to engage disadvantaged communities: Levels of engagement reached and how to increase it: A systematic review. *Health Policy.* 2023 Nov; 137:104905.
11. Warner ET, Huguet N, Fredericks M, et al. Advancing health equity through implementation science: Identifying and examining measures of the outer setting. *Soc Sci Med.* 2023 Aug; 331:116095.
12. Linden M, Linden U, Goretzko D, et al. Prevalence and pattern of acute and chronic multimorbidity across all body systems and age groups in primary health care. *Sci Rep.* 2022 Jan 7;12(1):272.
13. Van Aerde J, Gomes MM, Giuliani M, et al. Complex adaptive systems in CanMEDS 2025. *Can Med Educ J.* 2023 Mar 21;14(1):50–3.
14. Evans W, Meslin EM, Kai J, et al. Precision medicine: Are we there yet? A narrative review of precision medicine's applicability in primary care. *J Pers Med.* 2024 Apr 15;14(4):418.
15. Davies HP, Patel KC. General practice at the core of neighborhoods. *BMJ.* 2025 Jun 26;389:r1241.
16. Smith JD, Polaha J. Using implementation science to guide the integration of evidence-based family interventions into primary care. *Fam Syst Health.* 2017 Jun;35(2):125–35.
17. Curran GM, Bauer M, Mittman B, et al. Effectiveness-implementation hybrid designs. *Med Care.* 2012 Mar;50(3):217–26.

18. Asada Y, Kroll-Desrosiers A, Chriqui JF, et al. Applying hybrid effectiveness-implementation studies in equity-centered policy implementation science. *Front Health Serv.* 2023 Sep 8;3:1220629.
19. Bonfim D, Belotti L, de Almeida LY, et al. Challenges and strategies for conducting research in primary health care practice: An integrative review. *BMC Health Serv Res.* 2023 Dec 8;23(1):1380.
20. Marsden N, Star L, Smylie J. Nothing about us without us in writing: Aligning the editorial policies of the Canadian Journal of Public Health with the inherent rights of Indigenous Peoples. *Can J Public Health.* 2020 Dec 7;111(6):822–5.
21. Woodcock J, LaVange LM. Master protocols to study multiple therapies, multiple diseases, or both. *N Engl J Med.* 2017 Jul 6;377(1):62–70.
22. Sherman RE, Anderson SA, Dal Pan GJ, et al. Real-world evidence: What is it and what can it tell us? *N Engl J Med.* 2016 Dec 8;375(23):2293–7.
23. Beam AL, Kohane IS. Big data and machine learning in health care. *JAMA.* 2018 Apr 3;319(13):1317.
24. Wright B, O'Connor A, Fraher EP, et al. Family medicine research: Seizing the moment to advance the field. *BMC Health Serv Res.* 2024 Dec 20;24(1):1627.
25. Rigolot C. Transdisciplinarity as a discipline and a way of being: Complementarities and creative tensions. *Humanit Soc Sci Commun.* 2020 Sep 22;7(1):100.
26. Leavy P. Research design: Quantitative, qualitative, mixed methods, arts-based, and community-based participatory research approaches. New York: Guilford Publications; 2017.
27. Lim WM. What is qualitative research? An overview and guidelines. *Australas Mark J.* 2025 May 25;33(2):199–229.
28. Wallerstein N, Duran B, editors, et al. Community-based participatory research for health: Advancing social and health equity. Hoboken: John Wiley & Sons; 2017.
29. Tesema AG, Mabunda SA, Chaudhri K, et al. Task-sharing for non-communicable disease prevention and control in low- and middle-income countries in the context of health worker shortages: A systematic review. *PLoS Global Public Health.* 2025 Apr 16;5(4):e0004289.
30. Sylla B, Ismaila O, Diallo G. 25 years of digital health toward universal health coverage in low- and middle-income countries: Rapid systematic review. *J Med Internet Res.* 2025 May 29;27:e59042.
31. Berry HL, Waite TD, Dear KBG, et al. The case for systems thinking about climate change and mental health. *Nat Clim Chang.* 2018 Apr 3;8(4):282–90.
32. Best A, Berland A, Herbert C, et al. Using systems thinking to support clinical system transformation. *J Health Organ Manag.* 2016 May 16;30(3):302–23.
33. Creswell J, Plano Clark V. Designing and conducting mixed methods research. Thousand Oaks: Sage Publications; 2017.
34. Wagner C, Carmeli C, Jackisch J, et al. Life course epidemiology and public health. *Lancet Public Health.* 2024 Apr;9(4):e261–9.
35. Floridi L, Cowls J, Beltrametti M, et al. AI4People: An ethical framework for a good AI society: Opportunities, risks, principles, and recommendations. *Minds Mach.* 2018 Dec 26;28(4):689–707.

SECTION

2

Emerging Approaches in Primary Care Research

CHAPTER

3 Complexity

Theory and Application for Research

Trisha Greenhalgh

3.1 Introduction

3.1.1 Examples of Complexity

Box 3.1 shows some fictitious examples of complex phenomena in health systems. Example 1 (Anna) illustrates *logistical complexity* (multiple interdependent elements and requirements). Example 2 (Rahul) illustrates *clinical complexity* (multiple physiological feedback loops, pathological processes and comorbidities). It also features *socio-technical complexity*—the challenges of delivering care through a dynamic network of people (who are variably skilled and have particular beliefs and concerns) and technologies (which contain inbuilt assumptions about who will use them and how,[1] and which are fallible). Example 3 (Ayomide) is characterised by—in addition to logistical, clinical and socio-technical complexity—*political complexity*, in which values, priorities, resource allocation decisions and a country's troubled past loom large.

BOX 3.1 SOME EXAMPLES OF COMPLEX PHENOMENA IN HEALTH SYSTEMS

1. **Clinical rotas**: Anna, a manager, is in charge of organising the duty rota for a large community nursing service. Each staff member is contracted to work a certain number of day, evening and night shifts. Each locality must always have a senior person overseeing the work of frontline staff. Staff holidays, sickness and crises must be covered, sometimes at short notice. Anna must try to optimise continuity by ensuring that, where possible, a nurse works in the same local service on successive shifts. She must also ensure that trainees have the opportunity to accumulate clinical experience across several domains. All the nurses want to minimise their commute to work.
2. **Remote patient monitoring**: Rahul, a GP, works in a polyclinic. Partly because of limited slots for face-to-face appointments, the polyclinic has introduced a remote monitoring ('virtual ward') service. Patients with heart failure, for example, are to be

DOI: 10.1201/9781003652106-5

issued with weighing scales, oximeters and blood pressure machines, and asked to take daily measurements and complete a symptom checklist. Rahul's team, which includes trainee GPs and physician associates, will contact these patients by telephone regularly to collect data and make decisions about ongoing care, drawing on newly issued guidelines. But the change is not popular. Clinical staff say they have never monitored patients by telephone before, and they are questioning the guidelines. Pilot data suggests that the technologies are not 100% reliable and that some patients are misreading the displays (eg device upside down). It seems that an intervention intended to reduce clinical workload may have actually increased it, with threats to patient safety.

3. **Maternal and perinatal mortality in a low-resource setting**: Ayomide is an obstetrician in a sub-Saharan African country with a high maternal and perinatal mortality rate. The country, which has been impoverished by debt, civil war and famine, has a fragile health system. Transport links are poor, which means that many patients face a journey of several hours to reach their nearest community clinic (which is typically under-equipped and staffed by minimally trained people). Public understanding of health issues is low, and prevailing cultural practices mean that many women often present late in pregnancy (sometimes not until they are in labour). Ayomide spends much of her time dealing as best she can with emergencies that could have been avoided. She is angry that her government seems to rank the safe care of pregnant women and their babies below that of other policy priorities.

3.1.2 What Is It to Be Complex?

The different kinds of complexity outlined previously share a number of common features (Box 3.2).[2–6]

BOX 3.2 WHAT IS A COMPLEX SYSTEM?

Informed by work from previous authors[2–6]

A complex system consists of:

- *Multiple components*, linked to each other (these components—whether genes, cells, people, technologies or organisations—can be thought of as forming a *network*).
- *Interactions* that are not centrally controlled or predetermined, and hence have a degree of randomness about them.
- *Feedback loops*—data from one interaction influences subsequent interactions, either positively or negatively.
- *Non-equilibrium*—the system is open (ie connected to its environment), and hence can never achieve a stable, unproblematic balance.
- *Systems nested within systems*—each complex system is made up of (sub)systems and is in turn part of a larger system.

A complex system's behaviour is characterised by:

- *Self-organisation*—components of the network respond to local signals, producing a degree of structure and order.
- *Non-linearity*—a fixed input does not produce a fixed output. A small change in one part of the system may lead to a large change elsewhere in the system and vice versa.
- *Unpredictability*—nobody can foretell exactly what will happen in the system in the future.
- *Multiple scales*—because of the nested nature of systems and subsystems, change can emerge at (for example) the individual, group, organisational and societal levels and in short-, medium- and long-term timescales.
- *Historical path-dependency*—the system's behaviour is influenced by all the things that occurred in the past, both very recently and long ago. In that sense, the system has a 'memory'.

A complex system generates:

- *Patterns*—while exact prediction is impossible, recurring patterns can be discerned at all levels in the system.
- *Dynamic evolution*—the system changes over time in response to the interactions and feedback loops within it.
- *Adaptation*—as the environment evolves, so does the system.
- *Novelty*—the corollary of unpredictability is that some outputs of the system are unforeseen.
- *Resilience*—the system maintains its overall structure and function despite changes imposed by the environment.

These features should not be equated with harmony or optimum performance. It is said that a system is perfectly designed to generate the outputs (good or bad) that it is currently generating. In Example 3 in Box 3.1, for example, the system is perfectly designed to *perpetuate* the personal tragedies and societal inequities that have made Ayomide so angry. That system is 'resilient' chiefly in the sense that heroic efforts to improve the structures, processes and behaviours that contribute to high maternal and perinatal mortality in this challenging context may generate little in the way of improvement because the subsystems and components adjust accordingly.[7]

3.1.3 Complexity Theory Versus Complexity Thinking

The list of characteristics of a complex system (Box 3.2) reflect *complexity thinking*, but they do not amount to a theory. To theorise a particular instance of complexity, we need to be more explicit about what components and what interactions we are talking about. Cells, people, technologies, organisations and governments all react to external signals and exhibit interdependency, but they do so in different ways and for different reasons.

In the next section, I give four examples of how complex systems have been theorised: information systems, living systems, organisational systems and political systems. Each uses a different disciplinary lens (respectively, cybernetics; biology, ecology and human sciences; organisational sociology; and political philosophy). These examples, whose features are summarised in Table 3.1, are not intended to be exhaustive. I have chosen them because they have particular relevance for the study of healthcare and health systems. The four systems described are, of course, interrelated.

3.2 Theorising Complexity: Four Lenses

3.2.1 Information Systems (Cybernetics)

Cybernetics was the brainchild of mathematician Norbert Wiener, who defined it as "the science of control and communications".[8] It examines how systems adapt to changes in their environment and self-regulate. Weiner emphasised the similarities between mechanical and biological systems, focusing on concepts such as feedback, information and control. The thermostat in a room, for example, detects temperature; if the temperature is higher or lower than the set point, it triggers what Weiner would call 'effectors' (eg air vents, heaters) to bring the temperature back to the set point. Similarly, the human body's thermostat detects deviations from its biological set point and triggers physiological responses (eg sweating, shivering) to restore balance.

The original cybernetics literature ("first order cybernetics") came from early computer science, with brief mention of animal and biological systems.[8] Later, some cybernetics scholars, notably Gregory Bateson, tried to stretch the principles of cybernetics (in my view, somewhat too far) to explain diseases of the human mind and problems with social systems in what he called "second order cybernetics".[9]

3.2.2 Living Systems (Biology, Ecology and Human Science)

Consider the challenge facing Rahul (example 2 in Box 3.1). At first glance, remote monitoring seems an appealing solution to the problem of rising numbers of patients with long-term conditions and finite resources for monitoring them, but long-term conditions such as chronic heart failure are typically characterised by clinical complexity and variable ability of patients and carers to collect and submit the data needed for clinical decision-making.

An important feature of living systems is their ecological (multi-layered, interdependent) nature, comprising (for example) molecules, genes, cells, organs, individuals, families, groups, societies and so on.[10] To analyse a living system, and especially to explore *causation* in such systems, we need to analyse each layer in its own right, as well as examine the interactions among the layers and as these unfold over time. Box 3.3 summarises the complexity of heart failure and its management from the perspective of individual symptomatology and clinical findings, underlying myocardial and other organ damage, neurohormonal regulatory loops and drugs that moderate these, patient capability and compliance, family support networks, patient-clinician relationships, the organisation and delivery of remote monitoring services, staff acceptance of such new service models and the associated resource demands.

TABLE 3.1 Four Theoretical Lenses on Complexity

Lens (Disciplinary Origin); Key Authors	Key Concepts and Theories	Key Empirical Methods	When to Use This Lens	Published Empirical Examples
Information systems (cybernetics); Weiner ("first-order cybernetics"),[8] Bateson ("second-order cybernetics")[9]	System conceptualised as information flow in a [neural] network. Information is transformed at nodes ('governors'), which follow rules and constraints. As more nodes are added, the network adapts and evolves via feedback loops.	Mathematical modelling and simulation; [8] developing and testing artificial systems;[8] in-depth case study[66]	When information flow seems a dominant feature of the system	Schuurmans et al used case study methods to examine why an effort to reorganise out-of-hours cover for elderly residential homes in the Netherlands failed. The attempted change rerouted and reprocessed information pathways between professionals, leading to a buildup of stress via four mechanisms: fragmentation of information flows; accumulation of information; loss of richness of information; and slow-moving information flows.[66]
Living systems (biology, ecology, human sciences); Fustolo-Gunninck et al (clinical complexity),[6] Glass & McAttee (behavioural science),[67] Byrne (social science)[3]	System conceptualised as a nested hierarchy of levels of influence, evolving over time. Includes micro (eg genetics, neurohormonal effects, drug pharmacokinetics), meso (eg human behaviour and action), mezzo (eg family, workplace, community) and macro (eg economy, environment).	System dynamic modelling;[68] causal loop diagrams;[45,69,70] longitudinal ecological analyses (multi-level and followed over time)[67]	When studying clinical complexity, patient behaviour and how these are influenced by family, community and environment	In an early paper, Homer et al used system dynamic modelling to consider the multiple influences on antibiotic resistance; these included the emergence of resistant zoonotic pathogens due to poor animal husbandry practices and spread of these to humans; human expectations and behaviour (patients and doctors); research investment (or lack of it) in novel classes of antibiotic; surveillance infrastructure; and media attention.[71] More recently, causal loop mapping has illustrated the multiple and interacting causes of obesity.[72–74]
Organisational systems (organisational sociology); Scott (institutions),[11] Feldman (routines),[13] Czarniawska (narrative),[15] Weick (sensemaking),[17] Tsoukas ("don't simplify, complexify")[31]	System conceptualised as networks of organisational members who follow rules, are guided by norms (eg ethical standards) and enact routines. To understand organisational complexity, examine these rules, norms and routines. One technique is to collect and construct stories. To change an organisation, seek to change the rules, norms and routines.	In-depth 'n of 1' organisational case study (designed to capture a rich description of a unique case for its own sake)[48,75]	To support change (or explain lack of change) in an organisation or other formal setting	Love et al used Weick's theory of sensemaking to analyse mis-performance in three hospital mega-projects in Australia.[76] They showed that conventional logic-model theoretical lenses (project management, governance) were unable to account for key social and cultural influences that helped explain failures (eg delayed deliverables, exceeding budget). Weick and Sutcliffe used sensemaking to re-analyse data from a major UK inquiry into deaths in paediatric cardiac surgery, concluding that the prevailing organisational culture helped generate and perpetuate a clinically unsafe organisation.[77]

(Continued)

TABLE 3.1 Four Theoretical Lenses on Complexity (Continued)

Lens (Disciplinary Origin); Key Authors	Key Concepts and Theories	Key Empirical Methods	When to Use This Lens	Published Empirical Examples
Political systems (political philosophy): Easton (policy is based on values),[78] Laclau and Mouffe[20,79] (political identity is founded on difference)[20,79]	System conceptualised as competing interest groups who identify with a cause and use rhetoric to recruit others to that cause. Complexity relates to antagonisms ("us" versus "them") and values-driven conflicts between groups. To make progress, surface and deliberate on these conflicts, which can serve as useful "frictions".[20]	Deconstruction of texts and critical examination of charts,[50] algorithms and standards.[27] Collective deliberation using conflictual ("agonistic") approaches.[20]	When conflict among groups is a dominant feature of the system, and especially when interest groups present competing framings of the same issue	Hindmarsh used Mouffe's notions of difference and antagonism to analyse toxic clashes among interest groups relating to an Australian wind farm.[80] Local communities saw wind farms as spoiling a sense of place and showed limited recognition of their potential environmental benefits. Government and non-governmental actors framed the wind farm as a universal good and key contributor to climate targets; they had little awareness of why, or how strongly, communities felt negatively about it. These differences led to ongoing conflict and slowed progress.

BOX 3.3 THE COMPLEXITY OF HEART FAILURE AND ITS REMOTE MONITORING

Summarised from Greenhalgh et al 2017[81]

Heart failure is not a single disease but a clinical syndrome involving impaired ventricular filling or ejection. Symptoms (eg breathlessness on exercise) and signs (eg displaced apex beat) are harder to discern and interpret in people with high body mass index, older people and those with comorbidities (which are common). A firm diagnosis requires objective evidence of heart damage on investigations (echocardiography, MRI or isotope uptake studies), although these may not be available or affordable.

Heart failure is broadly classified into "heart failure with reduced ejection fraction" (HFREF), previously known as left ventricular systolic dysfunction, and "heart failure with preserved ejection fraction" (HFPEF), previously known as diastolic heart failure. In HFREF, myocardial damage (eg cardiomyopathy) reduces the proportion of blood pumped out with each contraction of the ventricle, which activates the renin-angiotensin system (RAS), producing a maladaptive increase in vascular resistance and fluid retention. Many popular drug therapies for HFREF (eg ramipril, losartan) are oriented to counteracting this RAS response.

In HFPEF, the primary insult is metabolic damage from hypertension, obesity or diabetes, which leads to thickening and stiffening of the ventricle, impaired relaxation during the cardiac cycle and an increase in filling pressure—which in turn leads to pulmonary and peripheral oedema. Patients with HFPEF comprise at least half of all heart failure cases and have a similar mortality, but research evidence on this condition is sparse. Treatment is mainly of the underlying causes. Therapies that improve prognosis in HFREF tend to be ineffective in HFPEF.

Patients with heart failure are often frightened, bewildered, socially isolated and variably able to self-manage (many are elderly). Remote monitoring technologies require fundamental changes to clinical roles and service models (eg regular appointments with a known and trusted heart failure nurse are replaced with an instruction to take measurements and enter data into a digital application). The more biomarkers and symptoms are monitored, the better informed clinical decision-making will be, but such "intensive" telehealth (multiple measurements, submitted frequently) places very high demands on patients, carers and staff and can be resource-intensive. Some virtual wards operate digitally and asynchronously ("cold" telehealth), but some use telephone calls ("warm" telehealth). Some services stick rigidly to models of telehealth that have been tested in randomised controlled trials, whereas others adapt and evolve according to patient and staff feedback.

The limited success of remote monitoring programmes in heart failure can be analysed in terms of key tensions in this complex system: between tidy, "textbook" heart failure (the classic HFREF patient) and the reality of multiple comorbidities (the under-researched and more complex HFPEF patient); between basic and intensive telehealth; between digitally savvy, well-supported patients and vulnerable, unsupported ones; between "cold" and "warm" telehealth; and between fixed and adaptive programmes.

3.2.3 Organisational Systems (Organisational Sociology)

Organisations are formal human systems. Healthcare organisations are also *institutions*: they exist for a social and ethical purpose, governed by three institutional pillars: (1) regulative (what we must do, eg legal requirements), normative (what we should do, eg professional standards and codes of conduct) and (3) cultural-cognitive (the patterns of what we routinely do).[11] To change an institution, professional leaders can exert coercive control, devise normative prescriptions to guide behaviour or change cultural-cognitive routines.[12] Routines are defined as repetitive patterns of interdependent action involving multiple actors;[13] they are a source of stability in organisations, but because they are enacted differently every time, they also contain within them the seeds of change (a practice meeting, for example, gradually evolves as some aspects of the routine are progressively strengthened and others attenuate).[14]

Sociologists of organisations have studied the framings, metaphors and stories that organisational members use to plan, describe and account for complex change.[15,16] Narrative is an important tool for studying causality in organisations, because such causality is multifaceted, non-linear and demands rich explanations and caveats. Karl Weick's theory of sensemaking, for example, includes a number of key concepts, including identity (a story being told about a desired—or undesired—change in an organization links to a sense of who we are, both individually and collectively), retrospection (the story makes sense of what has happened up to now, thus setting the stage for the change), future orientation (prospective unfolding over time as the story continues) and salient clues (stories told about early wins provide hope).[17] Sensemaking generates coherence and allows people to act.

3.2.4 Political Systems (Political Philosophy)

In a similar vein, political philosophy scholars have written about policy as being made of language and involving persuasion.[18,19] In this context, group narratives are explicitly values-based and often conflictual (ie emotionally laden and pitted against alternative narratives or framings of particular issues).[20]

Values and vested interests are an important aspect of complexity in human societies; they drive our actions and explain why we resist some changes passionately.[21] Values are embedded in standards, metrics and algorithms which, while they *appear* objective, actually serve the interests of some groups at the expense of others' interests.[22–24] Advocacy groups play an important role in surfacing these biases and challenging the standards, metrics and algorithms that most people take for granted.[25–27] Analyses that are overly focused on mathematical complexity may miss the important contribution of value complexity to stalled projects.[21,28]

3.3 Managing Complexity: Five Key Steps for Researchers

Despite much interest in the topic, there is remarkably little sound practical advice on how to study, manage and research complexity in healthcare and health systems. In this section, I suggest some principles and approaches which are relevant for both managing complexity and researching it.

3.3.1 Classify the Challenge: Simple, Complicated or Complex?

The most common error in managing complexity is to fail to recognise it. One approach to assessing a project's complexity is the Cynefin framework, developed by software engineer David Snowden (Figure 3.1).[29] *Cynefin* is a Welsh word that

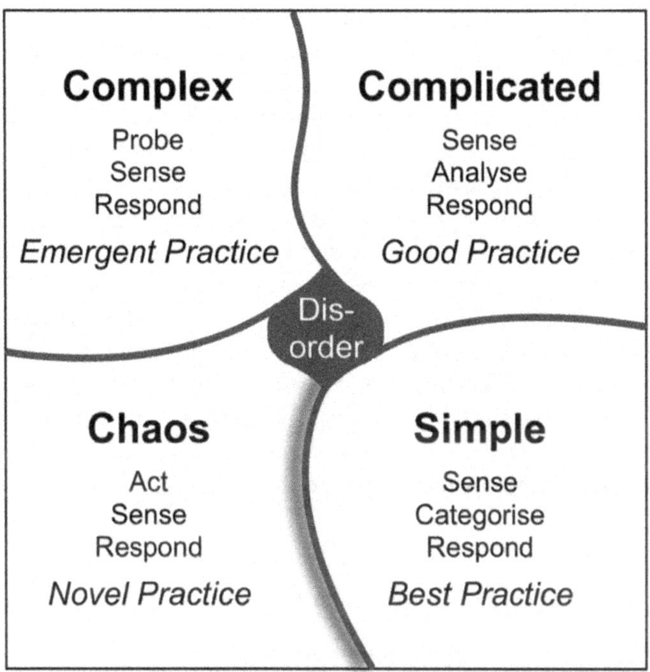

FIGURE 3.1 A version of the Cynefin framework (based on work by Snowden and Boone[29]), reproduced with permission from Puik and Ceglarek[64]

translates (approximately) to "place of multiple belongings"; it conveys a sense of balance, interconnectedness and sensitivity to local conditions and priorities.

Some problems are 'simple' or 'obvious' (bottom right in Figure 3.1); because they are predictable, off-the-shelf solutions work well. Simple problems can be addressed using the triad *sense* (estimate the project's requirements), *categorise* (work out what kind of problem it is), *respond* (select an off-the-shelf solution—there is usually a single 'best practice'). If, for example, you want to open a new bank account, it will not take the agent (whether human or algorithm) long to categorise your problem and link you to the application page.

In 'complicated' problems, some things are still predictable, and there may be off-the-shelf solutions, but there are more components and interactions. Cynefin recommends *sense* (as above), *analyse* (use existing 'good practices' or 'near enough' solutions, and recognise that there will not be a single, one-way-of-doing-things 'best practice'), *respond* (by tailoring and tweaking a solution to meet a particular use case). In example 1 in Box 3.1, many aspects of the rota problem are known, and good practices in human resource management can be adapted. Anna should tailor these practices to the local situation using her accumulated practical wisdom.

'Complex' problems are non-deterministic—that is, there are no off-the-peg solutions, and the strategy to deal with them changes as they unfold. Cynefin recommends a different triad: *probe* (estimate the project's requirements and add features), *sense* (get feedback on those features, understand barriers, get a sense of what features might be needed in the future), *respond* (respond to change, discover emergent solutions and iterate). I discuss this type of problem further later.

'Chaotic' problems are also non-deterministic but more so. This context usually comes about due to an emergency. Snowden and Boone suggest that, in chaos, all you can do is *act*—that is, instigate some novel action to change the situation and hope to shift the problem from (eg) 'chaotic' to 'complex'.[29]

The fifth category in Cynefin is 'disorder' (or 'confusion'), which means the problem has been misclassified and addressed with an inappropriate strategy. People who use banking as an example of how healthcare could be unproblematically automated are guilty of misclassifying a complex challenge as a simple one.

Organisational coach Ralph Stacey drew on Snowden and Boone's work to develop his certainty-agreement diagram.[30] His widely reproduced certainty-agreement diagram is reproduced in Figure 3.2. At the bottom left, the problem is simple—that is, close to certainty and close to agreement among all the stakeholders. At the top right, things are highly uncertain and stakeholders are far from agreement ('chaos'). Stacey's diagram is a useful heuristic, but we should note that later in his career Stacey himself rejected it as oversimplistic.

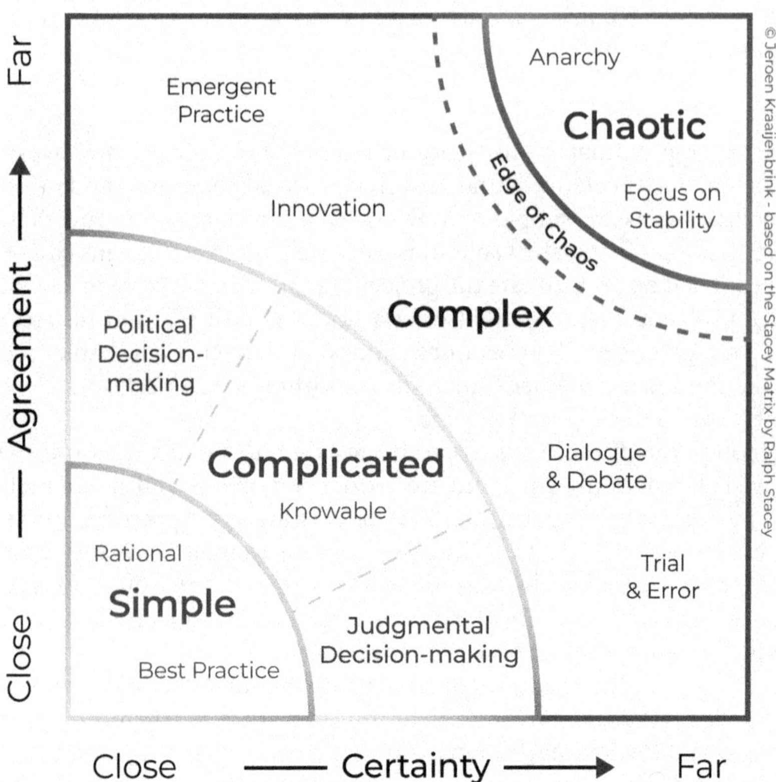

FIGURE 3.2 A version of the certainty-agreement diagram (based on early work by Stacey[30]), reproduced with permission from Kraaijenbrink[65]

The remainder of this section focuses on challenges that are 'complex' (the top left zone in Figure 3.1 and the diagonal in Figure 3.2).

3.3.2 Understand the System

3.3.2.1 Don't Simplify—Complexify

Sociologist Haridimos Tsoukas warns against the temptation to simplify complex systems in order to research them.[31] Rather, he says, we need to *complexify*—that is, engage with non-linearity, complex loops of causation and adaptation, and lack of predictability. Tsoukas proposes three requirements for addressing organisational complexity—(1) an *open-world ontology* (that is, seeing the world as subject to multiple interacting influences which must be described and studied in all their richness to reveal layers of influence), (2) a *performative epistemology* (that is, a focus on real-world action and on what becomes possible *through* action), and (3) a *poetic praxeology* (that is, writing up case studies in a way that values descriptive detail, apt metaphor and narrative coherence).[31]

Many methods that are widely used (and much-celebrated) in health services research—notably, randomised controlled trials and quasi-experimental approaches such as stepped-wedge—are based on an assumption of linear causality. I and others have argued elsewhere that efforts to develop and experimentally test "complex interventions" (ie interventions with multiple components delivered and coordinated by human agents) to generate a more or less transferable "effect size" are misplaced because it is primarily the *system*, not the intervention, that is complex and because interventions in complex systems by definition do not have fixed effects.[4,32–35] Similarly, studies that generate under-theorised lists of "barriers" and "enablers" are unlikely to be adequate to explore complex change in organisations, since they fail to acknowledge or explore the defining features of complexity (Box 3.2).[36] The next few sections suggest some ways of addressing these features.

3.3.2.2 Gather Many Different Kinds of Data

Because we need to look at complex phenomena from multiple different angles, we need multiple different kinds of evidence. The philosophical case for this approach ("evidential pluralism") has been made elsewhere.[37,38] Evidential pluralism links to the concept of epistemic justice—that no group of scientists has the right to claim that *their* methodology is inherently and universally superior to other approaches, although of course there are better and worse methods for addressing particular questions.

There is no universal formula to dictate your data sources or methods here: you will need to be guided by the needs of the project and by what is feasible. Broadly, you will need to obtain as many types and sources of data (administrative, financial, clinical, mathematical modelling, and perspectives of staff and patients) as you can.

Focus, in particular, on action (this is what Tsoukas means by "performative epistemology"[31]). Ethnography is a powerful tool here. Pay special attention to people who are closest to the delivery of healthcare, to patients, and to technologies.[39] How do these frontline actors frame the situation? What concerns and ideas do they have? Where appropriate, involve these actors in collecting and analysing data.

3.3.2.3 Look for Patterns

Complex systems are not deterministic (ie not fully predictable), but they do show patterns. Methods for detecting these patterns depend on the kind of complexity you are studying. For elucidating mathematical complexity, there are many computational approaches such as agent-based modelling or deep learning using AI.[2,5] When studying human disease, these methods can be combined with epidemiology to follow (and account for) change over time.[40]

For the socio-technical complexity of change in organisations and for the political complexity of value clashes, patterns may best be discerned by attending to language and narrative. In our study of workload in UK general practice, for example, we were struck by the recurrence of apocalyptic water metaphors in our early interviews ("deluge", "tsunami", "flood") to describe a perceived exponential increase in patient demand in recent years.[41]

3.3.2.4 Identify Tensions and Paradoxes

Tension and paradox are inherent to complex systems. We can rarely resolve these, but we can surface and explore them. In electronic patient records, for example, there is a tension between making data widely accessible and protecting patient privacy. The more "secure" we make these systems, the more likely it is that a clinician will be unable to access a patient's record. The correct balance between accessibility and privacy is not a generic truth that can be found in a textbook or guideline; it will emerge from reflection and discussion about the specific requirements and priorities of the project. Sometimes, when a complex project is "stuck", brainstorming the tensions and paradoxes can help get it moving again. Box 3.3 (final paragraph) shows some tensions in the complex system of remote monitoring of heart failure.

3.3.3 Represent the System

Representing complex systems in a format that people can grasp can bring coherence out of a situation that people find confusing, invite interpretations and hence be a bridge to effective action.[39,42,43] There are many ways of representing a complex system; the preferred one will depend on the audience.

3.3.3.1 Draw Maps

A popular way of representing complexity through visual means is causal loop diagrams.[44,45] Table 3.1 (column 4 of row 3) gives some examples. These diagrams are typically generated by combining qualitative data (eg experts' assumptions or hypotheses about causal links between variables) and quantitative data (eg epidemiological studies to test these hypotheses).[45] The resulting diagrams can be elegant and comprehensive, but they may be poorly understood by stakeholders and can even stall action if they convey the impression that most of the drivers of the problem are impossible to fix.[46]

3.3.3.2 Tell Stories

Narrative is an efficient tool for synthesising information about complex phenomena (particularly for depicting multiple causal influences).[42,43] Stories about needless suffering or inequality can inspire the moral imagination and ignite action to address these injustices.[43] Glenn Robert and his team use patient narratives to identify "emotional touch points" (eg things that make people angry or upset) in a journey through the health system to prioritise aspects of the system for improvement.[47]

In Box 3.3, narrative synthesis has been used to combine multiple interacting influences and levels into a meaningful account of what heart failure is and how it unfolds, the principles of managing it, how a remote monitoring system might work at organisational level, and why it might not work optimally for everyone. The same information could be conveyed in a causal loop diagram, but I prefer the narrative form because stories, as any toddler understands, are accessible, appealing, image-rich and inspiring.

Narrative helps us move beyond generalities and abstractions to understand the nuances of *particular* situations. "Anecdotes" are sometimes dismissed as poor-quality evidence because they are not generalisable, but there are good philosophical arguments for focusing on the particular and the specific when seeking to understand what is going on in an organisational case study.[48,49] For example, rather than saying "there was a lack of leadership", say "Dr Patel went on parental leave for 6 months. Her post was filled by a succession of locums and by two other partners taking on additional clinical work. The restructuring project initiated by Dr Patel was deprioritised until she returned."

3.3.3.3 Depict Competing Framings

Because complexity in human systems stems partly from clashes in values, which in turn support different framings of issues, it is important to depict each interest group's version of social reality. To some public health campaigners, facemasks during the COVID-19 pandemic were "protections", but to libertarians they were "restrictions".[50] Try to convey the different framings, including the assumptions underlying each position and the arguments, metaphors, symbols, images and data used to support it. Where data are presented in these framings, trace where the data came from and what 'realities' they create for whom.

3.3.4 Take Action

3.3.4.1 Muddle Through (Take an Emergent Approach)

The Cynefin framework (Figure 3.1) recommends that complexity is best approached in an emergent way (probe-sense-respond). In example 2 of Box 3.1 (remote patient monitoring for heart failure), there is no blueprint or formula we can give Rahul which, if followed, would guarantee the success of his project. Rather, he and his colleagues need to set a broad direction and then identify logistical, social and technical challenges and address these pragmatically by "muddling through" (working emergently and making pragmatic compromises)[51] and "tinkering" (fiddling and tweaking till things work).[52] Solutions are not off-the-shelf but *emergent*. The team could use sensemaking (eg generating a narrative, illustrated with example vignettes) to provide a sense of order (where we have come from and why; where we are now; where we hope to go next).[17,39]

The NASSS (non-adoption, abandonment, and challenges to spread, scale-up and sustainability) framework was designed to support an exploratory, emergent approach to technology projects in healthcare by considering the multiple domains in which complexity may be manifest (eg the disease, the technology, the value proposition, the intended adopters, the organisation and the wider system).[53]

3.3.4.2 Build Partnerships

Complex projects are delivered via partnerships, which must be organised and governed in a way that builds trust, shares power, assures psychological safety and supports collective action.[54] Consider approaches such as action research[55] or community-based participatory research.[54] If partnership outputs (milestones, deliverables) are prioritised over the relationship-building process, the change effort becomes oriented narrowly to a promised product at the expense of the long-term partnership synergies on which action depends—and hence, ultimately, ineffective.

3.3.4.3 Support Creative Action by Front-Line Actors

Whereas simple and complicated projects require competence (specific things that individuals know or are able to do), complex projects also require *capability*—the ability to adapt to change, generate new knowledge and continue to improve their performance.[56] Capability is enhanced through approaches such as exposing people to the challenge of unfamiliar contexts, giving feedback on performance and employing non-linear methods such as storytelling and small group, problem-based learning.[39,56] Psychological safety, in which even the most junior group members feel able to speak out and no-one is punished for raising concerns, helps develop and reinforce capability in the work setting.[57,58]

3.3.4.4 Acknowledge and Use Uncertainty

Scientific training typically teaches us to strive to eliminate uncertainty, but uncertainty and unpredictability are inherent to complex phenomena. Those who disregard uncertainty risk what Paul Han calls the "illusion of explanatory depth"—a strong but incorrect feeling of knowing arising when people feel they understand complex phenomena "with far greater precision, coherence and depth than they actually do".[59] Han defines uncertainty not as the absence of certainty but as "the attitude of committed neutrality that opens our eyes to our ignorance". Uncertainty can be of different kinds—for example, in relation to the relevance, completeness and trustworthiness of data, but also in relation to how actors make sense of those issues and what value they assign to them. Engaging with uncertainty requires human qualities such as humility, courage and flexibility.[59]

3.3.4.5 Harness Conflict

Political scientist Chantal Mouffe argues that conflicts are at the centre of politics.[20] To politicise an issue, she says, is to represent the world in terms of opposing "camps" with which people can identify. Mouffe distinguishes between *antagonism*, which she defines as a struggle between enemies in a war-like situation, and *agonism*, defined as conflict between adversaries who share a commitment to resolving the conflict through democratic means.[20] In Mouffe's vision of "agonistic pluralism", conflicts among interest groups are surfaced and openly discussed rather than hidden behind a veil of consensus (so-called "shared visions" can obscure silent dissent). To make progress on a contentious issue (think of assisted dying or vaccine hesitancy), all parties should try to understand where the other "sides" are coming from and why they feel so strongly about their position. Such conflictual engagement, says Mouffe, can provide "friction" that can lead to workable and acceptable multifaceted solutions.

3.3.5 Learn and Develop

3.3.5.1 Try Things Out and Monitor Their Impact

A learning health system gathers data on its own performance and uses those data to improve.[60] Clinical, administrative and financial data captured on computers (the kind we extract for audits) are important components of system learning, but we also need to capture data on the *human* dimensions of a project (eg Have staff made sense of proposed changes? Are the conflicting interest groups talking to each other?). When you have identified which data sources will give you a picture of progress, you can try things out on a small scale and measure their impact. Revisit and revise your map or narrative as new data emerge and situations change.

3.3.5.2 Deliberate Collectively

Group discussions, with patient and public involvement and informed by data and arguments, help the sensemaking process and guide us towards solutions that are right and reasonable.[61] Especially when multiple stakeholders hold opposing views about what the problem is and how to address it, all positions and all evidence need to be discussed and challenged. When researching such deliberation, clashes between different evidential paradigms should be treated as higher-order data.

3.3.5.3 Change Direction as Needed

If your complex project has been planned out in detail (eg with a tidy Gantt chart) before your study begins and you are committed to sticking rigidly to this plan come what may, you are probably trapped in the linear, deterministic thinking that still dominates the healthcare field. Research funders and ethics committees sometimes do not fully grasp this point and expect precisely such plans before approving a study.[62,63] You need to produce sufficient firm planning to persuade them that you will not drift aimlessly, but also commit to amending these plans in response to emerging data as your study unfolds. For example, set out what data you will collect to "probe" the system, and give examples of how particular findings could lead to a change of direction.

3.4 Conclusion

Complexity thinking in healthcare has been honoured more in the breach than in the observance. I hope the theoretical lenses and key steps to managing complexity covered in this chapter will help you as you strive to understand, influence and research complex systems.

References

1. Oudshoorn N, Pinch T. How users matter: The co-construction of users and technology. MIT Press; 2005.
2. Cilliers P. Complexity and postmodernism. London: Routledge; 1998.
3. Byrne D. Complexity theory and the social sciences: An introduction. Routledge; 2002.
4. Greenhalgh T, Papoutsi C. Studying complexity in health services research: Desperately seeking an overdue paradigm shift. *BMC Med.* 2018;16:1–6.

5. Ladyman J, Lambert J, Wiesner K. What is a complex system? *Eur J Philos Sci.* 2013;3:33–67.
6. Fustolo-Gunnink SF, de Boode WP, Dekkers OM, et al. If things were simple, word would have gotten around: Can complexity science help us improve pediatric research? *Pediatr Res.* 2024:1–10.
7. Black B. Belly woman: Birth, blood and ebola: The untold story. London: Neem Tree Press; 2022.
8. Weiner N. Cybernetics or control and communication in the animal and the machine. Cambridge: MIT Press; 2019 (1948).
9. Bateson G. Cybernetics & human knowing: A journal of second-order cybernetics auto poiesis. Imprint Academic; 2005 (1972).
10. Chen Y, Shi L, Zheng X, et al. Patterns and determinants of multimorbidity in older adults: Study in health-ecological perspective. *Int J Environ Res Public Health.* 2022;19(24):16756.
11. Scott WR. Institutions and organizations: Ideas and interests. London: Sage; 2008.
12. Scott WR. Lords of the dance: Professionals as institutional agents. *Organ Stud.* 2008;29(2):219–38.
13. Feldman MS. Organizational routines as a source of continuous change. *Organ Sci.* 2000;11(6):611–29.
14. Feldman MS, Pentland BT. Reconceptualizing organizational routines as a source of flexibility and change. *Adm Sci Q.* 2003;48(1):94–118.
15. Czarniawska B. A narrative approach to organizational studies. London: Sage; 1998.
16. Gabriel Y. Storytelling in organizations: Facts, fictions, and fantasies. Oxford: Oxford University Press; 2000.
17. Weick KE. Sensemaking in organizations. Thousand Oaks: Sage; 1995.
18. Majone G. Evidence, argumentation and persuasion in the policy process. New Haven: Yale University Press; 1989.
19. Fisher WR. Human communication as narration: Toward a philosophy of reason, value, and action. University of South Carolina Press; 1989.
20. Mouffe C. Agonistics: Thinking the world politically. Verso Books; 2013.
21. Greenhalgh T. Commentary: Without values, complexity is reduced to mathematics. *J Eval Clin Pract.* 2025;31(1):e14263. https://doi.org/10.1111/jep.14263
22. Adams Ve. Metrics: What counts in global health. Duke University Press; 2016.
23. Umoja Noble S. Algorithms of oppression: How search engines reinforce racism. New York: NYU Press; 2018.
24. Criado Perez C. Invisible women: Exposing data bias in a world designed for men. London: Penguin; 2019.
25. Ooms G. Navigating between stealth advocacy and unconscious dogmatism: The challenge of researching the norms, politics and power of global health. *Int J Health Policy Manag.* 2015;4(10):641.
26. Spencer G, Corbin JH, Miedema E. Sustainable development goals for health promotion: A critical frame analysis. *Health Prom Int.* 2019;34(4):847–58. https://doi.org/10.1093/heapro/day036
27. Greenhalgh T, Engebretsen E, Bal R, et al. Toward a values-informed approach to complexity in health care: Hermeneutic review. *Milbank Q.* 2023;101(3):646–74.
28. Wehrens R, Oldenhof L, Heerings M, et al. Integrating system dynamics and action research: Towards a consideration of normative complexity. *In J Health Policy Manag.* 2023;12.
29. Snowden DJ, Boone ME. A leader's framework for decision making. *Harv Bus Rev.* 2007;85(11):68.
30. Stacey R. Strategic management and organisational dynamics: The challenge of complexity (6th edition). London: Financial Times/Prentice Hall; 2010.

31. Tsoukas H. Don't simplify, complexify: From disjunctive to conjunctive theorizing in organization and management studies. *J Manage Stud*. 2017;54(2):132–53.
32. Moore GF, Evans RE, Hawkins J, et al. From complex social interventions to interventions in complex social systems: Future directions and unresolved questions for intervention development and evaluation. *Evaluation*. 2019;25(1):23–45.
33. McGill E, Er V, Penney T, et al. Evaluation of public health interventions from a complex systems perspective: A research methods review. *Soc Sci Med*. 2021;272:113697.
34. Shiell A, Hawe P, Gold L. Complex interventions or complex systems? Implications for health economic evaluation. *BMJ*. 2008;336(7656):1281–3. https://doi.org/10.1136/bmj.39569.510521.AD
35. Greenhalgh T, Russell J. Why do evaluations of eHealth programs fail? An alternative set of guiding principles. *PLoS Med*. 2010;7(11):e1000360.
36. Haynes A, Loblay V. Rethinking barriers and enablers in qualitative health research: Limitations, alternatives, and enhancements. *Qual Health Res*. 2024;34(14):1371–83. https://doi.org/10.1177/10497323241230890
37. Cartwright N. Rigour versus the need for evidential diversity. *Synthese*. 2021;199(5–6):13095–119. https://doi.org/10.1007/s11229-021-03368-1 [published Online First: 1 Nov 2021]
38. Shan Y, Williamson J. Applying evidential pluralism to the social sciences. *Eur J Philos Sci*. 2021;11:1–27.
39. Ancona D. Sensemaking: Framing and acting in the unknown. In: Snook S, Nohria N, Khurana R, eds. The handbook for teaching leadership. Thousand Oaks: Sage; 2012.
40. Rod NH, Broadbent A, Rod MH, et al. Complexity in epidemiology and public health: Addressing complex health problems through a mix of epidemiologic methods and data. *Epidemiol*. 2023;34(4):505–14. https://doi.org/10.1097/ede.0000000000001612 [published Online First: 30 May 2023]
41. Greenhalgh T, Shaw SE, Nishio AA, et al. Remote care in UK general practice: Baseline data on 11 case studies. *NIHR Open Res*. 2022;2.
42. Davidson B. Storytelling and evidence-based policy: Lessons from the grey literature. *Palgrave Comm*. 2017;3(1):1–10.
43. Denning S. The springboard: How storytelling ignites action in knowledge-era organizations. London: Routledge; 2012.
44. Cassidy R, Borghi J, Semwanga AR, et al. How to do (or not to do) . . . using causal loop diagrams for health system research in low and middle-income settings. *Health Policy Plan*. 2022;37(10):1328–36. https://doi.org/10.1093/heapol/czac064
45. Uleman JF, Stronks K, Rutter H, et al. Mapping complex public health problems with causal loop diagrams. *Int J Epidemiol*. 2024;53(4). https://doi.org/10.1093/ije/dyae091
46. McGlashan J, Hayward J, Brown A, et al. Comparing complex perspectives on obesity drivers: Action-driven communities and evidence-oriented experts. *Obes Sci Pract*. 2018; 4(6):575–81.
47. Robert G. Participatory action research: Using experience-based co-design to improve the quality of healthcare services. In: Ziebland S, Coulter A, Calibrese J, et al., eds. Understanding and using health experiences–improving patient care. Oxford: Oxford University Press; 2013.
48. Flyvbjerg B. Five misunderstandings about case-study research. *Qual Inj*. 2006;12(2):219–45.
49. Tsoukas H. Craving for generality and small-N studies: A Wittgensteinian approach towards the epistemology of the particular in organization and management studies. In: Buchanan D, Bryman A, eds. The Sage handbook of organizational research methods. London: Sage; 2009. p. 285–301.
50. Lupton D, Southerton C, Clark M, et al. The face mask in COVID times: A sociomaterial analysis. Melbourne: De Gruyter; 2021.

51. Lindblom CE. The science of "muddling through". *Public Adm Rev.* 1959;19(2):79–88.
52. Mol A, Moser I, Pols J. Care in practice: On tinkering in clinics, homes and farms. Transcript Verlag; 2010.
53. Greenhalgh T, Wherton J, Papoutsi C, et al. Beyond adoption: A new framework for theorizing and evaluating nonadoption, abandonment, and challenges to the scale-up, spread, and sustainability of health and care technologies. *J Med Internet Res.* 2017;19(11):e8775.
54. Jagosh J, Bush PL, Salsberg J, et al. A realist evaluation of community-based participatory research: Partnership synergy, trust building and related ripple effects. *BMC Public Health.* 2015;15(1):1–11.
55. Holmström P, Björk-Eriksson T, Davidsen P, et al. Insights gained from a re-analysis of five improvement cases in healthcare integrating system dynamics into action research. *Int J Health Policy Manag.* 2022;11(11):2707.
56. Fraser SW, Greenhalgh T. Coping with complexity: Educating for capability. *BMJ.* 2001;323(7316):799–803.
57. Edmondson AC, Lei Z. Psychological safety: The history, renaissance, and future of an interpersonal construct. *Annu Rev Organ Psychol Organ Behav.* 2014;1(1):23–43.
58. Dakin F, Rai T, Paparini S, et al. Supporting your support staff during crises: Recommendations for practice leaders to develop a relational workplace. *BMJ Leader.* 2023;7(Suppl 2):1–7. https://doi.org/10.1136/leader-2023-000780
59. Han PKJ. Uncertainty in medicine: A framework for tolerance. Oxford: Oxford University Press; 2021. p. 20.
60. Friedman C, Rubin J, Brown J, et al. Toward a science of learning systems: A research agenda for the high-functioning Learning Health System. *J Am Med Inform Assoc.* 2015;22(1):43–50.
61. Degeling C, Carter SM, Rychetnik L. Which public and why deliberate? A scoping review of public deliberation in public health and health policy research. *Soci Sci Med.* 2015;131:114–21.
62. Goodyear-Smith F, Jackson C, Greenhalgh T. Co-design and implementation research: Challenges and solutions for ethics committees. *BMC Mec Ethics.* 2015;16:1–5.
63. Lanham HJ, Leykum LK, Taylor BS, et al. How complexity science can inform scale-up and spread in health care: Understanding the role of self-organization in variation across local contexts. *Soci Sci Med.* 2013;93:194–202.
64. Puik E, Ceglarek D. The quality of a design will not exceed the knowledge of its designer: An analysis based on axiomatic information and the cynefin framework. *Procedia Cirp.* 2015;34:19–24.
65. Kraaijenbrink J. Strategy in the face of complexity. LinkedIn; 2023.
66. Schuurmans JJ, Felder M, Bal R, et al. Reorganizing medical care for older persons in times of scarcity: A cybernetics analysis of work pressure and organizational change. *Soci Sci Med.* 2024:117634. https://doi.org/10.1016/j.socscimed.2024.117634
67. Glass TA, McAtee MJ. Behavioral science at the crossroads in public health: Extending horizons, envisioning the future. *Soci Sci Med.* 2006;62(7):1650–71.
68. Darabi N, Hosseinichimeh N. System dynamics modeling in health and medicine: A systematic literature review. *Syst Dyn Rev.* 2020;36(1):29–73.
69. Baugh Littlejohns L, Hill C, Neudorf C. Diverse approaches to creating and using causal loop diagrams in public health research: Recommendations from a scoping review. *Public Health Rev.* 2021;42:1604352.
70. Cassidy R, Borghi J, Semwanga AR, et al. How to do (or not to do) . . . using causal loop diagrams for health system research in low and middle-income settings. *Health Policy Plan.* 2022;37(10):1328–36.
71. Homer J, Ritchie-Dunham J, Rabbino H, et al. Toward a dynamic theory of antibiotic resistance. *Syst Dyn Rev.* 2000;16(4):287–319.

72. Allender S, Owen B, Kuhlberg J, et al. A community based systems diagram of obesity causes. *PloS One*. 2015;10(7):e0129683.
73. McGlashan J, Johnstone M, Creighton D, et al. Quantifying a systems map: Network analysis of a childhood obesity causal loop diagram. *PloS One*. 2016;11(10):e0165459.
74. Savona N, Brown A, Macauley T, et al. System mapping with adolescents: Using group model building to map the complexity of obesity. *Obes Rev*. 2023;24:e13506.
75. Stake R. The art of case study research. London: Sage; 1995.
76. Love PED, Ika LA. Making sense of hospital project MisPerformance: Over budget, late, time and time again—why? And what can be done about it? *Eng*. 2022;12:183–201. https://doi.org/10.1016/j.eng.2021.10.012
77. Weick KE, Sutcliffe KM. Hospitals as cultures of entrapment: A re-analysis of the Bristol Royal Infirmary. *Calif Manag Rev*. 2003;45(2):73–84.
78. Easton D. Political system: An enquiry ito the state of political science. New York: Knopf; 1953.
79. Laclau E, Mouffe C. Hegemony and socialist strategy: Towards a radical democratic politic. Verso; 2001.
80. Hindmarsh R. Hot air ablowin! 'Media-speak', social conflict, and the Australian 'decoupled' wind farm controversy. *Soc Stud Sci*. 2014;44(2):194–217. https://doi.org/10.1177/0306312713504239
81. Greenhalgh T, A'Court C, Shaw S. Understanding heart failure; explaining telehealth: A hermeneutic systematic review. *BMC Cardiovasc Disord*. 2017;17:1–16.

CHAPTER

4

Use of Big Data in Primary Care Research

Karen Tu and Tokuharu Tanaka

4.1 Introduction

Primary care is considered the cornerstone of many high-performing healthcare systems.[1] Despite its central role and being the ideal place to study whole-person care, primary care research has historically been hampered by a lack of funding relative to specialty and hospital-based care.[2] Big data have been characterised as data that are high in volume, velocity, variety, veracity and value.[3] The use of big data has provided opportunities for exponential growth in primary care research over the past few decades.[2] For example, through the introduction of electronic medical records (EMRs), electronic recording of anthropometric measures, laboratory tests, medications and clinical narratives, combined with administrative healthcare utilisation data, patient-reported outcomes and digital health tools such as apps and wearable technologies.

4.2 Extensive Primary Care Research Opportunities with Big Data

Just as primary care is broad in scope, primary care big data research spans a wide variety of research areas. The vast amount of available EMR data and other big data related to primary care has unlocked new avenues for research, allowing researchers to explore a wide range of topics. Examples include:

- ***Symptom progression and disease recognition.***[4] Understanding how early symptoms evolve into diagnosed conditions.
- ***Quality of care assessments.***[5,6] Evaluating adherence to clinical guidelines and treatment effectiveness.
- ***Antimicrobial stewardship.***[7] Analysing patterns of antibiotic prescription to address concerns about antibiotic resistance.

DOI: 10.1201/9781003652106-6

- ***Polypharmacy***[8] ***and multimorbidity.***[9] Studying the effects of multiple medications and co-existing conditions on patient outcomes.
- ***Risk prediction models.***[10,11] Developing tools to predict the likelihood of disease progression or adverse outcomes.
- ***Vaccine safety and effectiveness.***[12,13] Evaluating how well vaccines prevent disease and their risks of adverse events in real-world primary care settings.
- ***Pharmacovigilance.***[14] Post-marketing surveillance of medication safety.
- ***Public health surveillance.***[15] Using primary care data for timely detection of outbreaks, exemplified by influenza surveillance systems in the United Kingdom (UK).
- ***Longitudinal cohort studies.***[16] Following patients over time with repeated observations.
- ***Medical education insights.***[17] Understanding physician training needs and decision-making patterns.
- ***Impact of COVID-19 on primary care.***[18] Analysing how the pandemic affected healthcare delivery and patient management.

At the Robert Graham Center in the United States, HealthLandscape[19] has paired big data with geographic information systems (GIS) to facilitate a better understanding of health and communities. HealthLandscape provides a suite of data visualisation tools to help primary care researchers find insights to improve healthcare. The Robert Graham Center is an excellent example of how primary care big data can be used to facilitate and inform policy decisions.

The UK has a well-established history of primary care EMR research, offering valuable lessons for other countries looking to establish similar databases.[20] The Nuffield Department of Primary Care at the University of Oxford[21] has recently converged several major primary care big data resources. They have convened the world's longest established and largest EMR database, and developed the UK's only prescribing database to build a big data analytics powerhouse. Notable databases include ORCHID, used to carry out disease surveillance, epidemiological, trial and prospective studies; Clinical Practice Research Datalink (CPRD), an observational database of primary care electronic health records for more than 35 million patients, which enables retrospective and prospective public health and clinical studies; and QResearch, a large consolidated database derived from the anonymised health records of more than 40 million patients to link general-practice derived and secondary care data.

The Nivel Institute in the Netherlands also has a longstanding history of using longitudinal primary care data for population health and health services research.[22] It combines general practitioner (GP) EMR, out-of-hours GP services, physiotherapy practices, exercise therapy practices, speech therapy practices and dietitian practices data in the Netherlands, which are linkable with other data sources such as secondary care, social care or social economic data.

4.2.1 Case Study: Canada's Experience in Advancing Primary Care Big Data Research

Initially, health services research in Canada concentrated on hospital data, where professional coders manually extracted and recorded information from paper-based hospital records. These coders documented key details such as the primary reason for hospitalisation, conditions that influenced the length of stay and comorbidities present in patients. By linking these records to postal codes and other data sources, researchers could associate these records with the patient's socioeconomic status and urban vs. rural residence.[23]

Hospital data proved to be highly accurate and invaluable for studying patient outcomes, particularly for conditions that required hospitalisation.[24] However, when it came to primary care, physician billing data were initially deemed unreliable for identifying disease conditions. Although these billing records contained diagnostic codes, the primary purpose of these codes was not clinical accuracy but administrative processing. Because physicians were required to submit only one diagnostic code per visit, and diagnoses could be based on clinical suspicion rather than confirmed evidence, the data lacked precision.

Despite these challenges, researchers developed validated algorithms combining hospital data and physician billing data to identify patients with disease conditions. Chart abstraction studies were carried out in primary care physician offices, whereby paper medical records were manually reviewed to enable the creation of a reference standard to validate algorithms for identifying chronic diseases such as diabetes[25] and hypertension.[26] These methods paved the way for the use of administrative data in primary care research, and facilitated the ability to study conditions commonly diagnosed and primarily managed in primary care settings.

4.3 The Transition to Electronic Medical Records in Primary Care

The early 2000s saw a major shift with the introduction of EMRs into family physician offices. This technological advancement not only revolutionised patient care but also further enhanced big data research in primary care. Although administrative data provides broad population-level coverage and includes information such as coded hospitalisations, physician billing records, emergency room visits and formulary medications dispensed from pharmacies, EMR data from family physician offices offers much more depth. It captures detailed patient-level information including structured data, such as physician billing codes and anthropometric measures; semi-structured data, including prescriptions, laboratory tests, smoking status and family and past medical history; and unstructured free text, such as progress notes, consult letters, hospital discharge summaries, emergency room records and diagnostic test reports.

4.4 Overcoming Key Challenges

Building a primary care EMR database comes with several challenges. These span from privacy concerns, ethical approvals, securing physician participation for data sharing, data extraction, data storage, data quality, cleaning and data governance. Ensuring patient confidentiality is a top priority, requiring researchers to implement robust de-identification methods that preserve data privacy while maintaining its research value.

If individual-level data are properly de-identified/coded to protect patient identities, then these databases generally meet the standard criteria for a waiver of consent. Requiring explicit patient consent would not only be impractical but would also introduce significant bias, making the database unrepresentative of the general population.

Legislation regarding these databases varies by country. Patients may be informed about data usage through posters displayed in clinic waiting rooms or by electronic means. These notices provide a contact number for patients who wish to have their data removed. This 'opt-out' rather than 'opt-in' approach is essential for maintaining the database's generalisability. Standardised coding and data-cleaning procedures are also essential to transform raw EMR data into a structured format suitable for analysis.

In the early days, extracting EMR data was a manual and labour-intensive process. It required physical visits to physician offices to access clinic servers and to run extraction programmes during off-hours to avoid disrupting clinical operations. Over time, technological advancements allowed for remote and automated data extraction, minimising disruption and improving efficiency.

One crucial principle in sustaining a research database is avoiding financial incentives for data contributors. While setting up an EMR database requires initial infrastructure, funding for hardware, software and staff, paying physicians for their data contributions could introduce ethical concerns and long-term sustainability issues. Instead, offering physicians confidential feedback on quality indicators and continuing medical education credits has proven to be a successful incentive model for recruitment and contribution.

A recognised shortcoming of primary care big data systems is limited standardisation and inconsistent recording of social care needs.[27] This poses a significant barrier to advancing research on multimorbidity and social determinants of health. Integrating social care variables with big data analytics is a critical next step in developing research on holistic, person-centred healthcare.

4.5 INTRePID: A Global Primary Care Big Data Consortium

In 2020, the emergence of the COVID-19 pandemic, a growing recognition of the common challenges faced in primary care worldwide and an increasing appreciation of virtual meeting software to facilitate international collaboration collectively contributed to the establishment of the International Consortium of Primary Care Big Data Researchers (INTRePID, www.intrepidprimarycare.org). The mission of INTRePID was to conduct international comparative research in primary care, foster collaboration, facilitate mentorship, exchange knowledge and promote capacity-building in primary care big data research worldwide.

4.6 Expanding Global Reach: Lessons Learned

Through its global expansion, INTRePID has learned several important lessons:

- ***Administrative data*** can provide significant research value even where comprehensive EMRs are not fully implemented.

- ***Local expertise and contextual knowledge*** are critical for accurately interpreting primary care data.
- ***Building trust and promoting sustainable, equitable collaboration*** is essential for fostering long-term international research relationships.
- ***Flexibility*** in identifying and using available data sources broadens the scope of global participation.

The experience of INTRePID underscores that countries at all stages of digital health development can meaningfully contribute to global primary care big data research, reinforcing the importance of inclusivity, adaptability and collaboration.

4.7 Expanding Big Data Research in Latin America

In the past decade, EMRs in primary care have gained traction across Latin America. Several countries have readily accessible administrative data that can contribute to big data research. Governments in countries such as Peru, Brazil and Colombia have implemented policies that facilitate data accessibility. For instance, in Peru, legislation mandates that government-held health data be made available to researchers upon request.[28] In Brazil, primary care data is open access, allowing anyone to download and analyse it.[29] Colombia has also enacted legal frameworks requiring public institutions to provide open access to government data, including a national open data portal that hosts thousands of datasets related to health and other sectors.[30]

While big data research in Latin American primary care has begun, there is still work to be done in assessing data quality and reliability.[31] However, with increasing interest in developing primary care EMR databases and ready access to administrative data, Latin America is poised to become a key player in the global expansion of primary care big data research.

4.8 Introducing Big Data Research in Africa

Expanding primary care big data research efforts in Africa presents unique challenges. Many African nations have yet to implement EMRs into primary care, and healthcare data infrastructure remains underdeveloped. During initial conversations with Kenyan colleagues, there was uncertainty about whether relevant data sources existed in Kenya. However, during a visit to a primary care clinic in Nairobi, Kenya, it was discovered that valuable healthcare data was already being collected for administrative purposes. Inside a designated 'data room', a young woman was entering patient visit details into a computerised government reporting system. Handwritten posters on the walls displayed quarterly reports for 2023, including the top 10 reasons for visits for patients under five and over five years old. This dataset was exactly what INTRePID had been seeking for a global comparative study on primary care visit patterns.[32] When asked how long they had been collecting these data, the clinic manager explained that for over 20 years, they had submitted patient data (including visit date, age, sex and reason for consultation) as part of a government requirement for reimbursement. This discovery demonstrated that even in settings where advanced EMR systems are lacking, meaningful primary care data may still exist and be able to be used for research.

Disease-specific databases such as those for HIV, tuberculosis and child and maternal health are often not integrated into broader primary care data systems, but District Health Information Systems (DHIS) exist in many African countries and have the potential to be used for primary care big data health services research.

Although the use of big data in African healthcare is still in its early stages, there is significant potential for growth. With increased expertise, experience and investment, African nations have the potential to harness big data to enhance primary care delivery across the continent.

4.9 The Future of Primary Care Big Data Research

Big data already exist in primary care across the globe, but they are not always recognised, structured or leveraged for research. Primary care big data research is most developed in Europe, North America and Oceania, but there is immense untapped potential worldwide.

The future of primary care research will likely be shaped by advancements in artificial intelligence (AI) and machine learning. AI-driven methods can enhance the analysis of free-text data, improve disease prediction models and generate real-time clinical insights. Additionally, as more countries adopt standardised EMR systems, make administrative data more accessible and develop platforms to link EMR data and administrative data, opportunities for global comparative research will continue to expand.

4.10 Conclusion

The journey of big data in primary care research has been transformative. From manually reviewing paper charts for administrative data validation studies to leveraging AI-driven EMR analysis, the field has evolved rapidly. Challenges remain in data standardisation, privacy protection and infrastructure development, but the benefits of utilising big data in primary care are undeniable. As international collaborations through initiatives like INTRePID grow, the future of primary care big data research looks brighter than ever, with the potential to improve healthcare outcomes on a global scale.

References

1. Starfield B. Is primary care essential? *Lancet*. 1994;344:1129–33. https://doi.org/10.1016/s0140-6736(94)90634-3
2. National Academies of Sciences, Engineering, and Medicine. Implementing high-quality primary care: Rebuilding the foundation of health care. Washington: National Academies Press; 2021. p. 448. [cited 9 Jun 2025; Available from: http://www.ncbi.nlm.nih.gov/books/NBK571810/]

3. Schulte T, Bohnet-Joschko S. How can big data analytics support people-centred and integrated health services: A scoping review. *Int J Integr Care*. 2022;22:23. https://doi.org/10.5334/ijic.5543
4. Rafiq M, White B, Barclay M, et al. A UK population-based case-control study of blood tests before cancer diagnosis in patients with non-specific abdominal symptoms. *Br J Cancer*. 2025;132:450–61. https://doi.org/10.1038/s41416-024-02936-9
5. Campbell SM, Braspenning J, Hutchinson A, et al. Research methods used in developing and applying quality indicators in primary care. *Qual Saf Health Care*. 2002;11:358–64. https://doi.org/10.1136/qhc.11.4.358
6. Månsson J, André M, Johansson E, et al. Enhancing primary care quality improvement through national data collection and validation: The primary care quality initiative in Sweden. *Scand J Prim Health Care*. 2025;1–11. https://doi.org/10.1080/02813432.2025.2490921
7. Schwartz KL, Langford BJ, Daneman N, et al. Unnecessary antibiotic prescribing in a Canadian primary care setting: A descriptive analysis using routinely collected electronic medical record data. *CMAJ Open*. 2020;8:E360–9. https://doi.org/10.9778/cmajo.20190175
8. Boateng I, Pascual CR, Grassby P, et al. The impact of polypharmacy on health outcomes in the aged: A retrospective cohort study. *PloS One*. 2025;20:e0317907. https://doi.org/10.1371/journal.pone.0317907
9. Ornstein SM, Nietert PJ, Jenkins RG, et al. The prevalence of chronic diseases and multimorbidity in primary care practice: A PPRNet report. *J Am Board Fam Med*. 2013;26:518–24. https://doi.org/10.3122/jabfm.2013.05.130012
10. Hippisley-Cox J, Coupland C. Development and validation of risk prediction equations to estimate survival in patients with colorectal cancer: Cohort study. *BMJ*. 2017;357:j2497. https://doi.org/10.1136/bmj.j2497
11. Clift AK, Coupland CAC, Keogh RH, et al. Living risk prediction algorithm (QCOVID) for risk of hospital admission and mortality from coronavirus 19 in adults: National derivation and validation cohort study. *BMJ*. 2020;371:m3731. https://doi.org/10.1136/bmj.m3731
12. Heins MJ, Spreeuwenberg P, Caini S, et al. Measuring the impact of influenza vaccination in the Netherlands using retrospective observational primary care, hospitalisation and mortality data. *Vaccine*. 2024;42:126244. https://doi.org/10.1016/j.vaccine.2024.126244
13. Faksova K, Walsh D, Jiang Y, et al. COVID-19 vaccines and adverse events of special interest: A multinational Global Vaccine Data Network (GVDN) cohort study of 99 million vaccinated individuals. *Vaccine*. 2024;42:2200–11. https://doi.org/10.1016/j.vaccine.2024.01.100
14. Lavertu A, Vora B, Giacomini KM, Altman R, Rensi S. A new era in pharmacovigilance: Toward real-world data and digital monitoring. *Clin Pharmacol Ther*. 2021;109:1197–202. https://doi.org/10.1002/cpt.2172
15. Cerqueira-Silva T, Marcilio I, de Araújo Oliveira V, et al. Early detection of respiratory disease outbreaks through primary healthcare data. *J Glob Health*. 2023;13:04124. https://doi.org/10.7189/jogh.13.04124
16. Darke P, Cassidy S, Catt M, et al. Curating a longitudinal research resource using linked primary care EHR data-a UK Biobank case study. *J Am Med Inform Assoc*. 2022;29:546–52. https://doi.org/10.1093/jamia/ocab260
17. Khamisy-Farah R, Gilbey P, Furstenau LB, et al. Big data for biomedical education with a focus on the COVID-19 era: An integrative review of the literature. *Int J Environ Res Public Health*. 2021;18:8989. https://doi.org/10.3390/ijerph18178989
18. Tu K, Sarkadi Kristiansson R, Gronsbell J, et al. Changes in primary care visits arising from the COVID-19 pandemic: An international comparative study by the International Consortium of Primary Care Big Data Researchers (INTRePID). *BMJ Open*. 2022;12:e059130. https://doi.org/10.1136/bmjopen-2021-059130
19. HealthLandscape. Robert graham center [cited 9 Jun 2025; Available from: www.grahamcenter.org/content/brand/rgc/maps-data-tools/healthlandscape.html]

20. Edwards L, Pickett J, Ashcroft DM, et al. UK research data resources based on primary care electronic health records: Review and summary for potential users. *BJGP Open.* 2023;7:BJGPO.2023.0057. https://doi.org/10.3399/BJGPO.2023.0057
21. Big Data. Medical sciences division, nuffield department of primary care health sciences, Oxford. [cited 9 Jun 2025; Available from: www.phc.ox.ac.uk/research/research-themes/big-data]
22. Vanhommerig JW, Verheij RA, Hek K, et al. Data resource profile: Nivel Primary Care Database (Nivel-PCD), The Netherlands. *Int J Epidemiol.* 2025;54:dyaf017. https://doi.org/10.1093/ije/dyaf017
23. Government of Canada Health Inequalities Data Tool. [cited 9 Jun 2025; Available from: https://health-infobase.canada.ca/health-inequalities/]
24. Williams JI, Young W. Appendix: A summary of studies on the quality of health care administrative databases in Canada. In: Goel V, Williams J, Anderson G, Blackstien-Hirsch P, Fooks C, Naylor D, eds. Patterns of healthcare in Ontario the ICES practice Atlas (2nd edition). Ottawa: Canadian Medical Association; 1996. p. 339–346. [cited 9 Jun 2025; Available from: www.ices.on.ca/publications/research-reports/patterns-of-health-care-in-ontario-2nd-edition/]
25. Hux JE, Ivis F, Flintoft V, et al. Diabetes in Ontario: Determination of prevalence and incidence using a validated administrative data algorithm. *Diabetes Care.* 2002;25:512–6. https://doi.org/10.2337/diacare.25.3.512
26. Tu K, Campbell NR, Chen Z-L, et al. Accuracy of administrative databases in identifying patients with hypertension. *Open Med.* 2007;1:e18–26.
27. Simpson G, Mutindi Kaluvu L, Stokes J, et al. Understanding social care need through primary care big data: A rapid scoping review. *BJGP Open.* 2022;6:BJGPO.2022.0016. https://doi.org/10.3399/BJGPO.2022.0016
28. Peru. Presidency of the Republic. Supreme decree no. 007-2024-JUS: Regulation of the law on transparency and access to public information. El Peruano; 2024. [cited 9 Jun 2025; Available from: https://cdn.www.gob.pe/uploads/document/file/6372106/5590378-decreto-supremo-que-aprueba-el-reglamento-de-la-ley-de-transparencia-y-acceso-a-la-informacion-publica.pdf]
29. Saúde MD. Sistema de Informação em Saúde para a Atenção Básica (SISAB). [cited 9 Jun 2025; Available from: https://sisab.saude.gov.br/]
30. Colombia. Ministry of information and communication technologies. Open data portal; Portal de Datos Abiertos. [cited 12 Jun 2025; Available from: www.datos.gov.co]
31. Lopes FRL, Monteiro KS, Santos S. How data provided by the Brazilian information system of primary care have been used by researchers. *Health Inform J.* 2020;26:1617–30. https://doi.org/10.1177/1460458219882273
32. Tu K, Lapadula MC, Apajee J, et al. Changes in reasons for visits to primary care after the start of the COVID-19 pandemic: An international comparative study by the International Consortium of Primary Care Big Data Researchers (INTRePID). *PLoS Glob Public Health.* 2024;4:e0003406. https://doi.org/10.1371/journal.pgph.0003406

CHAPTER

5

The Role of AI in Transforming Primary Care Research

Florian O Stummer and Thomas Frese

5.1 Introduction

Artificial intelligence (AI) has become a transformational influence in healthcare, fundamentally altering the processing, interpretation and application of data in clinical and research settings. The emergence of large language models (LLMs) and advanced machine learning (ML) architectures has facilitated enhanced sophistication in the synthesis of structured and unstructured health data, thereby bolstering diagnostic accuracy and personalised care strategies.[1–3] In primary care, a field characterised by intricate patient cases and ongoing management, AI is starting to transform both clinical workflows and the foundational approaches to research design and implementation.

AI's role in clinical decision support (eg triage systems, risk stratification tools and documentation automation) has garnered significant attention. Yet, its application in primary care *research* extends further, enabling methodological innovation through multimodal data integration, prompt-driven hypothesis generation, and dynamic simulation environments.[2,4] For instance, transformer-based models like BERT and Longformer allow for the encoding of extensive clinical narratives into semantically rich representations, thereby facilitating real-time extraction of population-level insights from electronic health records.[3] Furthermore, LLMs have demonstrated value in natural language processing (NLP) applications that automate chart review, detect adverse drug events or match patients to clinical trials with minimal manual oversight.

This growth necessitates rigour. Comprehensive assessments of AI models, especially chatbots and LLMs, have demonstrated significant variability in evaluation frameworks, highlighting the necessity for standardised criteria and clear model descriptions.[5] With increasing regulatory scrutiny, AI applications must be anchored in reproducibility, domain relevance, and clinical safety, particularly when utilised in decision-making contexts. Therefore, the first step is to analyse the ways in which AI improves primary care research via innovative approaches, tools, and paradigms. It emphasises the transition from passive data mining to reasoning-oriented systems

DOI: 10.1201/9781003652106-7

that replicate clinical cognition, examines case applications of AI-enhanced research in diverse worldwide contexts, and presents the nascent Mycelium of Thought paradigm as an experimental framework for collaborative AI–human reasoning. We aim to establish AI as a methodological catalyst in the advancement of primary care research by examining both empirical and theoretical advancements.

5.2 Conceptual Foundations of AI in Primary Care Research

AI comprises a wide array of computing methods designed to replicate human intellect, encompassing reasoning, learning, and decision-making. Fundamentally, AI is driven by ML and neural network models that allow systems to analyse extensive datasets, discern patterns, and generate probabilistic forecasts.[6] In healthcare, foundational models, pretrained on vast datasets, constitute the core of LLMs, which are being utilised in primary care research.[3]

The development of these core models demonstrates decades of advancement in algorithmic design, computational efficiency, and data accessibility. Transformer designs have transformed AI capabilities by facilitating bidirectional context comprehension and scalability learning across various tasks.[7] Encoder-based models such as BERT and hybrid systems such as BART have shown significant efficacy in biomedical applications, including clinical record analysis, risk classification, and patient phenotyping.[2] Transfer learning optimises these models by enabling pretrained systems to adjust to new, domain-specific datasets with minimal supplementary training, thus enhancing both accuracy and resource efficiency.

In the field of primary care, these AI functionalities must address distinct issues. Patient data is frequently disjointed, diverse, and documented in both organised and unstructured formats. Furthermore, the epistemic intricacy of primary care, characterised by uncertainty, multimorbidity, and socioeconomic determinants of health, necessitates models that are capable of integrating across modalities and reasoning through ambiguity.[8] The increasing emphasis on multimodal models, capable of concurrently processing text, images, audio, and genetic data, underscores the necessity for enhanced contextual intelligence.[3]

AI in primary care must go from static classification tasks to dynamic, reasoning-based frameworks. Recent advancements in explainable AI (XAI), modular inference, and collaborative decision-making[2] reflect human diagnostic reasoning and provide avenues for harmonising AI results with clinical intuition and ethical responsibility.

Thus, the conceptual foundation of AI in primary care rests not only on technical sophistication but also on epistemological alignment with the core values and complexities of generalist practice.

5.3 AI-Enabled Data Sources and Collection Tools

Electronic healthcare records (EHRs) provide the key data resource for the majority of AI research in primary care. They encompass structured data, such as ICD codes, laboratory findings, prescriptions, and encounter histories, alongside unstructured clinical narratives that provide valuable contextual insights. Contemporary LLMs employ embeddings to transform textual data into dense, multidimensional vectors that maintain semantic linkages, hence improving the model's capacity to identify clinical nuances.[1] Notwithstanding their utility, EHR systems frequently experience inadequate interoperability and variable data standards, which limit the scalability and generalisability of AI applications.[9]

The proliferation of wearable devices has created new opportunities for ongoing, passive health surveillance. These devices produce longitudinal datasets that record heart rate, sleep quality, physical activity and electrocardiogram (ECG) signals, which are essential for predictive modelling in chronic disease management.[10] Wearable data, when analysed by LLMs, can be combined with genomic, demographic or behavioural data to enhance risk classification and facilitate individualised therapies.[3]

The scalability of AI in primary care is contingent upon the incorporation of extensive public health data. Datasets such as MIMIC or national health registries provide essential real-world context for model validation and training. Federated learning, a technique enabling AI models to learn from decentralised data sources without sending raw data, offers a privacy-preserving solution that is particularly applicable to primary care networks.[2] This method facilitates learning from varied patient demographics while ensuring adherence to data protection laws, including GDPR and HIPAA.

The effective use of various data streams requires strong preprocessing tools. Natural language processing (NLP) components of LLMs can extract key-value pairs, resolve co-reference chains and identify clinical entities from unprocessed text.[7] Visualisation frameworks and metadata tagging augment the interpretability of multimodal datasets. Annotation platforms are progressively being created alongside AI tools to facilitate iterative human-in-the-loop training processes that ensure outputs conform to therapeutic standards.[5]

As the scope of primary care data broadens, the capacity of AI systems to integrate and respond to many data sources will be pivotal to their efficacy. Utilising EHRs, wearable data and public repositories via scalable, interoperable pipelines is essential for developing inclusive, responsive and contextually intelligent AI models for primary care research.

5.4 AI Methods in Primary Care Research

AI technologies in primary care research encompass a broad range, including conventional machine learning classifiers and sophisticated generative and reasoning-based systems. These approaches enable several functions:

1. Assessing illness risk
2. Analysing unstructured text
3. Categorising patient groups
4. Producing real-time suggestions

As primary care confronts intricate, multimorbid and contextually nuanced cases, the foundational AI methodologies must embody this diversity in both design and interpretability.

Supervised learning models have been utilised in primary care research for early disease diagnosis, risk stratification and outcome prediction. These models are developed using labelled datasets and refined for parameters including sensitivity, specificity and area under the curve (AUC). Convolutional neural networks (CNNs) have been utilised for imaging data to identify diabetic retinopathy, whereas gradient boosting trees have been employed for mortality prediction using EHRs.[2]

Recently, reinforcement learning (RL) frameworks have been implemented in primary care settings, where AI agents acquire knowledge through trial and error in dynamic situations. RL algorithms demonstrate potential in enhancing longitudinal treatment strategies by simulating disease trajectories and modifying recommendations accordingly.[3] Nonetheless, obstacles persist in delineating therapeutically significant reward functions and substantiating outcomes in practical studies.

Due to the narrative complexity of clinical records, NLP is crucial for extracting insights from unstructured text. Current AI systems utilise transformer-based models, such as BERT and BioMegatron, which are proficient at named entity recognition, relation extraction and clinical notes summaries.[1] These functionalities are particularly advantageous for recognising social determinants of health, adverse drug reactions and patient-reported outcomes derived from unstructured text fields.

Zero-shot prompting continues to be a prevalent method, enabling models to produce outputs for tasks not explicitly addressed during training. This method, however efficient, may jeopardise accuracy. More precise approaches encompass few-shot prompting, in-context learning and chain-of-thought prompting, wherein the model deduces incrementally prior to producing a conclusion.[2] These strategies improve interpretability and synchronise model outputs with the intricate logic frequently necessary in diagnostic reasoning.

Unsupervised learning methods are extensively employed to discern novel phenotypes and subpopulations within diverse primary care cohorts. Clustering methods, including k-means, hierarchical clustering and t-SNE dimensionality reduction, are frequently utilised to categorise patients according to symptom profiles, comorbidity patterns or utilisation histories. These classifications facilitate the formulation of customised interventions and the optimisation of resource distribution.[6]

LLMs such as GPT-4, Mistral, Claude, MedPalm, etc, signify a novel advancement in AI techniques, proficient in producing realistic responses, integrating information from many publications and engaging people in conversational exchanges. Nonetheless, these systems encounter constraints in clinical settings owing to hallucinations and inconsistencies when subjected to aggressive prompting.[11] Researchers have addressed this issue by employing instruction tuning and model alignment techniques, such as low rank adaptation (LoRA) and quantised LoRA (QLoRA), to fine-tune LLMs for domain-specific tasks while utilising minimal computing resources.[3]

In addition to generation, reasoning-based paradigms are currently being investigated for their capacity to replicate clinical cognition. These models emulate diagnostic processes, evaluate hypotheses, and assess alternative outcomes, indicating a transition from pattern recognition to intentional, context-sensitive reasoning.[1] The primary care-centred Mycelium of Thought (MoT) reasoning approach illustrates this shift by integrating modular, elucidative stages and adaptive feedback mechanisms that replicate the manner in which doctors navigate intricate cases.

A comprehensive assessment continues to be a significant barrier. Conventional measurements such as accuracy and F1 scores may hide clinically significant errors. AI in primary care increasingly use task-specific measures, such as BERTScore, BLEU, and confusion matrices, which are customised to clinical relevance.[7] Regulatory requirements necessitate clear model documentation, encompassing data lineage, tuning parameters, and interpretability attributes.

As AI methods in primary care evolve, their success will depend on balancing computational power with epistemic alignment, ensuring models not only function but also think in ways consistent with the values and complexity of generalist care.

5.5 Innovations in Research Design Using AI

The incorporation of AI into primary care research is transforming data analysis and fundamentally altering research design. Conventional paradigms, focused on fixed protocols, sequential processes, and hypothesis-driven approaches, are being enhanced by AI-driven systems that facilitate dynamic, adaptive, and real-time exploration. These improvements enable more adaptive, context-aware, and scalable research methodologies that correspond with the increasing complexity of primary care.

AI facilitates hybrid research methodologies that integrate prospective, retrospective, and real-time data streams. Simulation-based trials, wherein AI models produce synthetic data derived from real-world distributions, are employed to pretest hypotheses and enhance interventions prior to clinical implementation.[2] In adaptive trial designs, machine learning algorithms dynamically modify inclusion criteria, randomisation procedures or dose regimens based on interim assessments and prediction analytics.[12]

Furthermore, the incorporation of generative models into research design facilitates the development of synthetic control arms, which are especially beneficial when the recruitment of comparator groups poses ethical or practical difficulties. These AI-generated cohorts, based on historical EHR data, replicate baseline trajectories and enable researchers to more effectively identify the treatment effect.[10]

An important advancement is the application of rapid engineering not only for clinical duties but also as a methodological instrument in research. Researchers can utilise LLMs in interactive simulations, where prompts are systematically adjusted to investigate variable outcomes, patient responses or population-level behaviours across diverse intervention scenarios.[3] This methodology corresponds with the advent of instructional causality, wherein causal linkages are analysed via controlled linguistic interventions in AI models. Such frameworks enable quick cycle evaluation, wherein interventions are implemented, assessed, and modified in brief iterations. AI solutions aggregate feedback from digital health platforms, wearable devices or patient portals to facilitate near real-time modifications in study protocols.[12]

The capacity of AI to assimilate multimodal data, including clinical text, laboratory results, pictures, genomics, and sensor data, facilitates comprehensive representations of patient conditions, hence enhancing translational research across several fields. For instance, research including both behavioural indicators (eg activity data from wearables) and biological markers (eg genomic profiles) has been viable using LLM-driven fusion frameworks.[2] This integration not only improves internal validity but also expedites the translational process from observational results to intervention development.

These improvements are particularly pertinent to primary care, as research frequently needs to consider diverse patient demographics, comorbidities and regional healthcare environments. Integrating AI into study design enables primary care researchers to produce more sophisticated, representative and actionable insights, so facilitating a new era of responsive, patient-centred research.

5.6 Case Examples and International Applications

The practical implementation of AI in primary care research has advanced significantly in recent years, with global case studies offering important insights on feasibility, constraints and contextual adaptability. These examples illustrate the deployment of AI tools across several health systems to enhance diagnosis, documentation and decision-making, each influenced by local infrastructure, legislation and practice standards.

A notable instance is the application of LLMs to replicate medical board examination outcomes. Arvidsson et al[11] evaluated GPT-4 using Sweden's Family Medicine Board Exam and discovered that, although the model answered numerous questions correctly, it exhibited a deficiency in the nuance and contextual adaptation anticipated from certified physicians. This work highlights the capabilities and constraints of existing generative AI models: exceptional performance on standardised tasks may not ensure safe and trustworthy results in intricate, real-world clinical situations.

Weng et al[13] also emphasised the constraints of AI applications resulting from the omission of non-open-access data, such as proprietary exam databases, in model training. This limits AI's knowledge base and raises equitable issues regarding model performance across various disciplines and nations.

Conversely, in low-resource settings, AI is being evaluated for decision support in triage systems, where restricted access to physicians demands scalable, automated solutions. These tools are frequently underpinned by federated learning techniques that safeguard data privacy while facilitating cross-regional model training.[2]

Cross-national comparisons also disclose regulatory discrepancies. The European Union's AI Act requires responsibility distribution among developers and organisations for high-risk AI systems, while U.S. policies prioritise transparency and voluntary disclosure.[3] These disparities influence the speed and safety of AI adoption in primary care research, especially when studies incorporate patient-facing tools.

Collectively, these case examples reveal a landscape of rapid experimentation tempered by context-specific challenges. They affirm the need for flexible, locally adapted AI models and governance frameworks in primary care research worldwide.

5.7 Future Directions and Research Implications

As AI becomes more integrated into primary care research, the sector must transition from technological exuberance to deliberate incorporation. Future research directions are determined by technology innovation, epistemological coherence, trust establishment and regulatory transparency.

A predominant tendency is the shift from statistical pattern recognition to reasoning-based intelligence. Conventional AI systems have demonstrated proficiency in recognising connections among extensive datasets; nevertheless, they frequently lack effectiveness in scenarios requiring causal reasoning, ethical discernment and narrative integration. Recent advancements in quick engineering and few-shot learning demonstrate efforts to advance models toward higher-order cognition.[1,2]

The Mycelium of Thought (MoT) framework encapsulates this transformation. MoT denotes a modular, chain-of-thought prompting framework intended to replicate the sequential reasoning employed by clinicians in developing differential diagnoses or formulating research methodologies. MoT enhances LLMs by incorporating structured reflection, dynamic role-play and decision tree logic into prompts, so converting them from passive respondents into co-analysts proficient in diagnostic inquiry, research design or topic synthesis.[2] This paradigm improves interpretability and auditability while aligning with the cognitive ecology of generalist practice.

Integrating MoT into primary care research has multiple implications: (1) allowing AI to aid in hypothesis formulation from intricate EHR narratives; (2) enhancing real-time decision auditing in clinical trials; and (3) promoting interdisciplinary communication between researchers and data scientists via transparent reasoning pathways.

Future research settings will likely incorporate AI-driven platforms that enable multimodal research workflows, integrating structured data, text, sensor streams and patient-reported results. Federated learning will evolve to facilitate collaborative model training across geographically distributed, privacy-sensitive datasets.[3] Concurrently, low-code research assistants utilising LLM application programming interfaces (APIs) may democratise access to sophisticated analytical capabilities for underfunded primary care settings. The refinement of domain-specific LLMs (such as BioBERT, PubMedGPT or PMC-LLaMA) also opens new possibilities for specialised knowledge integration and task precision.[7]

The viability of AI in primary care research depends on strong governance. Issues including data leakage, performance degradation and bias transmission necessitate proactive frameworks for validation, transparency and equity.[5] Regulatory authorities in the EU and North America are starting to require comprehensive model disclosure and joint liability for AI-related damages; however, harmonisation across countries is still lacking.

To promote responsible innovation, researchers must incorporate evaluation metrics that extend beyond accuracy, including explainability, fairness and patient acceptability. AI co-authorship, audit trails and ethical review processes will become integral components of future research methodologies.

In conclusion, the future of AI in primary care research is not solely computational; it is also cognitive, collaborative and critical. Paradigms such as MoT highlight the forthcoming frontier: systems that engage in cognitive processes alongside humans, rather than solely on our behalf.

5.8 Conclusion

Artificial intelligence is initiating a new epoch in primary care research, marked by improved methodological accuracy, dynamic data integration and the development of reasoning-based systems. AI has enhanced the researcher's toolkit, facilitating intricate studies across diverse data sources, from electronic health records to wearable devices. Large language models today facilitate not only documentation and categorisation tasks but also hypothesis creation and real-time decision modelling.

This progress necessitates increased attention. Concerns of interpretability, equality and epistemic alignment necessitate thorough validation, interdisciplinary collaboration and strong governance frameworks. Future research will necessitate AI systems that are transparent, responsive and clinically informed, designed to enhance human judgment rather than only supplant it.

Reconceptualising AI as a co-reasoning partner rather than as a black-box instrument can enhance primary care research in terms of efficiency, depth, integrity and effect. As the industry advances, success will be characterised not only by innovation but also by a deliberate integration that respects the intricacies of primary care.

References

1. Shah K, Xu AY, Sharma Y, et al. Large language model prompting techniques for advancement in clinical medicine. *J Clin Med.* 2024;13(17):5101.
2. Du X, Zhou Z, Wang Y, et al. Generative large language models in electronic health records for patient care since 2023: A systematic review. *medRxiv.* 2024.
3. Timilsina M, Buosi S, Razzaq MA, et al. Harmonizing foundation models in healthcare: A comprehensive survey of their roles, relationships, and impact in artificial intelligence's advancing terrain. *Comput Biol Med.* 2025;189:109925.
4. Bracken A, Reilly C, Feeley A, et al. Artificial Intelligence (AI)–powered documentation systems in healthcare: A systematic review. *J Med Syst.* 2025;49(1):28.
5. Huo B, Boyle A, Marfo N, et al. Large language models for chatbot health advice studies: A systematic review. *JAMA Netw Open.* 2025;8(2):e2457879.
6. Maaz S, Palaganas JC, Palaganas G, Bajwa M. A guide to prompt design: Foundations and applications for healthcare simulationists. *Front Med.* 2025;11:1504532.
7. Scott IA, Zuccon G. The new paradigm in machine learning: Foundation models, large language models and beyond: A primer for physicians. *Intern Med J.* 2024;54(5):705–15.
8. Young RA, Martin CM, Sturmberg JP, et al. What complexity science predicts about the potential of artificial intelligence/machine learning to improve primary care. *J Am Board Fam Med.* 2024;37(2):332–345.
9. Abdulazeem HM, Meckawy R, Schwarz S, Novillo-Ortiz D, Klug SJ. Knowledge, attitude, and practice of primary care physicians toward clinical AI-assisted digital health technologies: Systematic review and meta-analysis. *Int J Med Inform.* 2025:105945.

10. Qin H, Tong Y. Opportunities and challenges for large language models in primary health care. *J Prim Care Community Health*. 2025;16:21501319241312571.
11. Arvidsson R, Gunnarsson R, Entezarjou A, Sundemo D, Wikberg C. ChatGPT (GPT-4) versus doctors on complex cases of the Swedish family medicine specialist examination: An observational comparative study. *BMJ Open*. 2024;14(12):e086148.
12. Afshar M, Gao Y, Wills G, et al. Prompt engineering with a large language model to assist providers in responding to patient inquiries: A real-time implementation in the electronic health record. *JAMIA Open*. 2024;7(3):ooae080.
13. Weng TL, Wang YM, Chang S, Chen TJ, Hwang SJ. ChatGPT failed Taiwan's family medicine board exam. *J Chin Med Assoc*. 2023;86(8):762–766.

CHAPTER

6

Empowering Primary Care Research Through Digital Tools and Applications

A Practice-Oriented Perspective

Buğu Usanma Koban and Mehmet Akman

6.1 Introduction

Digital health has emerged as essential research infrastructure within primary care, enabling the generation of real-world evidence, expanding study populations and enhancing methodological rigour. The COVID-19 pandemic proved the necessity and viability of digital tools for remote care, catalysing a shift in both clinical practice and research strategy.[1,2] In response, the World Health Organization's (WHO) 2023 Classification of Digital Health Interventions provides a structured paradigm (covering client-facing, provider-facing, health system management and data services) that this chapter employs to examine the role of digital tools in primary care research.[2] This focused scope deliberately excludes advanced artificial intelligence (AI) methodologies, which are examined in a separate chapter, allowing this discussion to remain centred on practical, field-level digital applications.

6.2 Digital Tools Enabling Primary Care Research

6.2.1 Electronic Health Records

Electronic health records (EHRs) are important resources for primary care research, providing longitudinal datasets that support cohort studies, quality monitoring and healthcare utilisation analyses. Organisation for Economic Co-operation and Development (OECD) data show that by 2021, more than 93% of primary care practices in member countries had functional EHR systems, with patient-accessible portals widely adopted.[3] However, data quality concerns remain; inconsistent coding and gaps in documentation frequently necessitate data-cleaning studies or mixed-method validation approaches.[4] Despite these barriers, pilot programmes

DOI: 10.1201/9781003652106-8

such as that introduced by the United Kingdom's (UK) National Health Service (NHS) have begun using EHRs to streamline consent and enhance equity in enrolment for clinical trials.[5]

6.2.2 Mobile Health Applications

Mobile health applications (mHealth apps) extend research into daily life, enabling chronic disease management, behavioural assessments and patient-reported data collection. For example, the Noom digital self-management app combined with human coaching resulted in significantly greater weight loss and sleep improvement compared to standard care in a South Korean primary care setting.[6] Systematic reviews have found that mHealth interventions can contribute to blood pressure control, HbA1c reduction, increased physical activity and improved patient satisfaction, along with enhanced clinical professional engagement.[7] Physician-facing apps, such as those used by Israeli GPs, improve clinical decision-making and information accessibility, with dual benefits for providers and patients.[8]

6.2.3 Geographic Information Systems

Geographic information systems (GIS) tools enable precise mapping of disease burden and healthcare access disparities. This system can be used not only for planning healthcare services during disasters and emergencies, but also for examining healthcare access in disadvantaged regions. It is particularly used in analysing spatial factors related to access to care, such as socioeconomic and environmental determinants.[9] By integrating spatial data into recruitment protocols and intervention planning, researchers can design equity-sensitive, geographically targeted studies.

6.2.4 Digital Survey Tools and Participation Platforms

Platforms such as REDCap, SurveyMonkey and Survey123 facilitate flexible, adaptive data collection capable of addressing multilingual needs and remote enrolment.[10] These tools support random assignment of survey versions or incentives, enable real-time monitoring of response rates, and support decentralised study architectures that can better include hard-to-reach populations.[11] One notable example in this context is the NIH-funded 'All of Us' research programme, a large-scale, multicentre data initiative that includes health information from more than 400,000 individuals. The database encompasses a wide range of variables, including medical conditions, medications and laboratory test results. This can facilitate rapid advancements in precision medicine by enabling researchers to conduct large-scale, data-driven analyses.[12]

6.2.5 Telemedicine and Remote Patient Monitoring

Telemedicine has become a cornerstone of primary care, particularly in response to COVID-19 restrictions, supporting remote consultations, chronic disease management and pragmatic clinical trials.[13,14] Its rapid adoption has transformed care delivery and expanded research opportunities, especially in decentralised or hybrid study designs. Remote patient monitoring (RPM) tools, such as home blood pressure monitors, glucometers and scales, enable longitudinal data collection beyond clinic walls. These technologies reduce participant burden, support real-world monitoring and strengthen the ecological validity of findings. Although AI-powered RPM is outside of this chapter's scope, conventional RPM systems have shown benefits in promoting patient self-management and reducing costs.[14] In Germany, digital health applications (Digitale Gesundheitsanwendung, DiGA), also known as "apps on prescription", are used to enhance the treatment of a wide range of illnesses by imparting information, providing context or guiding patients through exercises. In the United States, Medicare RPM collects and electronically transmits patient data from digital devices such as blood pressure monitors, blood glucose monitors and other wearable sensors.[14,15] As remote and digitally supported research models gain momentum, telemedicine and RPM are becoming essential components of primary care research infrastructure.

6.2.6 Additional Field Tools

Offline platforms such as open data kit (ODK) enable building powerful forms to collect data in the field. These allows for studies in low-connectivity environments, making them ideal for cluster designs and hybrid site-based/mobile data collection.[10] Dashboards offer real-time monitoring and quality assurance across multiple locations, while point-of-care testing tools (for example, for HbA1c or CRP) enable biochemical assessments in community settings and at the bedside.[16]

6.3 Methodological Innovations and Research Designs

6.3.1 Digitally Enhanced Recruitment and Decentralised Trials

EHR-linked platforms allow active, equitable recruitment outside of traditional clinic settings. In pilot studies using the NHS app, it matched eligible patients to ongoing studies.[17] Mobile and GIS-guided outreach expands representation among underserved communities, addressing systemic gaps.[11,16] Trial designs can include rolling enrolment, stepped-wedge models and adaptive consent workflows (see Chapter 17).[18]

6.3.2 Longitudinal Tracking and Repeated Measures

mHealth and RPM support high-frequency data capture, enabling pragmatic cohort studies and individualised n-of-1 assessments.[6] Remote symptom monitoring (for example, for post-stroke or diabetes management) enhances detection of outcome trends and adverse events, improving internal and external validity.[1]

6.3.3 Remote Intervention Delivery and Implementation Evaluation

Telemedicine enables decentralised trials and intervention delivery across distance. Evaluation frameworks such as RE-AIM (Reach, Effectiveness, Adoption, Implementation,

TABLE 6.1 Recent Digital Tool Implementations in Primary Care Research

Tool	Country	Study Design	Year	Key Outcome
Noom + coaching app	South Korea	RCT in 17 clinics	2020–21	Weight loss and improved sleep[6]
AccessMod	Afghanistan	Spatial cross-sectional	2023	Estimation of provinces underserved by primary care[21]
RPM interventions	US & EU	Systematic review	2016–21	Improved chronic illness outcomes[14]
NHS mobile recruitment	UK	Pilot integration	2023–25	Improved recruitment diversity[17]
DHIS2	Egypt	Oral health surveillance	2024	Feasible and sustainable method for collecting oral health data among preschool children[22]
mHealth behavioural health	US	Curriculum integration	2023–24	Improved behavioural health access[16]

US = United States; EU = European Union; UK = United Kingdom; RCT = randomised controlled trial; app = application; RPM = remote patient monitoring; NHS = National Health Service; DHIS2 = District Health Information Software 2

and Maintenance) and one developed by the UK Medical Research Council to evaluate complex interventions leverage digital logs and dashboards to monitor fidelity, adoption, reach and sustainability.[19] Digital metrics allow researchers to adapt protocols in near real-time, increasing methodological responsiveness.

6.3.4 Hybrid, Mixed-Methods and Spatial Study Designs

Researchers can embed qualitative sub-studies based on digital triggers, such as survey patterns or RPM flags, and combine survey results with GIS stratification to target hotspots. Hybrid cluster designs (combining digital and site-based data collection) and pragmatic trial models are well supported by existing digital infrastructures.[20] See Table 6.1 for recent implementation of various digital tools.

6.4 Ethical, Equity and Infrastructure Challenges

The use of digital tools in research raises critical ethical and infrastructure challenges. Data security requires robust encryption, anonymisation and compliance with international regulations such as the General Data Protection Regulation (GDPR) and Health Insurance Portability and Accountability Act (HIPAA).[23]

Digital literacy disparities may exclude vulnerable populations, requiring targeted training for both participants and research teams.[7,24] Implementation frameworks such as RE-AIM and the Consolidated Framework for Implementation Research (CFIR) offer structured approaches to evaluating the adoption, appropriateness and sustainability of digital interventions.[19] Finally, proactive recruitment strategies that target under-represented populations, combined with translation services and multisite digital deployment, are necessary to mitigate digital divides and ensure that research findings are generalisable across diverse patient populations.[25]

6.5 Future Perspectives and Recommendations

Primary care research should integrate WHO's digital health framework when designing studies, to ensure comprehensive coverage of digital interventions across client, provider, system and data domains.[2] Interoperable, user-centred platforms that integrate EHR data, telemedicine and patient-reported outcome measures (PROMs) will enable flexible research designs and data sharing. Investments in digital literacy training are essential to support both research teams and participants.[26] Telehealth and broader digital innovations have been shown to help close preventive healthcare gaps in rural and underserved communities.[27] Adoption of dynamic consent models will further enhance participant autonomy, allowing individuals to make informed decisions as research protocols evolve.[24] Simultaneously, alignment of funding mechanisms and regulatory frameworks will be essential to support the development, validation and scale-up of evidence-based digital research tools, as demonstrated by recent policy innovations from the National Institute for Health and Care Excellence (NICE), the US Food and Drug Administration (FDA) and other regulators.[28,29]

6.6 Conclusion

Digital tools, including EHRs, mHealth apps, GIS, telemedicine, RPM and digital surveys, represent powerful enablers of practice-oriented primary care research. Excluding AI methodologies previously earmarked for another chapter, this chapter has emphasised real-world applications, methodological innovations, country-level examples and critical ethical considerations. The future of primary care research depends on responsible integration of these tools, ensuring interoperability, inclusivity and structured governance, ultimately enabling equitable, high-quality evidence generation.

6.7 Disclosure

This chapter was developed with the assistance of generative AI tools, in compliance with the publisher's AI policy.

References

1. Pagliari C. Digital health and primary care: Past, pandemic and prospects. *J Glob Health.* 2021;11:01005.
2. World Health Organization. Classification of digital interventions, services and applications in health. 2023. [cited Apr 2025; Available from: https://iris.who.int/bitstream/handle/10665/373581/%209789240081949-eng.pdf?sequence=1]

3. OECD. Health at a glance 2023: OECD indicators. OECD; 2023. [cited Aug 2025; Available from: https://www.oecd.org/en/publications/health-at-a-glance-2023_7a7afb35-en.html]
4. Huang MZ, Gibson CJ, Terry AL. Measuring electronic health record use in primary care: A scoping review. *Appl Clin Inform*. 2018;9(1):15–33.
5. Wi CI, King KS, Ryu E, Natoli TL, Miller RP, Spiten MJ, et al. Application of innovative subject recruitment system for batch enrollment: A pilot study. *J Prim Care Community Health*. 2023;14. https://doi.org/10.1177/21501319231194967
6. Ju H, Kang E, Kim Y, Ko H, Cho B. The effectiveness of a mobile health care app and human coaching program in primary care clinics: Pilot multicenter real-world study. *JMIR Mhealth Uhealth*. 2022;10(5):e34531.
7. Arias López MDP, Ong BA, Borrat Frigola X, Fernández AL, Hicklent RS, Obeles AJT, et al. Digital literacy as a new determinant of health: A scoping review. *PLoS Digit Health*. 2023;2(10):e0000279.
8. Hernandez N, Castro L, Medina-Quero J, Favela J, Michan L, Mortenson WB. Scoping review of healthcare literature on mobile, wearable, and textile sensing technology for continuous monitoring. *J Healthc Inform Res*. 2021;5(3):270–99.
9. Stansberry TT, Tran L, Myers C. Using geographic information systems in health disparities research: Access to care considerations. *Res Nurs Health*. 2023;46(6):635–44.
10. Raja A, Tridane A, Gaffar A, Lindquist T, Pribadi K. Android and ODK based data collection framework to aid in epidemiological analysis. *Online J Public Health Inform*. 2014;5(3):228.
11. Bashshur RL, Howell JD, Krupinski EA, Harms KM, Bashshur N, Doarn CR. The empirical foundations of telemedicine interventions in primary care. *Telemed J E Health*. 2016;22(5):342–75.
12. Parente DJ. Leveraging the All of Us database for primary care research with large datasets. *J Am Board Fam Med*. 2024;37(Supplement2):S144–55.
13. Knop M, Mueller M, Niehaves B. Investigating the use of telemedicine for digitally mediated delegation in team-based primary care: Mixed methods study. *J Med Internet Res*. 2021;23(8):e28151.
14. Badr J, Motulsky A, Denis JL. Digital health technologies and inequalities: A scoping review of potential impacts and policy recommendations. *Health Policy*. 2024;146:105122.
15. Vudathaneni VKP, Lanke RB, Mudaliyar MC, Movva KV, Mounika Kalluri L, Boyapati R. The impact of telemedicine and remote patient monitoring on healthcare delivery: A comprehensive evaluation. *Cureus*. 2024. [cited Aug 2025; Available from: https://www.cureus.com/articles/227384-the-impact-of-telemedicine-and-remote-patient-monitoring-on-healthcare-delivery-a-comprehensive-evaluation]
16. Peyroteo M, Ferreira IA, Elvas LB, Ferreira JC, Lapão LV. Remote monitoring systems for patients with chronic diseases in primary health care: Systematic review. *JMIR Mhealth Uhealth*. 2021;9(12):e28285.
17. Fava VMD, Lapão LV. Provision of digital primary health care services: Overview of reviews. *J Med Internet Res*. 2024;26:e53594.
18. Phillips RL. Using geographic information systems to understand health care access. *Arch Fam Med*. 2000;9(10):971–8.
19. Unsworth H, Dillon B, Collinson L, Powell H, Salmon M, Oladapo T, Ayiku L, Shield G, Holden J, Patel N, Campbell M, Greaves F, Joshi I, Powell J, Tonnel A. The NICE Evidence Standards Framework for digital health and care technologies: Developing and maintaining an innovative evidence framework with global impact. *Digit Health*. 2021 Jun 24;7. https://doi.org/10.1177/20552076211018617
20. Nhavoto JA, Grönlund A. Mobile technologies and geographic information systems to improve health care systems: A literature review. *JMIR Mhealth Uhealth*. 2014;2(2):e21.

21. Mohammed RN, Khawari A, Shaguy JA, Abouzied A. A GIS-based approach to identifying communities underserved by primary health care services: An Afghanistan case study. *Front Public Health*. 2023;11:1209986.
22. Abdelrahman HH, Hamza M, Essam W, Adham M, AbdulKafi A, Baniode M. Electronic oral health surveillance system for Egyptian preschoolers using District Health Information System (DHIS2): Design description and time motion study. *BMC Oral Health*. 2024;24:807.
23. Vayena E, Blasimme A, Sugarman J. Decentralised clinical trials: Ethical opportunities and challenges. *Lancet Digit Health*. 2023;5(6):e390–4.
24. Lay W, Gasparini L, Siero W, Hughes EK. A rapid review of the benefits and challenges of dynamic consent. *Res Ethics*. 2025;21(1):180–202.
25. Bradway M, Årsand E. Diverse recruitment strategies are needed to reduce digital divide: Results from a workshop addressing digital divide and effects of pandemic restrictions. In: Séroussi B, Weber P, Dhombres F, Grouin C, Liebe JD, Pelayo S, et al., eds. Studies in health technology and informatics. IOS Press; 2022. [cited Aug 2025; Available from: https://ebooks.iospress.nl/doi/10.3233/SHTI220592]
26. Lin J, Bates SM, Allen LN, Wright M, Mao L, Kidd M. Integrating mobile health app data into electronic medical or health record systems and its impact on health care delivery and patient health outcomes: Scoping review. *JMIR Mhealth Uhealth*. 2025;13:e66650.
27. Simeon A-OA, Olayemi OA, Oluwaleke A, Aisha KI, Philip BK, Onyeka MU-E, et al. Bridging gaps in preventive healthcare: Telehealth and digital innovations for rural communities. *World J Adv Res Rev*. 2024;24(3):2861–72.
28. U.S. Food and Drug Administration (FDA). Digital health center of excellence. 2020. [cited 5 Aug 2025; Available from: https://www.fda.gov/medical-devices/digital-health-center-excellence]
29. NICE. Evidence standards framework for digital health technologies. 2022. [Available from: https://www.nice.org.uk/about/what-we-do/our-programmes/evidence-standards-framework-for-digital-health-technologies]

CHAPTER

7 Creative Methods for Primary Care Researchers

Kyle Eggleton

7.1 Introduction

Undertaking qualitative research is not solely about interviewing participants and developing themes from their responses. In fact, primary care researchers can use a vast array of different methods and methodologies in order to gather data and analyse that data. One such set of approaches are creative methods that elicit emotions, thoughts and feelings to describe personal experiences. Within this chapter, a range of creative methods are highlighted that primary care researchers may wish to use. The intent of this chapter is not to provide a detailed account of different methods, but rather to foster inspiration and prompt researchers to explore the wider body of literature.

Before incorporating creative methods into research, researchers must ask themselves whether the proposed methods are best suited for answering the research question and if the proposed methods align with the positionality of the researcher. Positionality is a critical component of not only qualitative approaches but research in general. Understanding our values, how we view the nature of reality and what we believe about knowledge influences our own generation of knowledge through research. Researchers are not neutral parties, observing participants dispassionately from a distance. We are active actors in the research process, bringing along our own biases, emotions, preconceived ideas and intents. Within creative methods, the researchers are generally engaged in the creation and visceral interpretation of data.

Creative methods align with my own positionality, and this is something that I sometimes bring into my research. I am a Pākehā (New Zealand European) male working as a general practitioner in a remote part of Aotearoa New Zealand (NZ). I am concerned about social injustice, health inequity and power. I view truth as being multifaceted and that all statements of truth are worthy of critique. I hold that subjectivity and experiences are shaped by privilege. My critical theorist paradigm has led me on a journey that has involved reflecting on the biases and privileges that I hold and how these shape my interactions with others. Creative methods have enabled me to undertake deep self-reflection and to engage with participants in ways that have fostered critical thinking.

DOI: 10.1201/9781003652106-9

Creative methods must fit the research question. Questions that require deep reflection or touch on emotive subjects or involve participants from 'vulnerable' or 'hard-to-reach' groups might be more suitable for creative approaches. Previously, my colleagues and I have also argued that creative methods allow researchers to collaborate with participants who might find it difficult to express concepts through 'talk' alone.[1] We have suggested that creative methods allow researchers access to ways in which participants see the world, and they can create shared meaning.

I have used all of the methods I describe in this chapter: photovoice, critical visual methods, poetry and creative writing. Within each section, I provide examples of how the method can be used, and where possible I have provided references with open access for further reading. Images are drawn from my own projects, which have not been published elsewhere.

7.2 Photovoice

Photovoice is a participatory technique that was originally described by Wang and Burris.[2] It involves participants taking pictures of scenes, objects or artefacts that answer a research question. The theoretical background of photovoice draws from critical consciousness literature and feminist theories.[2] Its intent is to enable people to represent their concerns to an audience via an image, to promote critical discussion with the audience and to reach policy-makers.[3]

Studies suitable for the photovoice method are research projects that might help shape policy, to teach others what is real in participants' lives or to help community members in shaping responses to an issue.[3] The general approach of a study using photovoice is:

- Identify an issue of concern (often a community concern).
- Recruit participants from within that community or who share that concern.
- Have a group discussion on the issue, discuss the process of taking pictures and the ethics of taking pictures (especially of other people).
- Give participants the time to take photos of the issue.
- Ask participants to select a photo(s) that they would like to present to a wider audience.
- Invite policymakers and the wider community to a meeting where participants share their pictures and encourage discussion.

In order to guide reflection on the photos, Wang posed a series of questions, represented by the acronym SHOWeD:[3]

- What do you **S**ee here?
- What is really **H**appening here?
- How does this relate to **O**ur lives?

- **W**hy does this situation, concern or strength exist?
- What can we **D**o about it?

Typically, discussions are recorded and transcribed, and themes are developed through a range of different analytical techniques.

7.2.1 Example 1: Rural Interprofessional Education Reflection

An example of a photovoice project is a study undertaken by our team trying to understand the experience and reflections of health students undertaking a rural health interprofessional programme in NZ. The programmes are located in predominantly Māori communities, and students are exposed to Māori culture. The local teaching teams invited students to participate in the project and discussed the aim. They paid particular attention to the ethics around taking pictures of other people, which was to be avoided, and culturally sensitive objects and locations, which were to be checked with a cultural advisor. Students discussed the photos they took in small groups and then selected a photo that best represented their reflection on their experience. Local community members and health professionals were invited to a group presentation, where students presented their photos and their meaning using the SHOWeD acronym. The discussions were audio-recorded, transcribed and then analysed through reflective thematic analysis.[4]

In Figure 7.1, the student is standing on a hill looking out over the rural town and the sky. Their reflection is of hope for a better future and a desire for people to be able to work together for the betterment of society. This represented a theme of hope for systemic change.

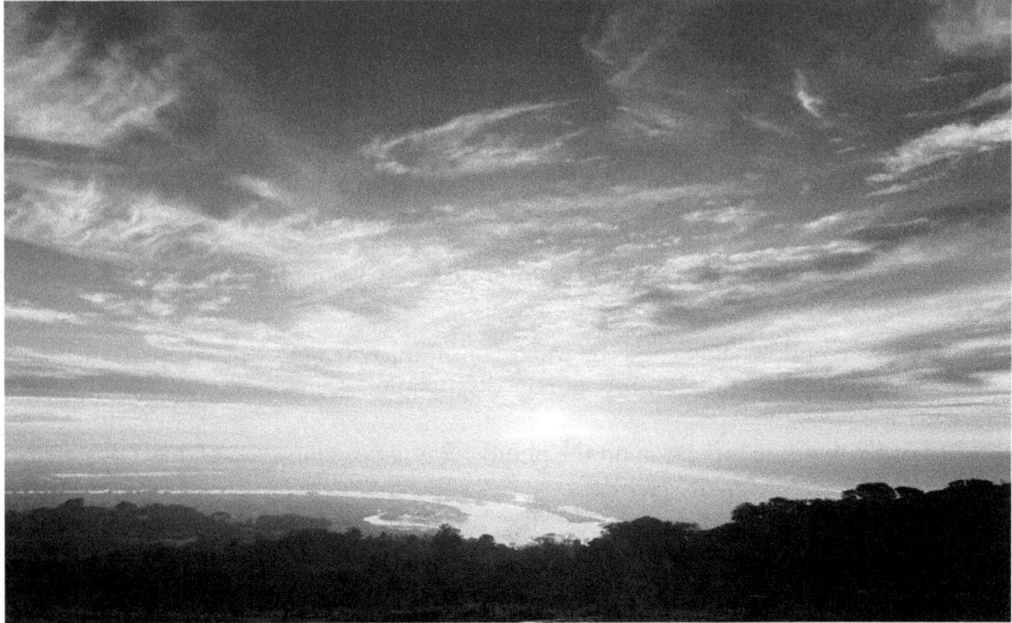

FIGURE 7.1 Photo of sky and town

7.3 Critical Visual Methods

Another visual approach is critical visual methods. This method draws from work by Rose that describes a framework for analysing drawings and paintings.[5] Within this method, participants are invited to draw or paint an image prompted by a question. This image is then jointly analysed by both participant and researcher. As such, critical visual methods represent another form of participatory research where participants are co-creators of knowledge.[1]

Drawing images can be a deeply reflective process. In addition, drawings can be rich in metaphor and meaning. In my own work, I have used drawings and a critical visual method to understand the experience of structurally disempowered groups on entering into primary care reception areas[6] and the forms of relationships enacted within a homeless support organisation. Drawing and critical visual methods have been used to reach 'hard-to-reach' populations.[7] However, my colleagues and I have argued that the drawing process alone does not reduce the power barrier between researcher and participant.[6] Rather, we suggest that clear positionality, reflective practices and culturally safe approaches are also critically important.[6]

Ethical considerations are important prior to using this method. One ethical issue relates to the discomfort that participants might feel in drawing. For example, in the primary care reception project, some participants felt like their art might be judged or that they were not artistic enough to draw. Participants should be reassured that it is not the quality of image that is examined. Rather, it is the meaning of that image to participants and the emotions that are invoked. There are also potential issues relating to drawing sensitive topics, and careful consideration should be made as to whether the unveiling of emotions might breach self-erected psychological barriers.

Rose's framework suggested three lines of questioning that should be posed to participants about the image.[5] These questions relate to:

- The production of the image, such as the circumstances or events surrounding it
- The image itself, such as the meaning of colour or objects
- The relationship between the image and the audience, for example, how would other people interpret the image?

The discussion around the generation and interpretation of the image is normally transcribed and analysed through a qualitative methodology.

7.3.1 Example 2: Reception Processes in Primary Care

An example of critical visual methods is a project examining primary care reception areas. The research aim was to understand the experience of people navigating reception processes and waiting rooms in primary care. Participants were recruited via agencies supporting people who have historically found it difficult to access primary care. Informed consent was gained from participants. In particular, the requirement to draw their experiences was discussed. Participants were interviewed, mostly in their homes, and were invited to draw three idealised pictures

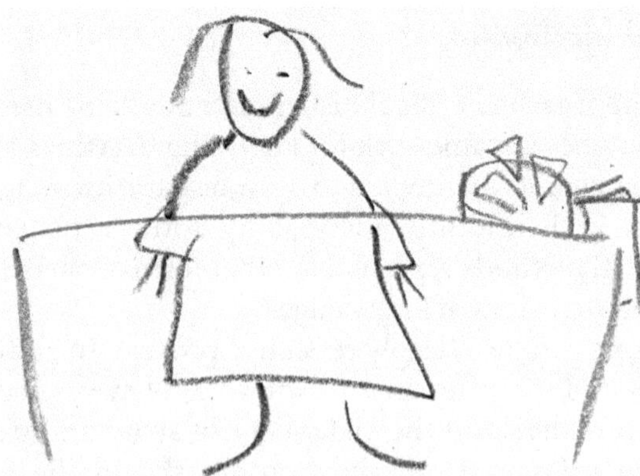

FIGURE 7.2 The receptionist desk

relating to making an appointment via a receptionist, engaging with a receptionist and waiting in a waiting room. During the drawing process, and on conclusion of the drawing, participants were asked questions relating to their experiences, including what the image represents, were there deeper meanings or metaphors in the image, why did they choose particular colours or materials, and how would other people view the image or interpret it. The interviews and drawing process took up to two hours, and the conversations were transcribed. A grounded theory method was used to analyse the data and themes generated.[8]

The primary finding from this project was that waiting rooms should be spaces that encourage relational permeability.[9] Receptionists should be able to navigate past their desks and engage with people waiting in the waiting room in a supportive and uplifting manner. In Figure 7.2, Fiona (not her real name) drew a desk with a receptionist behind it. She originally did not draw the receptionist's legs, but then changed her mind to indicate that she wanted the receptionist to be more visible and connected to her.

7.4 Poetry

Not all creative arts–based research involves the generation of images. Other creative methods include the written word. For example, poetry can be incorporated into research to generate an emotional response and increase engagement.[10] Although participant-generated poetry can be a source of data within health research,[11] it is normally used to present findings, share researcher interpretations or for autoethnographic reflections. These latter approaches are referred to as poetic inquiry. Brown describes poetic inquiry as a method that 'engenders moments of wonder, and stimulates deep, analytical thought'. [10] It can encourage researchers to move out of their own worldview and view the world through the lens of participants.[12]

Participant-voiced poetry uses data drawn from participants through interviews and represents these in poetic form. The researcher-generated poems are designed to embody the intent and meaning of participants. Although the poems should not portray the researchers' own experiences, they do capture the voice of the researcher in conjunction with the voice of participants. The construction of poems is influenced by the methodology of the study. Generally, data are analysed and themes or categories created. The researchers may use words from transcripts, in sequential order, to illustrate individual themes. This process is considered to be 'found-poetry'. In Brown et al's study on new doctors' transition into practice, the themes from the study are presented, along with supporting quotes and a poem.[12] For example, in a theme that describes how new doctors express their personal beliefs and values through patient-centred care, a poem was created to illustrate the theme.

The point of me waking up every day
Is that I know I am going to make someone feel better
Just holding someone's hand makes me feel more a doctor
Than anything I could do with drugs

Excerpt from *Just holding someone's hand* in Brown et al (p. 1243)[12]

Poetry that shares researcher interpretations can also be incorporated into studies. This often takes the form of using poetry to synthesise findings from a literature review. Similar to the 'found-poetry' technique described previously, researchers may select words from quotes in the literature to help construct a poem that would illustrate a particular concept. Quotes can include original participants' own quotes and the original researchers' interpretations. In an example from a literature review examining the experiences of caregivers of high-needs children who are transitioning to adulthood, three broad themes were described from the 19 studies identified.[13] The authors edited and blended original quotes and narratives to create free-verse poems. One example is a poem that illustrates a theme of retaining parental responsibility:

When you have a child with special needs,
It's not that you won't love them
It's that you'll love them too much.

Excerpt from *How is it possible to love a disabled child* in Slade et al[13] (p. 45)

The final form of poetry, which could be incorporated into primary care research, is autoethnographic poetry. This type of poetry is written by the researcher as part of an autoethnography and describes the researcher's experiences and reflections.[10] Field notes and journal entries generally form the source of the poem. Poetry writing in this context aids in reflexivity and development of ideas and concepts. This form of poetry writing is what I have used in my own research. In my PhD thesis, which explored how power and control of Māori primary care organisations was wielded by non-Māori entities and concepts, I wrote poems to help me express ideas that bubbled up. My poems drew from my experiences as a general practitioner working within a Māori primary healthcare provider. I would often tussle with thoughts and ideas as I navigated the research process, and I wrote poems to help me grapple with these concepts. The act of writing enabled me to lean into my emotions and process my experiences. An example of an autoethnographic poem is provided as follows, in which I reflect on a situation where I listened to a racist comment by a fellow general practitioner.

He stared at me intently, With fervent eyes.
Gleaming brightly.
And I watched his lips, Spit out the words,
Twisting darkly.

Excerpt from *My response to the racist* in Eggleton[14]

7.5 Creative Writing

There are a number of other ways beyond poetry of incorporating creative writing into research. One common example is using creative writing as an intervention and then analysing outcomes.[15,16] Using creative writing in this way generally focuses on exploring improvements in well-being or mental health. Another common way of using creative writing is to incorporate it into autoethnography. I have used this approach in my own research.

Using creative writing, as part of autoethnography, acts to present narratives and events in a more approachable and evocative fashion. It may bring the reader into the world of the researcher and highlights their internal dialogue. Stories can be of the researcher's own health journey, such as Sparkes' story of his fragile body and the impact on his self-identity.[17] Alternatively, they can be about the research journey of the researcher and the struggles that they have encountered, or the evolution of their thinking and praxis.[14] These struggles and emotional experiences are often drawn from the journals and field notes of the researcher.

When writing narratives, a tension can be created between presenting the 'truth' and protecting the confidentiality of others whose own stories become part of the researcher's story. Various strategies exist to manage this tension, such as creating composite characters who typify a multitude of people and collapsing events, which represent a common occurrence. The aim of autoethnographical writing is not necessarily to present factual information, but rather to present subjective and emotional experiences as factually as possible.

7.5.1 Example 3: Exploring How Non-Māori Control Māori Organisations

In this study, I used autoethnography to present concepts and ideas that I had encountered while undertaking my research. I focussed on experiences that had given me insight into the way in which I thought, my biases and the way in which my thinking evolved. I collected journal entries and generated a story that could reproduce my emotions. I did not base the characters on one single character, but instead used composite characters. Likewise, I used collapsing events to cluster experiences into one fictionalised account that remained true to the underlying facts. I wove the story throughout the thesis, bookending chapters both to introduce a general concept and to conclude my thinking on the topic. The story follows myself as I navigate a number of different interactions and conversations with patients, acquaintances and my alter ego.

An example from my writing in which I introduce concepts of feeling socially awkward, trying to articulate myself clearly and being shut down when I talk about social injustice and then relating my own personal experience back to the literature is as follows:

> *The noise from the stereo buffets me now, before I have a chance to respond to Simon and Jackie. Someone has turned the volume up because YMCA from the Village People is playing. Party goers start contorting their bodies into various letters of the alphabet while a lot of the men look awkwardly around, hoping that their partner is not going to drag them into the melee. Simon and Jackie look a little bemused and then turn back to me expectantly. In some ways the mechanism through which they have tried to shut me down reflects the ways in which Tauiwi [non-Māori] have always shut down Māori—through discourse and controlling the agenda.*

7.6 Conclusion

A vast array of creative methods can be used in primary care research. These methods can shift research from distanced representations of findings to evocative representations of the emotions of the findings. Selecting a creative method requires careful consideration of the researcher's positionality and ongoing reflectivity. Specific ethical issues with creative methods need to be taken into account. A good starting point for primary care researchers is to incorporate creative arts into everyday practice as a method on reflecting on interactions with patients/clients and colleagues and the thought processes that drive us.

I conclude with a found-poem derived from the text of this chapter.

> *Undertaking creative methods . . .*
> *Elicit emotions,*
> *Touches participants,*
> *Promote discussion.*
> *There is hope,*
> *In reflective approaches.*
> *Metaphors, colours.*
> *Waking thoughts,*
> *And exploring tensions*
> *That buffets us.*

7.7 Ethics

Ethics approval for the photovoice project was granted by the University of Auckland Human Participants Ethics Committee. Ethics number 27144.

Ethics approval for the primary care receptions project was granted by the University of Auckland Human Participants Ethics Committee. Ethics number 011176.

Ethics approval for the exploration of how non-Māori control Māori organisations project was granted by the University of Auckland Human Participants Ethics Committee. Ethics number 019988.

References

1. Kearns R, Eggleton K, van der Plas A, Coleman T. Drawing and graffiti-based approaches. In: von Benzon N, Holton M, Wilkinson K, Wilkinson S, eds. Creative methods for human geographers. London: SAGE Publications; 2021. p. 113–26.
2. Wang C, Burris MA. Photovoice: Concept, methodology, and use for participatory needs assessment. *Health Educ Behav.* 1997;24(3):369–87.
3. Wang CC. Photovoice: A participatory action research strategy applied to women's health. *J Womens Health.* 1999;8(2):185–92.
4. Braun V, Clarke V. Can I use TA? Should I use TA? Should I not use TA? Comparing reflexive thematic analysis and other pattern-based qualitative analytic approaches. *Couns Psychother Res.* 2021;21(1):37–47.
5. Rose G. Visual Methodologies: An introduction to researching with visual materials. SAGE; 2022.
6. Eggleton K, Kearns R, Neuwelt PM. Being patient, being vulnerable: Exploring experiences of general practice waiting rooms through elicited drawings. *Soc Cult Geogr.* 2017;18(7): 971–93.
7. Pain R, Francis P. Reflections on participatory research. *Area.* 2003;35(1):46–54.
8. Charmaz K. Constructing grounded theory: A practical guide through qualitative analysis. London: SAGE Publications; 2006.
9. Kearns RA, Neuwelt PM, Eggleton K. Permeable boundaries? Patient perspectives on space and time in general practice waiting rooms. *Health Place.* 2020;63:102347.
10. Brown MEL, Kelly M, Finn GM. Thoughts that breathe, and words that burn: Poetic inquiry within health professions education. *Perspect Med Educ.* 2021;10(5):257–64.
11. Lahman MKE, Geist MR, Rodriguez KL, Graglia PE, Richard VM, Schendel RK. Poking around poetically: Research, poetry, and trustworthiness. *Qual Inq.* 2010;16(1):39–48.
12. Brown MEL, Proudfoot A, Mayat NY, Finn GM. A phenomenological study of new doctors' transition to practice, utilising participant-voiced poetry. *Adv Health Sci Educ Theory Pract.* 2021;26(4):1229–53.
13. Slade K, Shaw RL, Larkin M, Heath G. Care-giving experiences of parents of young people with PMLD and complex healthcare needs in the transition to adulthood years: A qualitative poetic synthesis. *Arts Health.* 2025;17(1):39–56.
14. Eggleton K. Measuring the quality of Māori health providers: A critique of Tauiwi paradigms [PhD thesis]. [Auckland]: University of Auckland; 2020.
15. Mundy SS, Kudahl B, Bundesen B, Hellström L, Rosenbaum B, Eplov LF. Mental health recovery and creative writing groups: A systematic review. *Nord J Arts Cult Health.* 2022;4(1):1–8.
16. Porras-Segovia A, Escobedo-Aedo PJ, Carrillo de Albornoz CM, Guerrero-Jiménez M, Lis L, Molina-Madueño R, et al. Writing to keep on living: A systematic review and meta-analysis on creative writing therapy for the management of depression and suicidal ideation. *Curr Psychiatry Rep.* 2024;26(7):359–78.
17. Sparkes AC. The fatal flaw: A narrative of the fragile body-self. *Qual Inq.* 1996;2(4):463–94.

CHAPTER

8

Reflexivity in Primary Care Research

William L Miller and Benjamin F Crabtree

Confused resignation appeared on Dr Tapia's face as she thought about her recent patients. As a new general practitioner at a local village *barangay* (community) health centre in the Philippines, she was not prepared for the extent of fentanyl use on top of an already serious problem with "shabu" (methamphetamine hydrochloride) among young men.[1] "What's going on?" she wondered. "How should our practice respond?" As a family medicine resident in Manila, she had enjoyed participating with the Philippine Primary Care Studies on a network research project involving *barangay* health centres, so she e-mailed the investigators with her questions.

Now, one year later, Dr Tapia is part of a research team implementing a five-year grant using mixed methods and a community-based participatory approach. The research seeks to better understand the rise in substance use disorder in rural areas and to apply this information to design and test a practice an intervention to address the problem using a randomised cross-over design. The research team, led by a distinguished senior faculty from the university, includes several post-doc fellows with mixed-methods expertise, a biostatistician, clinicians and community health workers with little or no research experience and two primary care consultants from American academic health centres. The first part of the project uses in-depth and group interviews of substance users, rural community folk and practice members as well as surveys on current practice capacity. Using what is learned from these interviews, the research team will develop a practice-based intervention followed by implementation with a mixed-methods evaluation. At their initial research team gathering, Dr Beltran, one of the junior post-docs, who is well-trained in qualitative research methods, asks about the role of reflexivity in this project. Quite a fluffing and ruffling of feathers ensues. This chapter explores some answers to questions about reflexivity that this ruffling uncovered and the work of paying attention to the effect of researchers on the contexts and processes of knowledge generation.

We chose this case because it illustrates three characteristics of primary care research that impact how we think about reflexivity: (1) the setting of primary care, (2) the need for mixed methods and (3) the engagement of a collaborative team. Six

DOI: 10.1201/9781003652106-10

aspects of the primary care setting stand out. These include (1) the *comprehensiveness* of the field, where any person with any type of problem can present for care. Research involving an intervention on a particular problem such as substance use needs to account for any ripple effects on the care of people with other problems. This comprehensive scope and earlier contact within the natural history of an affliction mean a greater degree of (2) *uncertainty* in both diagnosis and treatment. Primary care demonstrates (3) *sensitivity to local conditions*, which leads to (4) greater *variability* regarding workforce, organisation and processes of care. These features suggest the importance of a (5) prudent and *pragmatic* approach in primary care and in the research design and methods used to understand it. Standardised research designs and one-size-fits-all interventions usually fit uncomfortably within the primary care setting. In addition, primary care clinical encounters emphasise (6) *collaborative decision-making*; thus, participatory research strategies and a more democratic knowledge production are encouraged to reflect this. All of these aspects of the primary care setting are present as Dr Tapia and her colleagues gather for their initial research meeting and ponder the role of reflexivity.

Who are you? Where are you doing your research? Who do those being studied think you are? Who do you work with? What are we doing? How do the answers to these questions influence the research outcomes? Do these questions matter for all research or only certain kinds? These are a few of the questions that arise when discussing Dr Beltran's question concerning reflexivity in primary care research. These questions are usually being asked and answered in a context that includes mixed methods and collaborative research teams.

Patients may receive primary care from an amalgamation of multiple professional, semi-professional and lay people. Patients accessing the formal healthcare system simultaneously use different primary care clinicians, medical sub-specialists, pharmacists, nurses and other healthcare professionals. Primary care researchers often must incorporate all of these modalities into research designs, requiring the integration of perspectives from multiple disciplines, including epidemiology, biostatistics, nursing, public health, anthropology, sociology, psychology and education. To develop the cross-disciplinary research that primary care needs, it is necessary to build safe collaborative space and teams, which requires reflexivity.

As Dr Tapia sat in one of the early meetings of the recently formed research team, it immediately became apparent why Dr Beltran had asked her question about reflexivity. The meeting had only just begun when the senior biostatistician sarcastically asked what the point was of including anecdotal interviews in their powerful parallel cluster randomised hybrid type 2 effectiveness implementation study. The junior team members like Dr Beltran felt powerless to speak up amongst the obvious hierarchy of physicians and senior biomedical investigators in the room. Pandemonium ensued as people hunkered down, using their own discipline-specific jargon and abbreviations as if the terms were part of common, everyday language. The nascent research team was in the "storming" stage of small group development (Table 8.1).[2] The team obviously needed help, but how do groups continue the conversation and reach agreement in an unfriendly environment?

Primary care research inevitably requires working in teams, and primary care generalist researchers must also know how to facilitate a group working through the

TABLE 8.1 Stages of Team Development and Reflexivity Activities to Facilitate

Stage	Team Member Experiences	Reflexivity Activities to Facilitate
Forming	Team members get acquainted and work to establish roles, rules, norms and expectations.	Engage in storytelling to make it personal and get out of a scientific rut. Acknowledge and discuss power and hegemony. Be transparent about budgets. Introduce norms for discussions, eg use of a talking stick.
Storming	Conflicts and disagreements arise among team members as they become competitive, protective and squabble over roles.	Clear the room of rhetorical stones, ie call out and discuss power heaping, jargon hurling and shaming. Use humour and silence. Discuss and acknowledge individual differences between being pragmatic and valuing reflection. Create and follow meeting agendas. When stuck, remember activities like passing around a talking stick, where someone can only talk when holding the stick.
Norming	The team has established norms and a sense of cohesion, found common ground, worked to develop a sense of safety, and agreed on methods for conflict resolution. Members have learned to step aside from disagreements to move forward.	Engage in periodic brainstorming and storytelling to maintain team cohesion. Engage in non-work-related group activities such as walks or group outings. Openly discuss authorship issues with a sense of shared abundance. In a less safe environment, develop consensus-building strategies that create a sufficient sense of safety to function.
Performing	The team is working collaboratively and effectively towards achieving shared common goals.	Regularly share experiences and discuss findings from different perspectives.
Adjourning	The end of the project is marked and the group is dissolved.	Engage in storytelling about the project and reflect on how team members changed over time.

stages of collaborative relationship. Challenging situations predictably arise, especially the power differentials in the hierarchy where junior faculty, post-docs and research staff do not feel safe speaking up; the dominance of positivism that keeps wanting to reduce the need for reflexivity; and conflicts between theories and paradigms, stymie progress. Overcoming these situations requires consensus-building skills, keeping a solution focus, maintaining a creative tension between outcomes and process, and staying flexible to group needs. Table 8.1 overviews the five stages of collaborative relationship development proposed by Tuckman and Jensen and some reflexivity activities that can be done to move towards being an effective team.[2]

With collaborative safe space sufficiently established, Dr Tapia's research team can address the issue of reflexivity, beginning with a better understanding of what it is. *Reflexivity* refers to the activities of using a critical eye to systematically pay attention to the research contexts and participants to better apprehend the effect of researcher(s) on the contexts and processes of knowledge construction.[3,4] This systematic attending focuses on four locations (see Figure 8.1): the personal (researcher and participant), the interpersonal, the contexts and the research methods.[5]

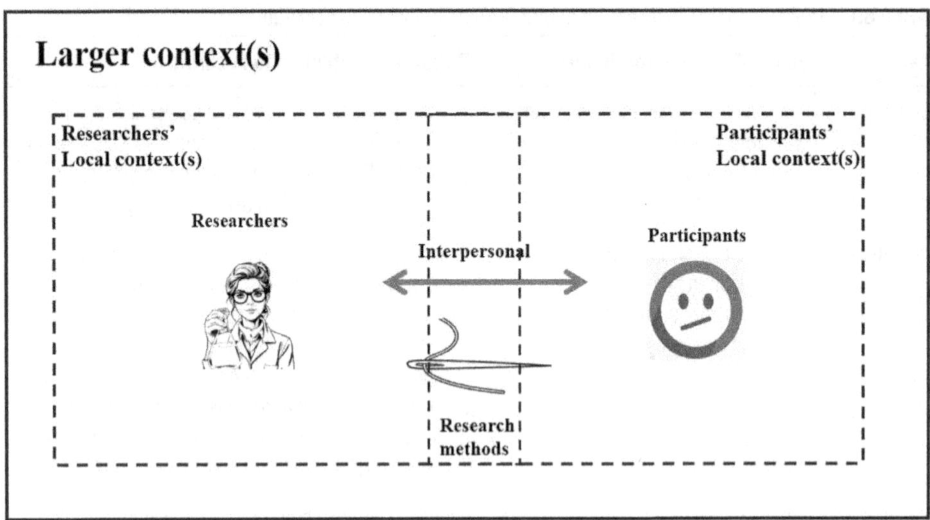

FIGURE 8.1 Locating reflexivity

Personal reflexivity explores the biases, assumptions, worldviews, identities, subjectivities (expression on researcher's face in Figure 8.1) and reactions of the researcher(s) as they engage in the research. The eyes of the researcher in Figure 8.1 represent their positionality or standpoint from which they conduct the research. What biases influence Dr Tapia as she begins her research? These biases can behave as traps of perception and understanding. Table 8.2 identifies many of the common biases and includes reflexivity questions that the research team can ask themselves to uncover and manage them.[7–16] Because of the diversity in Dr Tapia's research group, one can anticipate the discovery of many hidden biases and some meaningfully different worldviews. Worldviews are one's everyday personal set of beliefs and values used to make sense of the world, your operating system or way of seeing things.

Table 8.3 identifies some core value orientations[17] and beliefs and some reflexivity questions to help investigators explore how their worldviews are influencing the research process and outcomes.

Heuristics are cognitive "tendencies" wired into the brain as part of the human fast-thinking process.[7] Evolution has proven their value as tools for perception and understanding our world well enough to survive as a species. Thus, they serve as windows into valuable insights during the research process, but they can also mislead and become traps.[18] Reflexivity activates the slow-thinking processes in our brains to help with the discernment between window and trap. Table 8.4 names and describes several important heuristics and offers reflexivity questions for both opening the windows of understanding and discovering the traps.[7–9,19–20]

Interpersonal reflexivity includes how the researchers and participants view and affect each other, their respective roles and the influences of power in their relationships and on the evolving research. How do the participants see and understand the researchers, and how does that influence their responses and the researcher's behaviour?

TABLE 8.2 Biases as Traps of Perception and Understanding

Bias	Description	Reflexivity Questions
Affective	Aversion to that which evokes strong emotion	What information evokes the greatest emotion in me? How do I respond?
Commission	Predisposition to action; tendency when overconfident	Have I paid attention to all points of view? How might the proposed action be harmful?
Confirmation	Interpreting new information as validation of one's current beliefs	How might this new information change my current beliefs?
False priors (Implicit bias)	Bringing unproven biases into decision-making, eg gender bias, stereotyping—often implicit	What biases, especially racial and gender, might influence the interpretation? How does a reversal of the biases change the interpretation?
Introspective illusion	Wrongly thinking one has direct insight into their own thinking but that others don't	Do I think my insight is better than others? What's the evidence? How do others explain my thinking?
Narrative	Being drawn toward a particular outcome because it has a better story	How might different outcomes change the story?
Optimism	Overestimating the likelihood of positive things while underestimating the chance of negative	Have I overlooked any negative data?
Outcome	Preference for what you want to happen rather than what you believe will really happen	What do I want to happen? What do I believe will happen? What else might happen?
Overconfidence (egocentric)	Overestimating what you know and relying too heavily on it (self-serving bias)	What do others think? What information am I missing?
Social desirability	Presenting oneself in a way that is perceived to be socially acceptable (impression management and self-deception)	What is expected in this social and cultural situation? Am I willing to openly disagree with the participants or colleagues?
Sunk cost	Throwing good money after bad because so much has already been invested	Have I remembered the big picture, built creative tension, kept track of time and energy investments, been brutally honest and released personal attachments?
Visceral	Excessive emotional investment in your relationship with participant(s)	What would I think if I didn't know or care so much about this person?

Adapted and amended from: Crabtree & Miller. *Doing Qualitative Research*, 3rd edition.[6]

TABLE 8.3 Worldview and Reflexivity Questions

Worldview Category	Reflexivity Questions
Values Orientations	
Time	On what aspect of time do I focus—past, present or future? What about the research participants?
Relationship with habitat	How do I think humanity relates to its habitat—mastery, submission or harmony? What about the research participants?
Relationship with others	How do I believe individuals should relate with others—hierarchically, as equals, or according to their individual merit? What about the research participants?
Motivation for behaviour	What do I believe is the prime motivation for behaviour—to express one's self, to grow or to achieve? What about the research participants?
Human nature	What, in my opinion, is the nature of human nature—good, bad or a mixture? What about the research participants?
Beliefs	
Life and death	What are my beliefs about life and death?
Groups and societies	What are my beliefs and opinions about groups and societies?
What is important	What are my value judgements about what is worthwhile or important?
How the world is organised	What are my beliefs about how the world is organised and how it works?
How people should behave	What are my values or guideposts for how I think people should behave?
What is true and false	What are my beliefs about how people can or should decide what is true or false?
What is right and wrong	What are my opinions about what is positive or negative, right or wrong?
Who decides and how	What are my beliefs about how decisions should be made and who should make them?
Who succeeds and why	What are my beliefs about how human beings should act?

At least three different contexts require reflexivity: (1) the local world(s) of the researcher(s), (2) the local community settings for the participants and (3) the larger world context. Dr Tapia's local contexts include her *barangay* health centre, her home in a suburb 20 miles from the *barangay* and the university in Manila. The participants' contexts are the small, mostly rural villages where they live and work. How do those very different settings influence the research? And everyone involved in the research participates in and is influenced by the global context. As researchers, it is important to recognise that we are also doing science under the historical gaze of colonialism, and we need to pay attention to how coloniality sways the

TABLE 8.4 Heuristics as Windows and Traps of Perception and Understanding

		Reflexivity Questions	
Heuristic	**Description**	***Windows***	***Traps***
Anchoring	Tendency to use pre-existing or first-identified pieces of information to make sense of new data	What have I already identified that helps make sense of the new information?	What else have I uncovered that challenges the anchoring?
Association	Tendency to base decisions on previous similar situations	How is the new data similar to past experiences?	What's different or unique about this situation?
Attribution	Tendency to make assumptions about why people behave as they do	Why would I behave that way?	What's the evidence for attributing internal motivations to others?
Availability	Tendency to think that examples that readily come to mind are representative of the situation	Any examples from my past that might apply to this situation?	What other examples might muddy the understanding of the situation?
Framing	Tendency to decide based on the way information is presented	What understanding is highlighted by how the data is framed?	How would another way of presenting the information change my understanding?
Order effects	Tendency to better remember the first and/or last information received about the topic	What is the significance of what was noted first and last?	How does what I learned in the middle change my understanding?
Representativeness	Tendency to assess the probability of explanation by how it resembles similar data	How is current data like other datasets?	What doesn't fit about the explanation? What's different about this data?
Substitution	Tendency to substitute a simpler explanation in the face of complexity	Is there a simpler way to explain the complexity?	Have I preserved all the complexity in the data?

Adapted and amended from: Crabtree & Miller. *Doing Qualitative Research*, 3rd edition.[6]

research. Coloniality represents the enduring structures, systems and mindsets that emerged from imperial colonialism and persisted after the formal end of colonialism. They continue to shape the current global reality of the "universals" of Western modernity, Eurocentrism and global capitalism.[21] These mindsets are reinforced through neo-colonialism, the post–World War II use of power, pressure and technology to maintain dependence that is colonial-like, e.g., AI as a tool for neo-colonialism. Reflexivity requires that we explore for the features of coloniality and their influence in our research (see Table 8.5).

TABLE 8.5 Features of Coloniality

Feature ***Control of***	**Description**
Power/authority	Racialised power structures and hierarchies Control of institutions Armies and police and surveillance maintain security
Nature/economy	Exploitation of labour and natural resources and land appropriation Creation of dependence through unequal exchange, drain of wealth Structural violence
Gender/sexuality	Institutionalisation and enforcement of patriarchy
Knowledge/technology	Prioritisation of Eurocentric knowledge Suppression of Indigenous knowledges How knowledge is produced and disseminated Development of technology to support above
Culture/values	Imposition of language, religion, values Control of media

A fourth location for reflexivity resides in the methods. Each method, from an in-depth interview to a coefficient of determination in a regression model, nests within a paradigm and comes with underlying assumptions, limitations and a specific view of the world. Science is a way of knowledge generation, a meta method, which intentionally creates a space for the world to respond and creates a relationship between researcher and the participating world. The specific methods and paradigm deployed bound the generosity of that response. Paradigms are scientific worldviews. Reflexivity means knowing your paradigm and methods' blinders and wondering what lies beyond their view. Reflexivity is an expectation for qualitative methods, but it is often contested when proposed in reference to quantitative methods. At those times, remember that quantitative methods and the statistics used in them all have underlying assumptions, including independence of variables, homogeneity of variance, normality of distribution and linearity (straight-line relationship between independent and dependent variables). The categorisation of the variables is based on theory and the accompanying assumptions on how those hypothesised categories distribute and act with everything else in the world. Reflexivity in quantitative research asks us to recognise and identify those features, challenge them and explore alternative possibilities.[22]

Stimulated by the invigorating discussion that followed Dr Beltran's question on reflexivity, Dr Tapia and the group now wonder when and how to do reflexivity. They are surprised to learn that reflexivity happens throughout the research process (see Figure 8.2).[6]

It begins before the fieldwork when you explore the sources of your interest in this research question and make transparent the reasoning and experiences behind

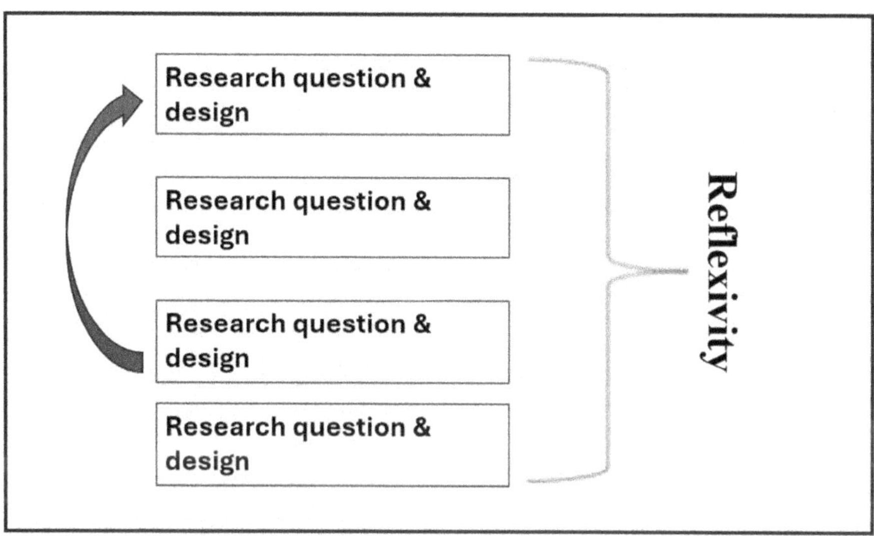

FIGURE 8.2 Research process and reflexivity

decisions about which methods and sampling strategies to use and who the team members will be. Dr Tapia notes her current thinking, past experiences and assumptions regarding substance use in the Philippines. What does she think the results will be and why?

The reflexivity continues during data collection, during analysis and interpretation, and again during dissemination of the results. As the team begins early analysis, reflexivity may result in changing later data collection strategies. The ongoing work of interpretation usually reveals hidden biases and assumptions, which necessitate a re-evaluation of prior analyses. The results should differ in some way from those expected, and how that happened and why, is one of the ways for explaining the role of reflexivity when preparing the manuscript/presentation for dissemination. Table 8.6 describes examples of reflexivity strategies for use during the research process. They are organised by the location for the reflexivity (see Figure 8.1). Because Dr Tapia's group is using a community-based participatory approach around the sensitive topic of substance use, it will be especially helpful to do frequent journaling, debriefing and assure peer support.[30]

Inspired by what they learned about reflexivity, Dr Tapia and the research team set aside a special meeting time where they each shared personal stories about substance use. The effect was powerful and drew the community members and the academics closer together. One of the community health workers wondered if more such sessions were forthcoming. Dr Beltran smiled. She reminded the group that reflexivity, like good medicine, is best in the proper dose. Reflexivity is a privilege that takes time and can become narcissistic, a never-ending hall of mirrors and a tool for anti-objectivity,[5] but used wisely, reflexivity becomes a source for transformation.

TABLE 8.6 Strategies for Reflexivity

Type	Strategy	Description
Personal (researcher)	Log/audit trails[23] Journaling[24] Personal memos[25] Narrative autobiography[5] (self-interview)	Physical audit trail documents key stages and methods' decisions; intellectual audit trail documents how investigators' thinking evolved. Regular self-reflective journaling to share personal and research experiences, opinions, feelings, reactions, thoughts, doubts and thrills. Brief communication in written or digital form on ideas, musings and impressions about self that arise during research process. Write autobiography highlighting personal experiences potentially related to research and your interest in it.
Personal (participant)	Member reflection[26] Participant debrief[26] Reading the margins[26]	Members/participants reflect in writing/recording on how they perceive the researchers and what's being researched. Participants are debriefed, in interviews, on how they view the researchers, their context and the research itself. Analyse the "marginal" data that highlights how participants are perceiving the research.
Interpersonal (research ensemble)	Reflexive vignettes[26] Circuit breakers[27] Reflexivity questions Expanding space	Brief evocative descriptions that highlight tensions that arise during research process, eg material, institutional, ethical tensions. Shared in a collaborative setting. Intermittent imposition of physical or thought actions, forcing shift to slow thinking when getting stuck, high tension, excessive fast thinking. Examples: do pro/con list; play break; ask questions to disconfirm or seek negative evidence in imagination; take a walk. Periodic review of questions in Tables 8.2, 8.3 and 8.4 to uncover traps of perception and understanding. Use of disclosure, feedback and exploration in research ensemble meetings.
Interpersonal (researcher-participant)	Interpersonal memos	Brief communication in written or digital form on ideas, musings and impressions about relationships that arise during research process.
Contextual	Context memos	Brief communication in written or digital form on ideas, musings and impressions about contexts that arise during research process.
Methods-related	Methods memos	Brief communication in written or digital form on ideas, musings and impressions about methods that arise during research process.

(Continued)

TABLE 8.6 Strategies for Reflexivity (Continued)

Type	Strategy	Description
Special situations	Dialogic engagement[4]	Strategic use of diverse thought partners and theory in a dialogic format. Partners can include ensemble colleagues and research participants.
	Investigator interviews[4]	Explicit depth interview of investigator(s) exploring motivation, relationship, influences and engagement with research. Transcripts shared in collaborative setting.
	Cultural Review[28]	Research ensemble sharing of past experiences and cultural understandings related to research topic. They inventory and examine the associations, incidents and assumptions that surround the topic in their minds.
	CAQDAS (analysis software) impact review[29]	Recurring explicit ensemble reflexive review of impact of analysis software, eg NVivo, Atlas.ti, on research process. Specifically, pre-research when choosing software, during research when adapting requirements of software and near end when exploring how process might have been different without the software.
	Retreats +/– facilitator	Half-day to four-day off-site events for all members of research team(s) and strategic guests with focused agenda, shared meals, multiple breaks and often incorporating several of the other tools in the table. Utilising an outside person to stimulate and facilitate more reflective conversations, manage tensions and conflicts, and assure psychological safety.

Adapted and amended from: Crabtree & Miller. *Doing Qualitative Research*, 3rd edition.[6]

References

1. Cordero DA Jr. Addressing the opioid crisis in the Philippines: Recognizing the severity and calling for proactive action. *Korean J Pain*. 2024;37(2):182–4.
2. Tuckman BW, Jensen MAC. Stages of small-group development revisited. *Group & Organization Studies*. 1977;2(4):419–27.
3. Holloway I, Biley FC. Being a qualitative researcher. *Qual Health Res*. 2011;21(7):968–75.
4. Ravitch, SM, Carl, NM. Qualitative research: Bridging the conceptual, theoretical, and methodological (2nd edition). Los Angeles: Sage Publications, Inc.; 2021.
5. Olmos-Vega FM, Stalmeijer RE, Varpio L, et al. A practical guide to reflexivity in qualitative research: AMEE Guide No. 149. *Med Teach*. 2022 Apr 7;1–11.
6. Crabtree BF, Miller WL. Doing qualitative research (3rd edition). Thousand Oaks: Sage Publications, Inc.; 2023.
7. Kahneman D. Thinking, fast and slow. New York: Farrar, Straus, and Giroux; 2011.
8. Preisz A. Fast and slow thinking; and the problem of conflating clinical reasoning and ethical deliberation in acute decision-making. *J Paediatr Child Health*. 2019;55(6):621–4.

9. Gorini A, Pravettoni G. An overview on cognitive aspects implicated in medical decisions. *Eur J Intern Med.* 2011;22(6):547–53.
10. Krumpal I. Determinants of social desirability bias in sensitive surveys: A literature review. *Quality & Quantity: Int J Methodol.* 2013;47(4):2025–47.
11. Taleb NN. The Black Swan: The impact of the highly improbable. New York: Random House; 2007.
12. FitzGerald C, Hurst S. Implicit bias in healthcare professionals: A systematic review. *BMC Med Ethics.* 2017;18(1):19.
13. Gopal DP, Chetty U, O'Donnell P, et al. Implicit bias in healthcare: Clinical practice, research and decision making. *Future Healthc J.* 2021;8(1):40–8.
14. Hugh TB, Dekker SWA. Hindsight bias and outcome bias in the social construction of medical negligence: A review. *J Law Med.* 2009;16(5):846–57.
15. Callaham ML, Wears RL, Weber EJ, et al. Positive-outcome bias and other limitations in the outcome of research abstracts submitted to a scientific meeting. *JAMA.* 1998;280(3):254–7.
16. Bolier M, Doulougeri K, de Vries J, et al. 'You put up a certain attitude': A 6-year qualitative study of emotional socialisation. *Med Educ.* 2018;52(10):1041–51.
17. Kluckhohn FR, Strodtbeck FL. Variations in value orientations. Evanston: Row, Peterson; 1961.
18. Klein JG. Five pitfalls in decisions about diagnosis and prescribing. *BMJ.* 2005 Apr 2;330(7494):781–3.
19. Bansback N, Li LC, Lynd L, et al. Exploiting order effects to improve the quality of decisions. *Patient Educ Couns.* 2014;96(2):197–203.
20. Ogdie AR, Reilly JB, Pang WG, et al. Seen through their eyes: Residents' reflections on the cognitive and contextual components of diagnostic errors in medicine. *Acad Med.* 2012;87(10):1361–7.
21. Mignolo WD, Walsh CE. On decolonialitiy: Concepts, analytics, Praxis. Durham: Duke University Press; 2018.
22. Jamieson MK, Govaart GH, Pownall M. Reflexivity in quantitative research: A rationale and beginner's guide. *Soc Personal Psychol Compass.* 2023;17(4):e12735.
23. Carcary M. The research audit trial—enhancing trustworthiness in qualitative inquiry. *The Electron J Bus Res Method.* 2009;7(1):11–24.
24. Ortlipp M. Keeping and using reflective journals in the qualitative research process. *Qualitative Report.* 2008;13(4).
25. Birks M, Chapman Y, Francis K. Memoing in qualitative research: Probing data and processes. *J Nurs Res.* 2008;13(1):68–75.
26. Rostron A. Who do they think we are? Reflexivity and participant constructions of the researcher. *J Manag Inq.* 2024;33(3):284–99.
27. Hogarth RM. Educating intuition. Chicago: University of Chicago Press; 2001.
28. McCracken GD. The long interview. Newbury Park: Sage Publications, Inc.; 1988.
29. Woods M, Macklin R, Lewis GK. Researcher reflexivity: Exploring the impacts of CAQDAS use. *Int J Soc Res.* 2016;19(4):385–403.
30. Karcher K, McCuaig J, King-Hill S. (Self-) reflection/reflexivity in sensitive, qualitative research: A scoping review. *Int J Qual Methods.* 2024;23:16094069241261860.

CHAPTER

9

Reporting Guidelines for Primary Care Research

Elizabeth Sturgiss and William R Phillips

Researchers must effectively report their work to contribute new knowledge, inform patient care and practice, influence healthcare systems and improve patient and population health outcomes. The reporting of primary care (PC) research largely determines how study findings are used by the PC community. Reporting, publishing and disseminating research findings are essential skills for PC researchers. This chapter presents the Consensus Reporting Items for Studies in Primary Care (CRISP), the first reporting guide for PC research.[5]

9.1 Reporting Guidelines to Support High-Quality Manuscripts

It is important to ensure that you report your research in a clear and logical way. The manuscript you write needs to provide enough detail for the reader to understand what you did in the study, what results you found, what these findings mean and how they might be relevant to their own context.

The needs of a researcher reading your report might be slightly different from those of a clinician. A researcher probably would like enough detail about study methods to replicate the research in their own system or population. A clinician might be more interested in the context of the research and how it might be similar or different from their own practice setting.

Research reporting guidelines have been developed to help investigators and authors report their research more effectively and efficiently. Reporting guidelines often include a checklist of essential items that should be included in reports to help readers assess study methods and research findings, review and synthesise results across studies, and implement interventions in practice, education and policy.

The EQUATOR Network is a global repository of research reporting guidelines that has catalogued more than 450 published research reporting guidelines. The guidelines are categorised by their focus on a specific study design, research method, disease or topic. Researchers might follow a checklist to help structure their report based on the study design, topic or technology. Some research may have more than one checklist that applies to their reports.

DOI: 10.1201/9781003652106-11

Many guidelines also have 'Extensions' that are amplified checklists tailored to specific study designs or topics. For example, the CONSORT guideline for randomised controlled trials[1] has multiple extensions that cover topics such as reporting surrogate endpoints,[2] reporting factorial randomised trials,[3] and reporting outcomes in trial reports.[4]

Because PC research uses such a diversity of methods to study such a wide range of topics, many research reporting guides are relevant to PC (Table 9.1). Some research

TABLE 9.1 Research Reporting Guidelines Commonly Used in Primary Care Research

Name	Focus	Website
STUDY TYPE		
CRISP Consensus Reporting Items for Studies in Primary care	Primary care research	https://crisp-pc.org
SQUIRE Standards for QUality Improvement Reporting Excellence	Quality improvement studies	https://www.squire-statement.org
AGREE Appraisal of Guidelines for Research and Evaluation	Clinical practice guidelines	https://www.agreetrust.org
RESEARCH METHOD		
SRQR Standards for reporting qualitative research	Qualitative research	NA
COREQ Consolidated criteria for reporting qualitative research	Qualitative research	NA
STARD Standards for Reporting of Diagnostic Accuracy	Diagnostic/Prognostic Studies	NA
STUDY DESIGN		
CONSORT Consolidated Standards of Reporting Trials	Randomised trials	https://www.consort-spirit.org
SPIRIT Standard Protocol Items: Recommendations for Interventional Trials	Study protocols for clinical trials	http://www.spirit-statement.org
STROBE Strengthening the Reporting of Observational Studies in Epidemiology	Observational studies	https://www.strobe-statement.org
PRISMA Preferred Reporting Items for Systematic Reviews and Meta-Analyses	Systematic reviews Meta-Analyses	http://www.prisma-statement.org

reports may find multiple reporting guidelines apply to their studies. Check guideline websites for current versions, guideline extensions and translations. For more information on these and other reporting guidelines, see the EQUATOR Network (Enhancing the QUAlity and Transparency Of Health Research: https://www.equator-network.org).

9.2 Reporting Guidelines Specifically for Primary Care

PC is the setting where most medical services are provided to most patients for most problems. It provides comprehensive care to all and first-contact care to unselected patients with undifferentiated problems. The unique nature of PC means that it rests upon a foundation of research with its own questions, perspectives and approaches, and its own needs for reporting.

PC research seeks to understand:

- Patients and their problems
- Health and illness as they occur in families and communities
- Processes of care and healing
- Social and environmental contributors, facilitators and barriers to care and health
- Clinicians, teams and systems of care in the PC setting.

PC research involves investigators from a wide variety of disciplines, professions and research traditions using the full spectrum of methods. Results are published in various journals and presented to diverse audiences. PC research must meet both high scientific standards and the needs of many users. Reporting and dissemination must meet the needs of researchers, practitioners, educators, policymakers, patients and communities. As with patient care, clinician training and service delivery, guidelines developed by more limited specialists with more focused points of view may not be appropriate or sufficient for PC research. High-quality reporting of studies done in, on, or about PC can help make the research more powerful in improving the care, health and lives of all.

Until recently, no reporting guidelines focused on the needs of PC researchers, practitioners and patients. PC is a distinct medical and scientific discipline with its own perspectives and methods to address the problems, patients, professionals and processes in PC settings. Evidence derived by other experts in other settings is helpful but not adequate to meet the needs of PC. The Consensus Reporting Items for Studies in Primary Care (CRISP) is the first research reporting guide developed by and for PC.[5] It is an exciting development in PC research that offers the potential to shape the future of research, reporting and application of new knowledge to improve patient care and health outcomes.

9.3 Consensus Reporting Items for Studies in Primary Care (CRISP)

CRISP is a new initiative in PC research that seeks to improve the reporting of PC research so that it is more helpful for clinicians, patients, researchers and others.

The uniqueness of PC and research in this setting means that bespoke reporting guidelines are better able to meet the needs of readers and researchers. The CRISP Checklist has been endorsed by the World Organization of Family Doctors (WONCA) and the North American Primary Care Research Group (NAPCRG) and is registered by the EQUATOR Network. The Checklist is also recommended to authors by many worldwide PC journals to improve published research reports.

CRISP is evidence-based, developed through a rigorous research programme that established the need for PC reporting guidelines via a scoping review of existing literature and guidelines,[6] a needs assessment of clinicians and patients,[7] and a survey of the international PC research community.[8] The final CRISP Checklist was established by consensus through an international Delphi survey to ensure the checklist was usable, relevant and met the needs of researchers, clinicians and patients.[9]

Research reporting guidelines have traditionally been developed by small groups of highly selected experts and are usually focused on a specific study design or method. CRISP also engaged experts from around the world and across relevant fields. CRISP took the view, however, that the necessary expertise was best sought from broad representation of those who create, use, apply and can benefit from PC research. These experts included researchers, clinicians, patients, community members, educators and policymakers. CRISP engaged 558 respondents from 29 nations across the two surveys, and the Delphi study included 89 panel members from 22 countries (Figure 9.1). This inclusive approach to its development helps CRISP be a useful guide for all producers and users of research across the varied international PC community.

9.4 The CRISP Checklist

The final CRISP Statement was published in October 2023.[5] A supplemental guide provides explanation and examples of applying the CRISP Checklist to PC research. You can download the CRISP Checklist and related documents, including regular updates, from the CRISP website: https://crisp-pc.org.

The final Checklist contains 10 main categories that cover the rationale for the research, details of the research context including the healthcare system and setting, description of the participants in sufficient detail for the reader to contextualise the findings and implications of the findings specifically for PC. CRISP is flexible to adapt to the variety of study designs and research methods in PC research; none of the checklist items is mandatory.

As of February 2025, 11 academic journals worldwide have added CRISP to their instructions to authors as a suggested tool to help research teams improve their research reports. To support the worldwide PC community, the CRISP Checklist is translated into a variety of languages. Current versions include Turkish, Chinese and French, with translations underway in Brazilian Portuguese, Spanish, German and Japanese.

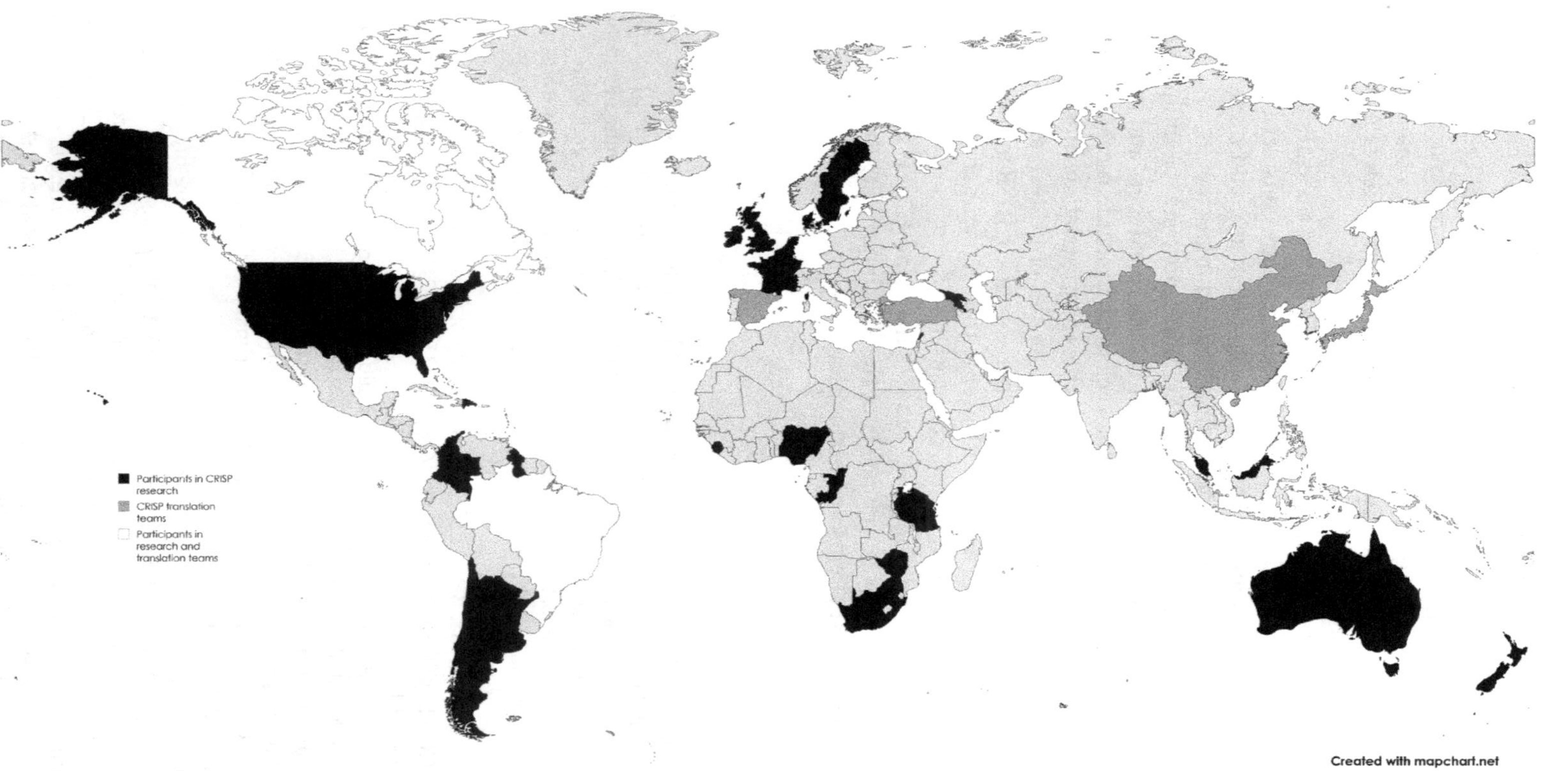

FIGURE 9.1 Participants and translation teams in the CRISP programme of research across the world

9.5 Using CRISP to Support Primary Care Research at All Stages

CRISP, as well as other research reporting guidelines that are focused on specific study designs and topics, can all support high-quality research at every stage of the research journey. CRISP is a PC-specific guide, which helps research reports deliver the elements that are unique and important to PC and therefore more likely to effect change in practice and policy.

For example, research teams can refer to CRISP in the early stages of planning their research design and protocol. This ensures they consider the rationale, relevance to the PC community, appropriate data elements and implementation considerations needed when writing the final research report.

Additionally, educators can use CRISP to demonstrate the unique aspects of PC research. This is particularly valuable for novice researchers and investigators from other specialties and disciplines. These elements include more detailed reports of context, reporting of new or continuing therapeutic relationships and how findings can impact the competing demands and priorities of PC teams.

Novice and more experienced researchers can use CRISP in the peer review process to ensure that reports are most useful and transmit enough detail about the elements most important to the PC community.

Finally, policymakers and grant funders may find CRISP useful to ensure that research accurately reflects the needs of the PC community to improve and assess the care provided to patients and populations.

References

1. Schulz KF, Altman DG, Moher D. CONSORT 2010 statement: Updated guidelines for reporting parallel group randomized trials. *Ann Intern Med.* 2010;152(11):726–32. https://doi.org/10.7326/0003-4819-152-11-201006010-00232 [published Online First: 24 Mar 2010]
2. Manyara AM, Davies P, Stewart D, et al. Reporting of surrogate endpoints in randomised controlled trial reports (CONSORT-Surrogate): Extension checklist with explanation and elaboration. *BMJ.* 2024;386:e078524. https://doi.org/10.1136/bmj-2023-078524 [published Online First: 9 Jul 2024]
3. Kahan BC, Hall SS, Beller EM, et al. Reporting of factorial randomized trials: Extension of the CONSORT 2010 statement. *JAMA.* 2023;330(21):2106–14. https://doi.org/10.1001/jama.2023.19793
4. Butcher NJ, Monsour A, Mew EJ, et al. Guidelines for reporting outcomes in trial reports: The CONSORT-outcomes 2022 extension. *JAMA.* 2022;328(22):2252–64. https://doi.org/10.1001/jama.2022.21022
5. Phillips WR, Sturgiss E, Glasziou P, et al. Improving the reporting of primary care research: Consensus reporting items for studies in primary care: the CRISP statement. *Ann Fam Med.* 2023;21(6):549–55.
6. Phillips WR, Louden DN, Sturgiss E. Mapping the literature on primary care research reporting: A scoping review. *Fam Pract.* 2021;38(4):495–508.
7. Phillips WR, Sturgiss E, Yang A, et al. Clinician use of primary care research reports. *J Am Board Fam Med.* 2021;34(3):648–60. https://doi.org/10.3122/jabfm.2021.03.200436
8. Phillips WR, Sturgiss E, Hunik L, et al. Improving the reporting of primary care research: An international survey of researchers. *J Am Board Fam Med.* 2021;34(1):12–21.
9. Sturgiss EA, Prathivadi P, Phillips WR, et al. Key items for reports of primary care research: An international Delphi study. *BMJ Open.* 2022;12(12):e066564.

CHAPTER

10

Reflecting on 50 Years of Practice-Based Research Networks

Lessons and Innovations

Anna Dania

10.1 PBRNs: Definition, Origins and Ecosystem

Practice-based research networks (PBRNs) are the research laboratories of primary care. They are longitudinal collaborations of researchers and clinical practitioners who are engaged in conducting research in, with and for primary care—cultivating evidence-based practice by addressing questions and problems that emerge from and matter in daily practice, and using rigorous research methods. PBRNs are learning communities that help translate research findings into evidence-based practice, which promotes quality improvement in primary care.[1–2]

Before research institutes or networks existed, individual practitioners conducted scientific inquiry to solve patient health problems. Over the past 125 years, five notable general practitioners—James Mackenzie, Will Pickles, John Fry, Frans Huygen and Curtis Hames—made key contributions shaping family medicine's evidence base.[3] More than 50 years ago, PBRNs emerged as organised efforts by collaborative groups of physicians. Since then, they evolved globally, exhibiting shared traits despite differences in infrastructure and national contexts.

The PBRN ecosystem serves as a hub for communication, interaction, knowledge sharing and reciprocity, functioning as a learning organisation. It fosters a collaborative, adaptive and community-centred milieu that accelerates the implementation of innovation. PBRNs are valued for their ability to translate emerging research questions into primary care data and research evidence that strengthens the family medicine evidence base and addresses real-world challenges driving meaningful and transformative change in primary care. In addition, PBRNs are well-positioned to swiftly gather and analyse data from diverse communities and practice settings to identify disparities, detect emerging issues and test interventions to advance health equity.[4–5]

This chapter highlights key lessons learned from this global experience of building and sustaining PBRNs.

DOI: 10.1201/9781003652106-12

10.2 Pathways to Building a PBRN

Previous research has underscored that PBRNs are built by setting a mission to fulfil (which may evolve over time) and cultivating long-lasting relationships, shared resources and a learning environment which develop foundational properties—essential for their progression, sustainability and maturity.[4,6] PBRNs were primarily initiated by academic departments of family medicine/general practice, recognising the value of research using real-world practitioner data.[7,8] These networks were often hosted by academic institutions throughout their evolution. Professional organisations and general practitioner colleges also played a crucial role, fostering PBRN development, supporting collaborative research and linking participation to professional education and growth. Some networks developed through partnerships within these organisations, involving academic departments from the outset or integrating them later.[4]

PBRNs typically undergo stages of development that sometimes assimilate the state of earlier PBRNs, albeit on a different timescale. Box 10.1 presents lessons from three models derived from pioneering early networks.

Practitioner motivation has been a critical component in the development and sustainability of PBRNs. The most compelling factors driving practitioner engagement were intrinsic motivations—particularly the desire to contribute to broader

BOX 10.1 LESSONS FROM THREE MODELS DERIVED FROM PIONEERING EARLY PBRNs

The 'Dutch model' was based on the continuous registration of patients' health problems, with relationships built around data recording and data coding, and quality cycles that built camaraderie.[7] In this model, the professional organisations played an important role to influence support from the government for the PBRNs.

The 'British model' supported primary care research and development, where the relationships were based on research capacity-building activities providing access to expertise and resources to practitioners to support their individual interests. These two models were based on academic departments and promoted higher degrees of education and academic appointments. Some British networks were based on the skills of remunerated and centrally coordinated research practices, whereas others operated as practitioner-academic cooperatives with research-designated teams. In this model, the state served as the driving power behind the development of PBRNs in primary care,[14] but the Weekly Returns Services (WRS) started as an initiative of the Royal College of General Practitioners (RCGP).

The 'American model' adopted an egalitarian approach where academics from the family medicine departments recruited practitioners advancing ideas and resources sharing to build a surveillance network (using the WRS data collection model) and collaborative research on topics important for primary care, which were otherwise not attainable, relatively quickly, and with sufficient data volume.[9] In this model, professional organisations played a supportive role recognising the value of practice-based research for the family physician's growth.[9]

All three models included physicians' research training and involvement of physicians in research as principal investigators (PIs) or co-PIs when possible.

efforts aimed at improving patient care and the inherently altruistic ethos of family medicine. In addition, collegial relationships were identified as significant, as previously discussed.[9]

Active involvement of practitioners in academic dialogue concerning research and implementation emerged as a powerful motivating factor. Empowering, collaborative and intellectually stimulating environments fostered a sense of ownership and led to the development of studies that were closely aligned with practice needs, which generated meaningful outcomes and improvement in patient care. Practitioner disengagement often resulted from poor communication around research priorities, as well as from an overemphasis on academic outputs at the expense of practical relevance.[9]

Both material and non-material incentives played essential roles in fostering practitioner commitment. Recognised professional development opportunities, such as continuing professional development credits, and participation in quality improvement (QI) audit cycles were situated at the intersection of intrinsic motivations and reciprocal benefits. Moderate financial compensation was regarded as a form of recognition for practitioner contributions, and over time, structured remuneration for participation has become a standard practice in many PBRNs—particularly those with top-down governance. In the current landscape, the pathways for establishing a PBRN can be categorised into four approaches, which are often interrelated (Box 10.2).

BOX 10.2 FOUR APPROACHES IN BUILDING PBRNs

Relationship-Building Through a Research Activity

This approach involved:

- Engaging in forums and research panels to identify and pursue shared research interests fosters team spirit and builds confidence through 'small wins' achieved through collaborative research.
- Involving residents or trainee doctors in PBRN activities, fostering a research culture among the new generation of physicians.
- Deploying surveys to gather insights on practitioners' motivation, characteristics, research interests, training needs and available resources to support research that is meaningful for the practitioners and sustainable relationships.
- Practitioners' empowerment through research capacity building was a next step in this approach.[4,9]

Building Team Spirit Through Common Professional Activities and Then Start Research

This approach included:

- Forming peer networks focused on practice improvement before expanding into research.
- Building relationships through professional training initiatives that also set research goals.[22]

- Promoting resource-sharing and intellectual exchange[23] to empower practitioners to engage in research.
- Practitioner research capacity-building activities was also a next step here.

Research Capacity-Building Approach

This approach focused on developing research skills in primary care, and in some countries (e.g., UK, Australia), it has been a key priority for policymakers, supported by dedicated funding. Research capacity-building included the following initiatives:

- Structured training or research programmes or research specific training
- Online workshops
- Opportunities for professional development (e.g., academic appointments)
- Career promotion through advanced academic curricula
- Partnering with other more research-experienced networks[14]

Data-Driven Approach

This approach initially was based on the effort for larger and more diverse research datasets for generalisable findings, securing patient confidentiality and regulatory compliance. The infrastructures of these networks depended on their mission and might be based on, for example, routinely recording practice data and development of centralised repository[7] data-sharing from distributed practice databases[24] or from PBRN-partner databases,[25] or academic groups contributing national datasets for international comparative studies.[26]

Depending on the network's mission, these PBRNs also incentivised their partners by providing health information technology (HIT) tools that support research and/or QI activities, learning healthcare system (LHS) facilitation, other learning initiatives.[25]

10.3 Essential Components of PBRNs

10.3.1 Human Resources

Leaders of PBRNs are often recognised 'research enthusiasts' committed to improving primary care, advancing knowledge and influencing policy. They typically hold academic positions or are experienced clinicians or had prior PBRN engagement.[10,11] Their roles are vital for network sustainability, and they are characterised by qualities such as commitment, responsiveness, effective communication, motivation, action orientation and agility. Successful leaders build and maintain relationships within the network and with external stakeholders, communicating clearly, building trust, inspiring collaboration, listening sensitively and translating ideas into actionable plans.

Empowering clinicians through research capacity building is key to supporting PBRN operations, expanding intellectual capital and ensuring long-term sustainability. These investments give rise to distinct roles that support research integration at the practice level:[6]

- Clinician-researchers are clinicians with advanced academic skills and specialised training, who contribute to fostering a research-oriented culture within networks. They are pivotal figures in PBRNs, bridging community practice with academic research and blending practical wisdom with research expertise, observation and curiosity.
- Researchers-in-residence are experts who bring complementary expertise to practice managers and clinicians, bridging the gap between research and practice. They apply evidence in real-world settings or generate new insights in areas with limited or context-specific knowledge. Using participatory approaches, they collaborate with frontline teams and managers to co-create and implement innovative services and improvements in real time.[12]
- Clinician champions are a broader group of clinicians, who possess strong research capabilities but remain primarily focused on clinical care while actively contributing to research governance and implementation in their settings.
- Practice facilitators originated in the United Kingdom (UK) and evolved into a more sophisticated model in United States (US) PBRNs, working to improve practice performance and support team-based QI by guiding teams and understanding their values and preferences. They facilitate system-level changes, share resources, lead QI efforts, provide project-specific training and serve as liaisons and conveners. They support practices facing research demands, foster learning communities, maintain motivation through ongoing communication and act as regional health connectors, strengthening ties between primary care and public and community health to advance practice improvement.[13]
- British networks established Research Designated Teams with protected time for active research involvement. Their education includes research training, supervision and partnership development. Members of these practices earn advanced research qualifications (eg MSc, MD, PhD). Their multidisciplinary teams embed practice-relevant, collaborative research into daily work, influencing practice improvements and informing local and regional strategies. These research-focused teams also serve as testing grounds for ideas, often leading to larger grants and supporting sustainability through ongoing research and funding.[14,15]

10.3.2 Relationships

Building a PBRN requires a core of dedicated academics and practitioners committed to collaboration. Maintaining strong, long-lasting relationships is essential to the foundation and sustainability of PBRNs.

Central to PBRNs and their greatest and most important asset is that the relationship between academics and practitioners is grounded in mutual respect, trust and appreciation, cultivating a collaborative and collegial environment. Over two decades, this approach has expanded to include patient and community groups, healthcare stakeholders, social service providers and various professional organisations, who are increasingly involved in the network's governance and agenda development, fostering similar values in these relationships.[6,16]

This growing involvement has led to the development of PBRNs with multiple stakeholder engagement from the outset[17] and results in the implementation of innovative methodologies for conducting research and translation, ensuring that all stakeholders work together toward a mutual understanding of cultures, concepts, interests, roles, responsibilities and actions in their joint efforts.[18]

10.3.3 Shared Resources and Properties

Shared resources refer to both tangible and intangible assets essential to a network's infrastructure and operations. These resources include:

- Contributions of scientific knowledge and expertise from academics, alongside real-world practice experience from practitioners
- The organisational framework for network governance, including steering committees, advisory boards, fundraising efforts, financial resource management and administrative support for daily operations, HIT applications and support
- Research methodologies, training and educational materials, scientific literature, collective intellectual contributions and jointly developed intellectual properties and innovations
- Research data, data management systems and databases[6]

Research demonstrates that the availability of readily accessible expertise is a key motivator for practices to engage in PBRNs, particularly when this expertise addresses broader practice needs in addition to research-related issues.[6] Properties refer to the innovations that emerge collectively through PBRN activities, while the learning environment serves as the operational and organisational structure that generates and disseminates innovations across diverse stakeholder groups.[4]

10.4 The Learning Environment of PBRNs

The learning environment within PBRNs typically encompasses the establishment of learning communities (eg communities of practice), the implementation of learning health systems and activities designed to build research capacity, in addition to data audit and QI audit cycles for practitioners. It may also involve the exposure of trainee doctors and the active participation of residents in practice-based research activities to cultivate a research culture among young practitioners and promote professional development as researchers.[6]

Interactions within the learning environment of PBRNs, particularly when engaging stakeholders such as patients and community members, facilitate research and translation relevant to clinical practice, patient/community needs and/or QI.[4,6] Consequently, innovations emerging from PBRNs, including insights from evidence implementation and best practices, contribute to the development of shared resources that benefit not only the entire network but also a diverse range of external stakeholders. Among these are category academic institutions and faculties that collaborate with PBRNs, leveraging their role as experimental grounds connected with the community. Through these partnerships, PBRNs have demonstrated the capacity to nurture a broader cross-disciplinary learning environment, advance knowledge across these stakeholder groups and expand their recognition as contributors to knowledge beyond the field of family medicine/general practice into multiple academic disciplines.[6,9]

10.5 Organisational Infrastructure, Funding and Governance

Early-era and novice PBRNs typically implemented an informal and low-cost governance model hosted by university departments or professional organisations. Governance typically included a director, a steering committee for oversight and a coordinator. Funding came primarily from academic institutions and professional organisations, supplemented by external project funders.[4,6] In countries such as Australia and the UK, national entities provided strategic investments and sustained research capacity-building programmes. Strengthened research capacity and recognition that PBRN research is relevant to real-life problems of primary care resulted in greater success in obtaining competitive grants, further contributing to network sustainability.[6]

In response to sustainability challenges, PBRNs adapted business models based on their strengths, which can be categorised as either data-driven (eg leveraging 'big data' or reusing data for multiple studies), capacity-driven (eg providing expertise or specialised resources for external projects) or partnership-driven (eg partnering with academic institutions, community organisations and industry).[6,19]

Later, the 'meta-networks' (networks of PBRNs) also came into the US and UK with more sophisticated infrastructures, often resembling non-profit organisations with salaried executive directors, boards, committees, subcommittees and task forces—depending on their structure and complexity.[9,19,20] These infrastructures aim to ensure sustainability through more profound innovations or more generalisable results.

PBRN governance types can be characterised as top-down, bottom-up or a mixed model that engages the entire organisation, sometimes called a 'whole system approach'.[21] However, in practice, these types are not always distinct in implementation, leading to subcategories such as the top-down collaborative approach.

Importantly, the national health landscape is a key factor in shaping a network's infrastructure and development. Aligning the network's focus with the evolving healthcare system, demographic shifts, health needs and financial resources—while organising governance and research capacity to address these changing demands—is both crucial and challenging.[6]

10.6 Innovations within PBRNs

Innovations were developed to support PBRN infrastructure and operations while addressing stakeholder priorities, especially those of the community. PBRN innovations have shaped the discipline of family medicine/general practice, influenced academic curricula, enhanced clinician education, improved care delivery and informed communities, policymakers, funders and other healthcare stakeholders—offering new perspectives on primary care. They can be categorised into two main groups: (1) process and technique innovations, and (2) other innovations, including intellectual, technological, methodological and socially accountable innovations.[6]

Box 10.3 outlines the first category and provides some examples.

BOX 10.3 INNOVATIONS OF PBRNS

Innovations in Processes and Techniques

- Development and adjustment of research methodologies for:
  - Data collection (card studies—a field-tested approach for collecting data in clinical settings) to the continuous recording of reasons for encounters in primary care practices, data collection using various electronic tools and the use of EHR data for research.[7,27]
- Research studies employing original research methodologies (such as surveys, observational studies, qualitative research methods, randomised controlled trials, comparative effectiveness research), or adapting methodologies to real-world clinical conditions (such as by implementing pragmatic randomised controlled trials).[5,28,29]
- Approaches for setting research priorities (such as community participatory methods for generating research ideas,[5,30] multiple stakeholder consultation,[16,17] and bidirectional decision-making through open-ended surveys and group discussions).[31]
- Dissemination and implementation (D&I) approaches that advance evidence adoption, enable real-time evaluations of novice primary care models and generate new practice-based evidence to accelerate implementation.[32]
- Quality improvement (QI) implementation and evaluation:
  - New methodologies for practice quality improvement (QI) by translating research discoveries that can be categorised in:
    - Collaborative models that utilise collective knowledge, skills and resources[19]
    - Continuous practice QI through quality audit cycles and benchmarking of clinician and practice performance
    - Participatory methods to better engage community stakeholders in research and practice QI such as community-based participatory research (CBPR)[5] and patient engagement panels[33] and a mix of nominal group technique (NGT) and protovoice[34]
  - Recommendations for practice and policy development (such as the PBRN Research Good Practices [PRGPs] for PBRN infrastructure building, study development, data management and dissemination policies,[28] a toolkit to guide the development and execution of multi-site clinical trials within PBRNs,[28] and set of recommendations to succeed research with policy impact[9] and approaches for direct policy development)[35]

References

1. Mold JW, Pasternak A, McCaulay A, Manca D, Rubin G, Westfall J, et al. Definitions of common terms relevant to primary care research. *Ann Fam Med.* 2008 6(6):570–1.
2. Agency for Healthcare Research and Quality. Practice-based research networks. 2016. [cited 11 Apr 2025; Available from: https://pbrn.ahrq.gov]
3. Green LA, Hickner J. A short history of primary care practice-based research networks: From concept to essential research laboratories. *J Am Board Fam Med.* 2006;19(1):1–10.
4. Dania A, Nagykaldi Z, Haaranen A, Muris JWM, Evans PH, Mäntyselkä P, et al. A review of 50 years of international literature on the external environment of building Practice-Based Research Networks (PBRNs). *J Am Board Fam Med.* 2022;35(4):762–92.
5. Nease DE, Westfall JM, Wilson E. Practice-based research networks: Asphalt on the blue highways of primary care research. *J Am Board Fam Med.* 2024 37:S129–32.
6. Dania A, Nagykaldi Z, Haaranen A, Muris JWM, Evans PH, Mäntyselkä P, et al. The sustainability of practice-based research networks across the globe: Insights from a worldwide qualitative study. *BMC Health Serv Res* (in press). 2025.
7. van Weel C. The continuous morbidity registration Nijmegen: Background and history of a Dutch general practice database. *Eur J Gen Pract.* 2008;14:5–12.
8. Green LP, Pace W, Carroll J, Peek C. Looking back to move forward: Future horizons for PBRNS extending learnings from the first 40 years of ASPN-NRN. *Ann Fam Med.* 2024;22(Supplement 1):5898.
9. Peek CJ, Reed FM, Calonge N, Nutting PA, Hickner J, Pace WD, et al. Looking back to move forward: Reflections of PBRN directors. *J Am Board Fam Med.* 2024;37(5):955–68.
10. Pitkethly M, Sullivan F. Networking Four years of TayRen, a primary care research and development network. *Prim Health Care Res Dev.* 2003;4(4).
11. Van Weel C, Smith H, Beasley JW. Family practice research networks: Experiences from 3 countries. *J Fam Pract.* 2000 49(10):938–43.
12. Marshall M, Pagel C, French C, Utley M, Allwood D, Fulop N, et al. Moving improvement research closer to practice: The researcher-in-residence model. *BMJ Qual Saf.* 2014;23(10).
13. Nagykaldi Z, Mold JW, Robinson A, Niebauer L, Ford A. Practice facilitators and practice-based research networks. *J Am Board Fam Med.* 2006;19(5):506–10.
14. Carter Y, Thomas K. Research opportunities in primary care (1st edition). Oxford: Radcliffe Medical Press; 1999. 256p.
15. Cooke J, Nancarrow S, Dyas J, Williams M. An evaluation of the "designated research team" approach to building research capacity in primary care. *BMC Fam Pract.* 2008;27(9):37.
16. Gaglioti AH, Walston D, Guzman CEV, Dera NT, Ortiz C, Wright LSC, et al. A practical approach to establishing a practice-based research network stakeholder engagement infrastructure. *J Am Board Fam Med.* 2019;32(5):695–703.
17. Peters S, Chakraborty SP, Barton C, Sturgiss EA, Mazza D, De Leon-Santiago M, et al. Building a practice-based research network for healthcare integration: A protocol paper for a mixed-method project. *BMJ Open.* 2022;12(6).
18. Norman N, Bennett C, Cowart S, Felzien M, Flores M, Flores R, et al. Boot Camp translation: A method for building a community of solution. *J Am Board Fam Med.* 2013;26(3):254–63.
19. NIHR. Income distribution from NIHR RDN Industry Portfolio Studies. [cited 11 Apr 2025; Available from: https://www.nihr.ac.uk/income-distribution-nihr-rdn-industry-portfolio-studies]
20. NIHR. Support for delivering research. [cited 11 Apr 2025; Available from: https://www.nihr.ac.uk/support-and-services/support-for-delivering-research]

21. Thomas P, Griffiths F, Kai J, O'Dwyer A. Networks for research in primary health care. *BMJ.* 2001;322. 588–90.
22. Sardell A. Clinical networks and clinician retention: The case of CDN. *J Comm Health.* 1996;21(6).
23. Mold JW, Peterson KA. Primary care practice-based research networks: Working at the interface between research and quality improvement. *Ann Fam Med.* 2005;3(Suppl 1).
24. Kristoffersen ES, Bjorvatn B, Halvorsen PA, Nilsen S, Fossum GH, Fors EA, et al. The Norwegian PraksisNett: A nationwide practice-based research network with a novel IT infrastructure. *Scand J Prim Health Care.* 2022;40(2):217–226.
25. DARTNet Institute—networks. [cited 11 Apr 2025; Available from: https://dartnet.info/Networks.htm]
26. NTRePID International consortium of primary care big data. [cited 11 Apr 2025; Available from: https://www.intrepidprimarycare.org/]
27. Stabler ME, Westfall JM, Nease DE, Raymond J, Jobse B, Daudier Z, et al. A pilot comparison of clinical data collection methods using paper, electronic health record prompt, and a smartphone application. *J Am Board Fam Med.* 2025;38(1):46–55.
28. Dolor RJ, Schmit KM, Graham DG, Fox CH, Baldwin LM. Guidance for researchers developing and conducting clinical trials in Practice-Based Research Networks (PBRNs). *J Am Board Fam Med.* 2014;27(6):750–8.
29. Nagykaldi Z. Practice-based research networks at the crossroads of research translation. *J Am Board Fam Med.* 2014; 27:725–9.
30. Westfall JM, VanVorst RF, Main DS, Herbert C. Community-based participatory research in practice-based research networks. *Ann Fam Med.* 2006;4(1):8–14.
31. Fisher M, Brewer SE, Fernald DH, Holtrop JS, Nederveld A, O'Leary ST, et al. Process for setting research priorities: A case study from the State Networks of Colorado Ambulatory Practices and Partners (SNOCAP) consortium. *J Am Board Fam Med.* 2019;32(5):655–62.
32. DeVoe JE, Likumahuwa-Ackman SM, Angier HE, Huguet N, Cohen DJ, Flocke SA, et al. A Practice-Based Research Network (PBRN) roadmap for evaluating COVID-19 in community health centers: A report from the OCHIN PBRN. *J Am Board Fam Med.* 2020;33(5):774–8.
33. Warren NT, Gaudino JA, Likumahuwa-Ackman S, Dickerson K, Robbins L, Norman K, et al. Building meaningful patient engagement in research: Case study from ADVANCE clinical data research network. *Med Care.* 2018;56(10 Suppl 1):S58.
34. Nederveld A, Duarte KF, Broaddus-Shea ET. Growing PEACHnet: Building a Practice-Based Research Network in Western Colorado. *J Am Board Fam Med.* 2022;35(1):115–23.
35. Golden RE, Klap R, Carney D V., Yano EM, Hamilton AB, Taylor SL, et al. Promoting learning health system feedback loops: Experience with a VA practice-based research network card study: VA card study promotes learning health system. *Healthc.* 2021;8(Suppl 1):100484.

SECTION

3

Extending the Realm of Primary Care Research

CHAPTER

11

Research Implications of Genomics in Personalised Primary Care

Braulio Mark Valencia, Jialing Lin, Chris Dietz, Peter Brown, Rafal Chomik, Shona Bates, Patricia Mary Davidson, Marc R Wilkins and Michael Kidd

11.1 The Genetic Basis of Health and Disease States

Among the many medical terms used in primary care, *genetics* and *genomics* are perhaps the least commonly mentioned—if they are mentioned at all. This is likely due to the assumption that they are often related to rare congenital disorders, which are not the most prevalent in primary care. However, common symptoms in primary care, such as fever, coughing or fatigue, are driven by regulatory mechanisms shaped through millions of years of evolution and encoded in our DNA as *genes*.[1] These responses—referred to hereafter as *traits*—do not result from the expression of a single *gene*, but rather from the coordinated activity of tens or even hundreds of genes across multiple pathways in different organs, with the number increasing with the complexity of the response.

Although the specific function or influence of these *genes* could be irrelevant in clinical practice, primary care workers encounter them daily, expressed as *traits*. Interestingly, *traits* differ among individuals (eg diverse severity in flu infections in an aged care facility) and even in the same individual under different circumstances (eg glucose control with or without stressful life events). This variability is explained by differences in *gene expression* resulting from underlying *genetic* differences in every individual and, perhaps more importantly, environmental factors that regulate *gene expression* directly (eg temperature, oxygen levels) or indirectly (eg *epigenomics*).[2] This complex interplay between *genes* and environment explains why, in response to the same trigger, some individuals develop "textbook" manifestations, whereas others show mild or subclinical features, and some develop unusual manifestations.

Thus, far from being unrelated, *genetics* and *genomics* play an essential role in both determining and understanding the variability observed in clinical practice

DOI: 10.1201/9781003652106-14

and will be crucial for personalised primary care. Understanding the basic concepts of *genetics* and *genomics* is vital to grasp the complexity and challenges of personalising primary care.

11.1.1 Ischemic Heart Disease Example

Given its significant impact on mortality and life expectancy, let us use ischaemic heart disease as a case scenario.[3] Among its many modifiable, biological, environmental and social determinants,[4] the formation of atherosclerotic plaques is a central event.[5] Although dyslipidaemia is a significant risk factor and a key therapeutic target, there is no linear causation between abnormal lipid levels and atherosclerosis. Rather, plaque development arises from the complex interplay of multiple mechanisms, including dyslipidaemia, which interact with environmental exposures in complex and probably uncharacterised ways to produce diverse *traits* observed in clinical practice (Figure 11.1). Key contributors, such as dyslipidaemia, hypertension and endothelial dysfunction, each driven by heritable and acquired mechanisms, interact in multifaceted ways and are further shaped by the environment. This complexity helps explain the broad spectrum of *traits*. Note that the heritable components can contribute to disease prediction even within such a biologically and environmentally intricate landscape.

Each of these mechanisms has acquired and *heritable* underpinnings. From a *heritable* perspective, although less than 2% of dyslipidaemia cases harbour rare *gene variants* with large effects (eg familial hypercholesterolaemia), most cases lack these variants. Their abnormal lipid levels are explained by the cumulative influence of

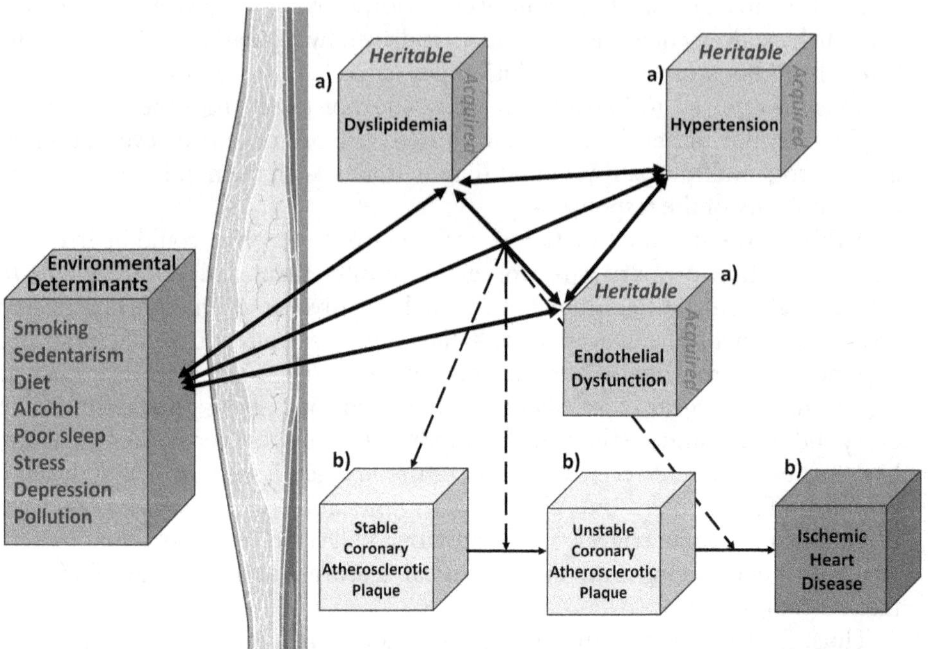

FIGURE 11.1 Pathogenesis of atherosclerosis

more than 250 common *genetic variants* or *single-nucleotide polymorphisms (SNPs)* across at least 11 different *genes*.[6] This is also the case in other atherosclerotic mechanisms (depicted in Figure 11.1) and is likely the same in other prevalent conditions in primary care, including infections, metabolic diseases, degenerative conditions and physiological processes. Consequently, understanding the *heritable* components of health and disease *traits* is essential to understanding personalised care needs.

Thus, to efficiently tackle the research implications of *genomics* in personalised primary care, it is critical to comprehend key concepts and terminology of human *genetics* and *genomics*, which are highlighted in italics throughout this manuscript and summarised in Table 11.1 for clarification, particularly if the terms are unfamiliar or entirely new.

TABLE 11.1 Key Terms and Definitions in *Genomics* and Personalised Care

TERM	CONCEPT
Genome	Vast DNA library stored in all nucleated cells, containing genes and non-coding regions. This information is based on four "characters" or nucleotides called purines (A = adenine, G = guanine) and pyrimidines (T = thymine, C = cytosine), primarily arranged into two complementary chains in a double-helix structure and other secondary and tertiary structures highly compacted in chromosomes. Humans have a 3 billion nucleotide pair genome, with ≤1% of these pairs forming genes.
Gene	Nucleotide sequence containing the basic instructions to build the structural or functional molecules required for the development, reproduction and maintenance of cells in health and disease states. A gene comprises *exons* (nucleotide sequences with part of these instructions), *introns* (nucleotide sequences without instructions) and regulatory regions located before and after the gene.
Ribonucleic acid (RNA)	Short, single-stranded molecule composed of four nucleotides (A, G, C and U = uracil) similar to DNA. Several forms of RNA exist, with messenger RNA (mRNA) being the most functionally significant. mRNA serves as a transcribed copy of a gene, using sequences of three nucleotides (codons) to direct the synthesis of proteins.
Trait	Any observable or measurable feature in organisms influenced by heritable or non-heritable mechanisms, including skin pigmentation, lipid levels or immunoglobulin types.
Inheritance	Mechanisms by which traits are passed from parents to offspring.
Heritability	Proportion of a trait variance attributable to genes. In other words, the contribution of genes to the trait.
*Genetics**	1. Branch of science studying the mechanisms and consequences of inheritance. 2. Study of the structure, function and regulation of genes, and how these affect traits or their heritability. 3. Frequency, distribution and effect of alleles in populations. 4. Part of medicine that involves diagnosing, managing and counselling individuals with genetic disorders and their families. 5. Genetic testing is the targeted analysis of DNA (eg chromosomes, genes, variants) associated with normal or diseased traits.

(Continued)

TABLE 11.1 Key Terms and Definitions in *Genomics* and Personalised Care (Continued)

TERM	CONCEPT
*Genomics**	1. Systematic study and characterisation, including structure, function and evolution of an organism's genome. 2. Study of variations of genomes within and between populations and the forces shaping these variations. 3. Use of genome-wide data to inform diagnosis, prognosis, treatment and prevention of diseases.
*Epigenomics**	1. Study of heritable changes in gene function that occur without gene variants. 2. Molecular mechanisms that regulate gene activity and chromatin structure without altering DNA sequence. 3. The interface between the genome and the environment that influences, in a reversible way, the expression of genes.
Gene variant (or genetic mutation)	Any detectable and permanent change in the DNA, whether or not it causes changes in traits. This change involves the substitution of specific nucleotides in any region of genes or structural changes (deletions, duplications, translocations) in small or large sequences.
Allele	Essentially the same as a gene variant; however, given its frequency in a determined population and its impact on traits, alleles can be labelled as common, low-frequency or rare variants. Commonly, rare variants have a pathogenic effect on traits.
Allele frequency	Allows for the classification of alleles as normal variants or rare variants. Common allele variants have frequencies >5%, low-frequency variants are between 1–5%, and rare variants are <1%. These are population-specific.
Size effect (of an allele)	The effect of an allele on a trait. Using statistical terms, a trait's risk (eg odds ratio, hazard ratio) if an allele is inherited.
Single-nucleotide polymorphism (SNP)	Allele with a frequency of >1% in a specific population is considered a SNP. Thus, a SNP in South Asians could be a rare allele in Caucasians.
Gene expression	It is also a trait. It encompasses the transcription of DNA into RNA, RNA modifications, the translation of RNA into a polypeptide, and subsequent post-translational protein modifications. Thus, genes are expressed as molecular (eg C-reactive protein in response to infections) or observable traits (eg height).
Gene regulation	A diversity of processes that influence the differential gene expression in cells. It could be genomic regulation mediated by nearby (promoters, enhancers, silencers) or distant regions (trans-regulation). It could be epigenomic, if regulated by chemical modifications in DNA (eg methylation), RNA (adenylation), polypeptides (adenylation or phosphorylation) or in proteins packaging DNA (eg histone phosphorylation). Non-coding RNA could regulate gene expression by interfering with transcription or translation.
Genetic architecture (Figure 11.2)	Results from two main parameters: (1) allele frequency, or how common a genetic variant is in the population, and (2) effect size, which is the magnitude of its influence on the trait, often measured as an odds or hazard ratio.

(Continued)

TABLE 11.1 Key Terms and Definitions in *Genomics* and Personalised Care

TERM	CONCEPT
Monogenic or Mendelian inheritance (or genetic architecture)	Transmission of single-gene traits in a predictable pattern. This means that a single allele has a significant size effect on traits. Alleles involved in monogenic conditions have a low or rare frequency.
Polygenic inheritance (or genetic architecture). Also known as complex traits.	Many genes and their alleles influence the transmission of traits, contributing with additive effects. This means that a single allele has a minimal effect on traits. Even with all genes and alleles quantified, their impact is partial as the environment influences the trait. Alleles involved in complex traits are common in different populations.
Next-generation sequencing (NGS)	Sequencing technology that, compared to traditional sequencing, allows for rapid and accurate sequencing of millions of DNA or RNA fragments. NGS uses short-reading (200–500 nucleotide-length fragments, which are later reassembled) or long-reading technologies (entire chromosomes in a single read). Some long-reading technologies can also be used as "point-of-care" to characterise DNA, RNA and epigenetic features, such as methylation or adenylation.
Whole-genome sequencing (WGS)	Sequencing of the ~3 billion nucleotides in an individual's genome. This is achieved using different NGS approaches.
Genome-wide association study (GWAS) analysis	Technique centred on characterising all common allele variants (>5% frequency) and a significant number of low-frequency variants (1–5% frequency) in the entire genome. Depending on the method, this number ranges from 680,000 to 5 million alleles. Although it encompasses the whole genome as WGS, it primarily focuses on alleles. To consider an allele as statistically associated, p-values are expected to be $<5x10^{-8}$, significantly more stringent than the conventional $p<0.05$.
Whole-exome sequencing (WES)	Similar to WGS, WES uses NGS to sequence all exons (see definition of *gene*) contained in a gene or panel of genes required explicitly by the corresponding medical specialist (eg clinical geneticist).
Omics	Simultaneous characterisation of different molecules in a comprehensive way, including DNA (genomics), epigenomic modifications (epigenomics), RNA (transcriptomics), proteins (proteomics), lipids (lipidomics) or metabolites (metabolomics). In most cases, except for tumours or specific immune cells, genomics can be performed on any tissue or fluid, providing the same information. In contrast, the other omics require tissue-specific (eg lung) and context-specific (eg pneumonia) sampling.
Systems biology	Interdisciplinary approach that focuses on the systematic study of complex interactions within biological systems to understand how genes, proteins, cells and other components work together to produce traits. Given the magnitude and diversity of data from each element, advanced computational and bioinformatic tools are required.

* Multiple definitions for a single term depending on the context.

11.2 Human Diseases from a Genetic Perspective

As outlined previously, *genes* influence human *traits* in two ways or by two modes of *inheritance* (Figure 11.2). The first is *Mendelian* (or *monogenic*) *inheritance*, where a single *allele* has a significant influence on a *trait*, such as whether a person manifests a condition or remains asymptomatic. The second is *polygenic*, in which the cumulative effect of many common *alleles* or *SNPs* across multiple genes contributes to a quantitative *trait* (eg HDL cholesterol levels, height or blood pressure). This relationship between *alleles* and *traits* is referred to as *genetic architecture.*[7] Pathogenic *alleles* with large *effect sizes*, such as those causing cystic fibrosis or spinal muscular atrophy, are often subject to negative selection and remain at low frequencies or are rare within the population. In contrast, *SNPs* tend to have smaller *effect sizes* with higher *allele frequencies* than do pathogenic *alleles*, but their frequency may vary significantly between populations. As noted, *alleles* and *traits* have a significant population connotation, highlighting two gaps in *genetics* and *genomics* research with implications in personalised primary care.

Whether normal or disease-related, human traits are predominantly *complex traits*. They are influenced by many common *alleles*, each with a small effect (*SNPs*), along with environmental factors. Although the *effect size* of individual *SNPs* is minor, their combined impact determines the different heritability of each trait (eg type 1 diabetes vs. type 2 diabetes). In contrast, *monogenic* conditions are caused by rare *alleles* that have a significant individual effect and can cause disease on their own. *Oligogenic* conditions fall in between, involving a few *alleles* with intermediate *effect size* that work together to influence the *trait* or with a significant environmental contribution.

Most *genomic* studies have been conducted on individuals of European ancestry, limiting our understanding of *genetic architectures* in other ethnic groups. Second, *alleles* do not necessarily exert the same effects across populations, making it challenging to extrapolate clinical insights to different ethnic backgrounds.[8] In addition

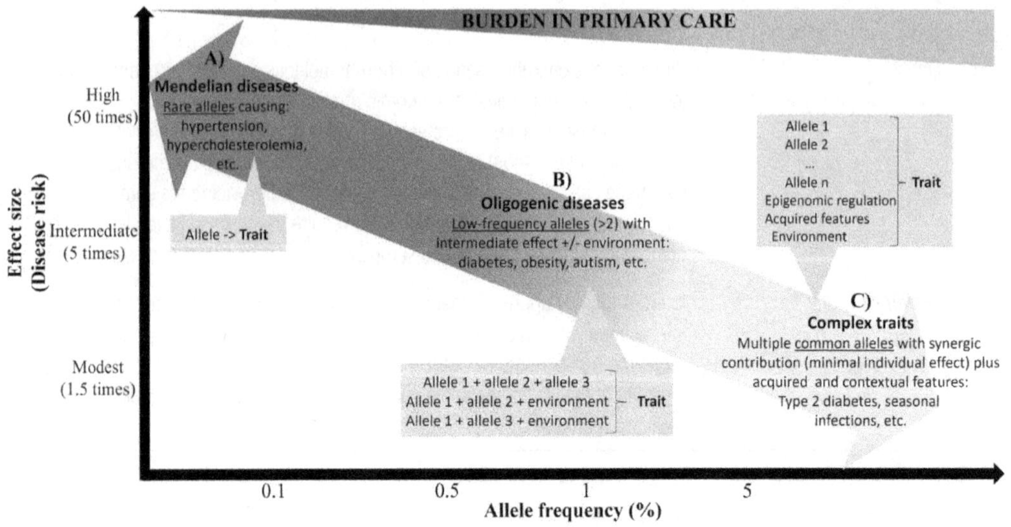

FIGURE 11.2 Human traits and their genetic architecture

to these gaps, *complex traits* pose an additional challenge: *genetic* factors explain a proportion of a *trait*, while environmental influences account for the rest. A classic example is height, which has a substantial *heritable* component but is also shaped by environmental factors such as prenatal and childhood nutrition.[9,10] This interplay of *genetics* and environment also applies to prevalent non-communicable and communicable diseases. For instance, COVID-19, despite being caused by the same virus, shows a wide range of *traits*, from asymptomatic infection to severe, life-threatening illness. Despite *rare alleles* being associated with life-threatening manifestations in a minority, age, comorbidities, access to care and multiple *genetic* determinants influence infection outcomes in the majority of cases.[11] Thus, the existing biological and population evidence suggests that most human features, including prevalent multimorbid conditions that require primary care, are likely *complex traits*. Although investigating *complex traits* presents considerable methodological, logistical and financial challenges, tackling them represents exciting opportunities to develop high-impact and sustainable personalised primary care.

11.3 An Optimal Approach to Achieve Personalised Primary Care

For nearly two decades, healthcare has aspired to realise the vision of "4P medicine": personalised, preventive, predictive and participatory care. This model has become a standard of care for rare or very rare conditions with monogenic inheritance, while remaining largely unrealised for complex traits, despite these accounting for most of the global disease burden. Concepts such as 4P medicine, precision medicine and personalised medicine emerged alongside the rise of *systems biology*, a paradigm shift from traditional reductionist approaches that study one variable at a time to hypothesis-free, integrative data-driven models that primarily focus on mapping the interactions of multiple molecular pathways to explain biological phenomena.[12] Interestingly, the foundations of *systems biology* were conceptually outlined as early as 1628 in Latin.[13] Thus, *systems biology* provides a far more suitable framework for understanding *complex traits* than do reductionist approaches, which are better suited to *Mendelian* conditions.

Consider, for example, a patient presenting with painless jaundice. Relying solely on liver function tests may miss the broader spectrum of underlying causes, including extrahepatic diseases. The standard medical practice involves a systems-based approach, accounting for the interplay of multiple physiological pathways and comorbid conditions to identify the most likely diagnostic and therapeutic plan. As personalised primary care spans diagnosis, treatment guidance and prognosis, limiting it to targeted *genetic testing* or *whole-exome sequencing (WES)* is unlikely to meet the diverse clinical needs of *complex traits*. Instead, comprehensive genomic approaches are more likely to meet these demands, including *whole-genome sequencing* (*WGS*) or *genome-wide association study* (*GWAS*) analyses. These tools are better suited to uncover the intricate, multilayered biological mechanisms that could drive the diseases frequently encountered in primary care.

However, because *complex traits* are also shaped by environmental factors, even the most comprehensive approaches remain inherently limited: they capture only the individual's genomic makeup while overlooking critical external influences.

Thus, while often considered central to personalised medicine, *genomics* alone will have limited power to fully support personalised care, given the multifactorial nature of *complex traits*. Even comprehensive genomic characterisation may be insufficient, as epigenomic mechanisms also contribute to heritability and can influence phenotypic expression independently of DNA sequence.

11.4 How Genomics Is Currently Supporting Clinical Practice

The accelerated development of *next-generation sequencing (NGS)* has significantly enhanced accuracy, simplified procedures and, perhaps most notably, drastically reduced costs. At the end of the Human Genome Project in 2003, sequencing a *whole genome* using traditional sequencing methods cost hundreds of thousands of US dollars. Today, *GWAS* is now available for US$100–600 per sample.[14] *WGS* can be performed for approximately US$200–600 per sample, substantially narrowing the cost gap between these two technologies. With the continued improvement of *NGS* and the development of novel sequencing approaches, *WGS* costs are expected to decline even further, raising the prospect that GWAS may become increasingly redundant in the near future. Nonetheless, the application of NGS in clinical settings remains focused on sequencing selected genes rather than entire *genomes*, echoing the more constrained scope of *genetic testing* available since the 1990s.

Despite significant improvements in accuracy and turnaround time offered by *NGS* over traditional *gene testing* methods, their integration into clinical care remains largely confined to specialised areas, such as rare disease diagnostics, oncology and pharmacogenomics, using targeted sequencing but not genomic characterisation. For example, targeted *gene* panels and *WES* have significantly improved diagnostic yield and clinical decision-making in rare and inherited conditions.[15]

In oncology, tumour profiling—either at a *genomic* or gene-targeted level—is standard for personalised therapies based on actionable mutations, such as those reported in breast (BRCA1/2), lung (EGFR), and colon (KRAS) cancers.[16] In pharmacogenomics, *alleles* in 29 *genes* have been linked to therapeutic efficacy and adverse drug reactions.[17] Similarly, *NGS* can support reproductive medicine through non-invasive prenatal testing, carrier screening and preimplantation diagnosis of inherited conditions, especially those with significant morbidity and mortality.[18] However, contrary to the optimistic view that *genomics* is on the verge of widespread clinical implementation, we primarily witness the refinement of traditional *genetic testing* through *NGS*. It is essential to distinguish that *NGS* encompasses diverse sequencing technologies, whereas *genomics* refers to a broader, systems-level approach to understanding and applying genome-wide data.

11.5 Implementation of Genomic Medicine in Healthcare

Some existing applications can be translated to primary care (eg pharmacogenomics or prenatal testing), but the implementation of "genomic medicine" or "precision medicine" in primary or secondary healthcare has not been achieved. Derived from

GWAS, polygenic risk scores (PRS) represent the most promising approach for near-term translation into clinical practice. A *GWAS* aims to identify individual *SNPs* that meet stringent significance thresholds. PRS go beyond and aggregate the effects of many SNPs, using more permissive statistical thresholds and other bioinformatic methods, to construct the best cumulative score.[19] PRS have demonstrated modest or moderate risk stratification power, equivalent to 20–40% of the trait's predictability.[20] This is expected, as PRS capture only the heritable component of *complex traits* and do not account for environmental, lifestyle or other non-genetic contributors.

Further, the predictive accuracy of PRS varies across traits, mainly depending on their *heritability*. Traits with high *heritability*—such as type 1 diabetes—tend to yield more accurate predictions,[21] whereas those with low *heritability*—such as Parkinson's disease—offer limited risk stratification.[22] PRS are developed in one cohort and require validation in an independent cohort to confirm their predictive utility, but many published PRS lack such external validation.

Additionally, due to the discussed genetic variability across populations, PRS developed in one ancestral group, such as those derived from European populations, do not perform similarly when applied to individuals from different ethnic backgrounds. For example, PRS that show high predictive accuracy of breast cancer in Europeans have limited utility and reduced predictive power in African or African-descended populations.[8] Another major criticism of PRS is the inclusion of well-known demographic risk factors (eg age, sex and BMI) within predictive models, where the contribution of genetic variants is often marginally relative to these non-genetic factors, raising concerns about their utility in clinical settings.

However, these criticisms can be addressed through meta-genomic risk scores (metaGRS), a meta-analysis of PRS improving the predictive accuracy by enhancing statistical power, increasing ancestral diversity, broadening outcome definitions and more reliably isolating the heritable component of *complex traits*.[23] As a result, metaGRS tackle accuracy and generalisability across diverse populations. Multiple metaGRS have now been developed and validated for a range of diseases, including coronary artery disease,[24] breast cancer,[25] prostate cancer,[6] type 2 diabetes,[27] and ischaemic stroke.[28] A common benefit across these studies seems to be the ability to effectively identify individuals at elevated risk of early-onset complications, enabling proactive detection and the implementation of timely preventive measures.

11.6 Gaps and Challenges to Achieving Personalised Primary Care

Precision medicine was defined nearly two decades ago as a framework integrating inherited and acquired traits, lifestyle factors and environmental exposures to enable personalised approaches to disease prevention and healthcare delivery.[29] Despite the proliferation of definitions in recent years, this early formulation captures the fundamental challenges and essential elements discussed in the preceding sections. Its broad, integrative scope offers a flexible foundation that can readily adapt to future scientific advances and clinical innovations. In the context of *systems biology*, this definition is particularly significant as it tackles essential components of *complex traits*:

1. **Contextualises the contributions of genomics**: As previously discussed, inheritance is governed by both *genomic* and *epigenomic* mechanisms. Even with complete characterisation of a trait's *genomic* architecture, predictive accuracy remains limited without a corresponding *epigenomic* component. Although emerging long-read sequencing technologies (eg Oxford Nanopore, PacBio) can characterise *epigenomic* features such as DNA methylation and will be incorporated among *genomics* to tackle *heritability* in all its extension, a comprehensive *epigenomic* profile requires different approaches, such as characterising *histone* modifications (see Table 11.1, gene regulation) and non-coding RNAs affecting gene expression (*transcriptome*) and protein composition and abundance (*proteome*). Unlike the *genome*, which is static and mainly immutable, the *epigenome* is dynamic, modifiable and organ specific. It is influenced by various external factors, including lifestyle, environmental exposures and chemical agents. Consequently, a reliable *epigenomic* characterisation will require repeated, context- and time-specific analysis across tissues to capture biologically meaningful changes.
2. **Highlights the relevance of individual, non-heritable features**: The *transcriptome* and *proteome* are also *complex traits* that result from heritable and non-heritable mechanisms and can be measured in healthy and diseased states. Thus, by analysing gene expression (via *transcriptomics*), protein structure and abundance (via *proteomics*), post-translational modifications (eg through *glycoproteomics*), and other molecules such as lipids and metabolites (via *lipidomics* or *metabolomics*), and integrating these data with genomics and epigenomics, it becomes possible to distinguish the heritable and non-heritable components of individual complex traits—such as those illustrated in Figure 11.1—thereby reinforcing the value of a systems biology approach. Among these, *transcriptomics* is currently the most accessible for clinical translation, as it can be addressed using *NGS*. In contrast, due to methodological complexity, high cost and the lack of scalability, most other *omics* technologies remain limited to specialised research environments. As a result, their implementation, even in basic research, is currently confined to well-resourced, high-throughput laboratory settings. This situation can be easily reversed, considering the remarkable progress of NGS over the last decade.
3. **Highlights the relevance of environmental features**: Although lifestyle and environmental exposures can be assessed through validated questionnaires (eg physical activity, stress levels, sleep quality) or objective measurements (eg blood lead levels, radiological evidence of asbestos exposure), most external factors remain unknown and unmeasured due to the lack of comprehensive, timely and standardised quantification. This limitation may partly explain why environmental factors are often overlooked in basic research and could be a reason for the lack of replication of laboratory discoveries in real-life situations. Nonetheless, environmental exposures also exert measurable effects at the molecular level, such as inducing post-translational protein modifications (eg pesticides), altering the composition of commensal microbiota across anatomical sites (eg indiscriminate antibiotic usage) or supplying beneficial or noxious molecules to humans (eg short-chain fatty acids or microplastics). Although multiple *omics* have been employed to characterise environmental influences at a molecular level, *epigenomics* holds

TABLE 11.2 6P Medicine in Primary Care

Component	Health Care That
Personalised	Tailors diagnostics, treatments and follow-up strategies to what is most effective for each individual, based on their unique genomic profile, medical history and environmental exposures
Preventive	Implements interventions aimed at reducing the likelihood or severity of disease, shifting from a reactive model of care to one focused on prevention and harm minimisation
Predictive	Forecasts disease risk before the onset of symptoms by leveraging genomic data, biomarkers, family history and digital health information
Participatory	Empowers individuals to manage their health actively, fostering a stronger patient–clinician partnership and promoting shared decision-making, informed consent and health literacy
Precise	Leverages the molecular resolution and computational capabilities provided by multi-omics, artificial intelligence and big data to refine personalisation in healthcare and move decisively beyond the one-size-fits-all model
Proactive	Enables anticipatory action well before traditional preventive approaches by leveraging the precision component for early risk detection, continuous monitoring and timely intervention

greater potential for translation into clinical practice.[30] Thus, the quantification of environmental influences is no longer out of reach and can be incorporated into both basic and primary care research.

Unlike the barriers faced two decades ago, delivering 4P medicine in primary care is now increasingly attainable. Its conceptual and methodological foundations are well-established and accessible, but translating these into practice still presents significant challenges and substantial opportunities. Among these, the sheer volume and complexity of data generated pose significant demands on computational infrastructure and require a highly specialised workforce for data integration, analysis and interpretation. Yet this complexity is also a powerful opportunity. Multi-omics approaches offer molecular-level *precision* by enabling the simultaneous characterisation of heritable, acquired and environmental determinants of health and disease. Such approaches enable healthcare to move beyond prevention towards a truly *proactive* model, allowing for earlier and more accurate detection than current preventive strategies permit. To realise this vision, personalised primary care must evolve beyond the 4P framework and adopt a more comprehensive 6P medicine paradigm, reflecting the full potential of modern systems biology and digital health integration (Table 11.2).

11.7 What Should the Research Agenda Look Like to Advance 6P Medicine in Primary Care?

Table 11.3 outlines practical ways practitioners can contribute to the development of 6P medicine in primary care. The agenda presented here is a general and non-exhaustive reference, but it can offer a valuable opportunity to engage with future health systems, develop a passion for research and transform present challenges into actionable steps toward patient-centred care and professional excellence.

TABLE 11.3 Research Agenda to Build 6P Medicine in Primary Care

Action	**Examples**
Translate evidence-based interventions into primary care	Conduct studies to evaluate the effectiveness, cost-benefit and scalability of evidence-based genomic interventions in primary care settings, including: • Primary care–relevant pharmacogenomic panels, encompassing drug classes such as cardiovascular agents, antidepressants, antibiotics and antivirals, analgesics, anticoagulants and gastric acid–reducing therapies.[17] Complete lists and details (gene, alleles, inheritance mechanism) are available at: https://www.pharmgkb.org/guidelineAnnotations • Post-hoc and prospective studies of metaGRS in coronary artery disease,[24] breast cancer,[25] prostate cancer,[26] type 2 diabetes,[27] and ischemic stroke[28]
Enhance genomics literacy in primary care workers and consumers	As genomic medicine will become an integral part of healthcare, primary care researchers must be equipped with a solid understanding of key genomic concepts and methodologies—not only to apply them effectively, but also to communicate complex information clearly to patients. This can be achieved through the following approaches: • Conducting quantitative studies to evaluate knowledge, attitudes and practices related to genomics among primary care researchers, frontline staff and undergraduate trainees • Developing updated curricula and targeted educational interventions that deliver practical genomic literacy, with a focus on formative assessment and real-world applicability • Designing communication-focused interventions to equip primary care researchers with strategies for explaining complex genomic information in ways that support patient autonomy and informed decision-making • Investigating the impact of genomic integration on shared decision-making, including how it may enhance or complicate patient-provider interactions in the primary care context
Support translational genomic research into primary care	Foster the integration of genomics into primary care through a bidirectional approach that bridges research and clinical practice by: • Encouraging the incorporation of genomics into routine primary care, despite current uncertainties around its practical implementation Standardising data collection within electronic health records (EHRs) can support long-term tracking of health outcomes and improve trait characterisation • Promoting and incentivising the active involvement of primary care researchers in multidisciplinary research teams—including bioinformaticians, geneticists, clinicians and genetic counsellors—to ensure that research questions align with the priorities and contextual realities of primary care • Supporting the participation of primary care researchers in multi-centre consortia to facilitate the replication and scaling of findings across diverse healthcare settings. This is particularly critical for ensuring the inclusion of underrepresented non-European populations in genomic research. • Integrating genomic research with data on social determinants of health to enable a more comprehensive understanding of how genetic risk interacts with lifestyle, environmental exposures and socioeconomic conditions

(Continued)

TABLE 11.3 Research Agenda to Build 6P Medicine in Primary Care (Continued)

Action	Examples
Ethical, regulatory and funding preparedness	Develop robust ethical, legal and regulatory frameworks to support the responsible integration of genomics into primary care by: • Engaging key stakeholders—including policymakers, healthcare professionals, researchers and consumers—to identify existing gaps and barriers in the implementation of genomics in primary care • Establishing clear protocols for the secure and ethical collection, storage and governance of genomic data, including instances where its immediate interpretation is not feasible • Advocating for targeted funding to support genomics research that directly addresses the priorities, challenges and realities of primary care practice

11.8 Conclusion

Realising the vision of 6P medicine in primary care requires a shift into systems biology and omics-driven research to address the complex interplay of heritable, acquired and environmental determinants that define complex traits (Box 11.1). Primary care researchers have an opportunity to proactively shape the research agenda by focusing on the conditions most relevant to their practice, by leading and participating in initiatives that generate evidence for personalised primary care. Although undergraduate and postgraduate education equips healthcare workers with a systems-level perspective at the organ and physiological levels, this lens must now expand to the molecular level. Understanding the principles of omics technologies and the capacity to manage and interpret large-scale data are essential skills for delivering personalised care in the digital age. The path ahead is undoubtedly challenging, but it is also an exciting opportunity to redefine the role of primary care in a new era of precision health.

BOX 11.1 TAKE-HOME MESSAGES

- Primary care predominantly addresses *complex traits* rather than *monogenic conditions*.
- The contribution of *genomics* to *complex traits* is variable and, in most cases, remains poorly understood. Even under this uncertainty, it is not expected to explain the entirety of any *complex trait*.
- A 6P primary care (personalised, preventive, predictive, participatory, precise and proactive) requires the integration of heritable factors (*genomics* + *epigenomics*), acquired characteristics and environmental exposures.
- Unlike *genomics*, which are static and require only a one-time characterisation, other *omics* (eg *epigenomics, transcriptomics, proteomics*) are dynamic, context-dependent,

and often require organ-specific and periodic interpretation. Thus, *genomics* alone is not sufficient to fulfil the 6P model.

- *Genomics* are often conflated with *next-generation sequencing*; however, their distinction is crucial. Current applications of "genomic medicine" are still limited to *monogenic* conditions and highly specialised clinical settings, making its use in primary care both limited and conceptually imprecise.
- Pharmacogenomics and polygenic risk scores currently represent the most promising *genomic* tools with near-term potential for translation into primary care.
- Some *omics*—such as *genomics*, *transcriptomics* and *epigenomics*—are gradually progressing toward feasibility in primary care, but the volume and complexity of *omics* data still demand advanced computational infrastructure and a skilled workforce with differentiated competencies across the healthcare system.

References

1. Hart BL. Biological basis of the behavior of sick animals. *Neurosci Biobehav Rev.* 1988;12(2):123–37. https://doi.org/10.1016/s0149-7634(88)80004-6
2. Miko I. Phenotype variability: Penetrance and expressivity. *Nat Educ.* 2008;1(1):137.
3. Global burden of 288 causes of death and life expectancy decomposition in 204 countries and territories and 811 subnational locations, 1990–2021: A systematic analysis for the Global Burden of Disease Study 2021. *Lancet.* 2024;403(10440):2100–32. https://doi.org/10.1016/s0140-6736(24)00367-2
4. Khoja A, Andraweera PH, Lassi ZS, et al. Modifiable and non-modifiable risk factors for Premature Coronary Heart Disease (PCHD): Systematic review and meta-analysis. *Heart Lung Circ.* 2024;33(3):265–80. https://doi.org/10.1016/j.hlc.2023.12.012
5. Stone PH, Libby P, Boden WE. Fundamental pathobiology of coronary atherosclerosis and clinical implications for chronic ischemic heart disease management: The plaque hypothesis: A narrative review. *JAMA Cardiol.* 2023;8(2):192–201. https://doi.org/10.1001/jamacardio.2022.3926
6. Gilliland T, Dron JS, Selvaraj MS, et al. Genetic architecture and clinical outcomes of combined lipid disturbances. *Circ Res.* 2024;135(2):265–76. https://doi.org/10.1161/circresaha.123.323973
7. Timpson NJ, Greenwood CMT, Soranzo N, et al. Genetic architecture: The shape of the genetic contribution to human traits and disease. *Nat Rev Genet.* 2018;19(2):110–24. https://doi.org/10.1038/nrg.2017.101
8. Hayat M, Chen WC, Babb de Villiers C, et al. Genome-wide association study identifies common variants associated with breast cancer in South African Black women. *Nat Commun.* 2025;16(1):3542. https://doi.org/10.1038/s41467-025-58789-0
9. Bicknell LS, Hirschhorn JN, Savarirayan R. The genetic basis of human height. *Nat Rev Genet.* 2025. https://doi.org/10.1038/s41576-025-00834-1
10. Jelenkovic A, Sund R, Yokoyama Y, et al. Genetic and environmental influences on human height from infancy through adulthood at different levels of parental education. *Sci Rep.* 2020;10(1):7974. https://doi.org/10.1038/s41598-020-64883-8
11. Słomian D, Szyda J, Dobosz P, et al. Better safe than sorry: Whole-genome sequencing indicates that missense variants are significant in susceptibility to COVID-19. *PLoS One.* 2023;18(1):e0279356. https://doi.org/10.1371/journal.pone.0279356
12. Kitano H. Perspectives on systems biology. *New Gener Comput.* 2000;18(3):199–216. https://doi.org/10.1007/BF03037529

13. Auffray C, Noble D. Origins of systems biology in William Harvey's masterpiece on the movement of the heart and the blood in animals. *Int J Mol Sci.* 2009;10(4):1658–69. https://doi.org/10.3390/ijms10041658
14. Wetterstrand KA. DNA sequencing costs: Data from the NHGRI Genome Sequencing Program (GSP). 2025. [cited 19 Jun 2025; Available at: www.genome.gov/sequencingcostsdata accessed 11 Jul 2017; 19 Jun 2025]
15. Hong J, Lee D, Hwang A, et al. Rare disease genomics and precision medicine. *Genomics Inform.* 2024;22(1):28. https://doi.org/10.1186/s44342-024-00032-1
16. Casolino R, Beer PA, Chakravarty D, et al. Interpreting and integrating genomic tests results in clinical cancer care: Overview and practical guidance. *CA Cancer J Clin.* 2024;74(3):264–85. https://doi.org/10.3322/caac.21825
17. Sadee W, Wang D, Hartmann K, Toland AE. Pharmacogenomics: Driving personalized medicine. *Pharmacol Rev.* 2023;75(4):789–814. https://doi.org/10.1124/pharmrev.122.000810
18. Zemet R, Van den Veyver IB. Impact of prenatal genomics on clinical genetics practice. *Best Pract Res Clin Obstet Gynaecol.* 2024;97:102545. https://doi.org/10.1016/j.bpobgyn.2024.102545
19. Koch S, Schmidtke J, Krawczak M, Caliebe A. Clinical utility of polygenic risk scores: A critical 2023 appraisal. *J Community Genet.* 2023;14(5):471–87. https://doi.org/10.1007/s12687-023-00645-z
20. Lambert SA, Abraham G, Inouye M. Towards clinical utility of polygenic risk scores. *Hum Mol Genet.* 2019;28(R2):R133–R42. https://doi.org/10.1093/hmg/ddz187
21. Sharp SA, Rich SS, Wood AR, et al. Development and standardization of an improved type 1 diabetes genetic risk score for use in newborn screening and incident diagnosis. *Diabetes Care.* 2019;42(2):200–7. https://doi.org/10.2337/dc18-1785
22. Nalls MA, Blauwendraat C, Vallerga CL, et al. Identification of novel risk loci, causal insights, and heritable risk for Parkinson's disease: A meta-analysis of genome-wide association studies. *Lancet Neurolog.* 2019;18(12):1091–102. https://doi.org/10.1016/S1474-4422(19)30320-5
23. Di Lenarda F, Balestrucci A, Terzi R, et al. Coronary artery disease, family history, and screening perspectives: An up-to-date review. *J Clin Med.* 2024;13(19). https://doi.org/10.3390/jcm13195833
24. Inouye M, Abraham G, Nelson CP, et al. Genomic risk prediction of coronary artery disease in 480,000 adults: Implications for primary prevention. *J Am Coll Cardiol.* 2018;72(16):1883–93. https://doi.org/10.1016/j.jacc.2018.07.079
25. Mavaddat N, Michailidou K, Dennis J, et al. Polygenic risk scores for prediction of breast cancer and breast cancer subtypes. *Am J Hum Gene.* 2019;104(1):21–34. https://doi.org/10.1016/j.ajhg.2018.11.002
26. Huynh-Le M-P, Karunamuni R, Fan CC, et al. Prostate cancer risk stratification improvement across multiple ancestries with new polygenic hazard score. *Prostate Cancer Prostatic Dis.* 2022;25(4):755–61. https://doi.org/10.1038/s41391-022-00497-7
27. Mars N, Koskela JT, Ripatti P, et al. Polygenic and clinical risk scores and their impact on age at onset and prediction of cardiometabolic diseases and common cancers. *Nat Med.* 2020;26(4):549–57. https://doi.org/10.1038/s41591-020-0800-0
28. Abraham G, Malik R, Yonova-Doing E, et al. Genomic risk score offers predictive performance comparable to clinical risk factors for ischaemic stroke. *Nat Commun.* 2019;10(1):5819. https://doi.org/10.1038/s41467-019-13848-1
29. Council NR. Toward precision medicine: Building a knowledge network for biomedical research and a new taxonomy of disease. Washington: The National Academies Press; 2011.
30. Lieberman-Cribbin W, Domingo-Relloso A, Navas-Acien A, et al. Epigenetic biomarkers of lead exposure and cardiovascular disease: Prospective evidence in the strong heart study. *J Am Heart Assoc.* 2022;11(23):e026934. https://doi.org/10.1161/jaha.122.026934

CHAPTER

12

Integrating Health Sectors

Primary Care, Public Health and Community Care Research

Sabrina T Wong, Ginetta Salvalaggio, Monica Aggarwal, Lynden Crowshoe and Stephanie Montesanti

12.1 Introduction

Over the past century, health systems worldwide have undergone significant transformations, characterised by diverse governance, organisational and funding structures and service delivery models. Despite different health system approaches, the global impact of the COVID-19 pandemic has been profound. Interestingly, the pandemic was mostly agnostic to health system arrangements, whether measured in health outcomes (numbers of cases, deaths, disability), healthcare utilisation (numbers of vaccinations, COVID-19 diagnostic tests, hospitalisations, intensive care unit admissions), health human resource burden or broader social, economic, and political impacts.[1] Additionally, the pandemic both revealed and worsened many long-standing health system issues, especially systemic inequities. For instance, racialised populations, Indigenous peoples and those living in under-resourced or geographically isolated communities consistently faced higher risks of infection, more severe outcomes and reduced access to timely and culturally safe care.[2] These disparities were often compounded by intersecting health threats (eg climate displacement, drug toxicity, housing precarity) that are more likely to impact equity-deserving groups.

Within the field of health research, the pandemic had extensive impacts. Some research labs and clinical trials were forced to shut down, while research-related travel to communities was restricted. Researchers involved in community-based and participatory studies experienced restrictions related to community–academic partnerships, delaying or stopping ongoing initiatives. Other researchers focused efforts on addressing urgent gaps in studying COVID-19-related health and social impacts. Despite these disruptions, the pandemic also sparked unprecedented collaboration across governments, funders, clinicians, researchers and communities, all of whom devoted attention to finding solutions to address the pandemic. Some focused efforts on vaccine development and on studies to understand the seroprevalence of SARS-CoV-2 and immune correlates of infection.[3] Researchers formed new collaborations across different sectors, such as

DOI: 10.1201/9781003652106-15

with industry, to support the development of new diagnostic tests and treatments, with geography and engineering to inform wastewater surveillance for SARS-CoV-2, and mathematical modelers and immunology researchers to develop and refine testing approaches.[4] Communities also collaborated with frontline care providers to champion contextually and culturally appropriate local responses, inviting researchers into this process.[5,6] These needs prompted researchers to build partnerships with policy- and decision-makers, healthcare leaders and public health (PH) officials, amongst others; it also highlighted the importance of considering the intersections among health, PH, social care, education and other sectors of society.

What clearly has been reinforced, given the worldwide COVID-19 pandemic experience, is that greater integration and strengthened collaboration are necessary between PH and primary care (PC). Pandemics, health syndemics and poly-crises are too complex to be managed individually by either sector. PC is foundational, as it provides integrated and accessible health services delivered by clinicians who are responsible for addressing the majority of an individual's health needs. It is based on ongoing, trust-based relationships with patients and delivered within the context of their families and communities.[7] Although most often provided in clinics or offices, PC can extend beyond these walls to include hospice, home, nonprofit and community settings. Abiding by primary healthcare principles,[8,9] we broadly define PC as encompassing the full spectrum of first-contact healthcare models that focus on 'comprehensive, person-centred care sustained over time along with primary healthcare initiatives that incorporate health promotion, community development and addressing the social determinants of health'.[10] In contrast, PH is an organised activity of society to promote, protect and improve, and when necessary, restore the health of individuals, specified groups or the entire population. It is a combination of sciences, skills and values that function through collective societal activities and involve programmes, services and institutions aimed at protecting and improving the health of all people. The integration of PC and PH, and research therein, can strengthen both sectors' ability to fulfil their missions and connect with the community to foster a collaborative, interdisciplinary activity aimed at improving population health.

However, a lack of infrastructure and human resources for both PC and PH makes it challenging to achieve the quintuple aim: equity, improved care, health, experiences and lower system costs. In particular, Indigenous peoples across several countries continue to experience disproportionate burdens of disease and persistent health disparities, compared to non-Indigenous people.[11,12] To address unmet needs and inequities, we need to expand access to high-quality, comprehensive PC and strengthen the capacity of PH systems. Furthermore, research on the healthcare settings wherein most people receive care—PC and PH—needs serious attention. Notably, PC research in the United States received 0.2% of overall research funding,[13] which is undoubtedly a similar situation across many countries.

Despite their central role in shaping population health, many countries spend a small percentage of their health dollars on PH and PC.[14] Meanwhile, the politicisation of PH has intensified.[15] Recently, PH officials have been blamed and publicly harassed for their leadership during the COVID-19 pandemic, expert scientists have been dismissed from vaccine advisory boards over partisan ideology, and worsening outbreaks of communicable diseases such as measles are occurring due to misinformation about vaccine safety and efficacy.[16] Against this backdrop, greater collaboration between PC and PH has been promoted internationally as a strategy to overcome challenges related to underspending,[17,18] combat disinformation and strengthen trust and dialogue among individuals, organisations and communities. Indeed, a core feature of the World Health Organization's (WHO) vision of primary healthcare in the 21st century is collaboration between PC and PH as a cornerstone for achieving equitable, resilient health systems. Moreover, the World Health Assembly endorsed a resolution to sustain regular and meaningful social participation in decision-making and processes for health, including empowering people and communities as part of a primary healthcare approach.[19] In this chapter, we build on that vision by offering insights into how integration between PC and PH can be strengthened and by identifying key priorities for future research.

12.2 Methods

In writing this chapter, we draw primarily on our Canadian context, while acknowledging that the process of strengthening integration between PC and PH needs to be adapted to other geographic contexts. We are guided by the Royal Society of Canada research report,[20] which outlines three of 12 recommendations for producing and using health research:

1. Strengthen Indigenous health research and break down systemic barriers to its conduct;
2. Develop mechanisms to produce novel research; and
3. Enhance research use across the health research ecosystem.

These recommendations are based on knowledge exchange sessions and surveys conducted with participants from G7 countries (Canada, France, Germany, Italy, Japan, United Kingdom, United States), Australia and New Zealand. The participants included leaders from funding agencies, research institutes, PH, health and social policymakers, researchers and members of the public.[20] The three recommendations are categorised under the WHO's framework for health research systems.

We draw on extensive knowledge and expertise as PC, PH and policy researchers, alongside clinical disciplinary knowledge and diverse cultural backgrounds. Two federal funding agencies, the Canadian Institutes of Health Research (CIHR) and the Strategy for Patient Oriented Research (SPOR), have invested in research networks across Canada. This includes the Canadian PC Research Consortium, which brings together researchers, decisions-makers, patients and communities, and the only pan-Canadian electronic medical record data repository of PC and practice-based research and learning networks.[21] In addition, CIHR's Network Environments for Indigenous Health Research (NEIHR) is the Indigenous Primary Health Care and Policy Research (IPHCPR) Network, which builds capacity and fosters collaboration in PC for innovation and research aligned with Indigenous values and knowledge systems, and promotes a research-to-practice and policy platform.[22] Together, we offer these areas of future research that could strengthen PC and PH. We also acknowledge that in order to strengthen ways of working to produce new insights, creating an ethical space that allows for Indigenous and Western spheres of culture and knowledge to come together in respectful dialogue is always needed to understand and instigate change within PC and PH systems[23] and at the coalface, in communities.

12.3 The Case for Strengthening Integration between PC and PH

The COVID-19 pandemic highlighted the disproportionate impact of the disease on low-income and racialised communities—the most vulnerable people in our society. Worldwide, studies show a clear association between racialisation and poverty and the risk of COVID-19 positivity, intensive care unit admissions, hospital admissions and mortality rates.[24,25] As noted by several scholars, these health disparities are deeply embedded in a long history of systemic inequities. These include holding essential and frontline jobs that increase the risk of exposure to infectious disease; greater prevalence of chronic conditions; reduced access to healthcare or essential services; living in crowded or substandard housing conditions; facing racism and discrimination; gaps in literacy, language and technology; living in rural areas; and being at greater risk of exposure as essential workers in high-risk occupations.[26–28] The lessons learned from the pandemic underline the importance of investing in and building integrated PC systems that provide a diverse range of comprehensive services for equity-deserving populations that are informed by equity-oriented approaches.[29] This requires strong partnerships between PH and PC that focus on improving population health and effectively responding to future pandemics, health syndemics and poly-crises.

Both PC and PH are key sites for population health interventions that address the social determinants of health to reduce inequities.[30–33] Strengthening collaboration across PC and PH for increased multisectoral action can occur through an equity-oriented approach.[34] For example, the UK's successful response to COVID-19 vaccine rollout rested on PC networks helping to operate more than 4,000 accredited vaccination sites across seven regions of the National Health Service and 153 local authorities.[35]

12.4 Emerging Areas of Research for Strengthening PC and PH

12.4.1 Community-Embedded, Participatory Approaches

The WHO's definition of health is explicit that health is not just the absence of disease or infirmity (https://www.who.int/about/governance/constitution) and includes physical, mental and social well-being. This definition underscores that many determinants of health lie outside the current boundaries of formal healthcare services, and thus using a social well-being lens in future research can offer innovative ways to improve health at the individual and population levels. Amartya Sen's Capabilities framework[36] of functionings, capabilities, agency and freedom is substantial and among the most closely examined. This framework importantly notes that well-being depends on a combination of functionings—the various things people may value doing and being—and capabilities, which are the opportunities to enjoy functionings. The work of Martha Nussbaum[37] reflects one of the most fully developed frameworks for specifying functional capabilities—real opportunities contextualised within the individual's personal and social circumstances. Importantly, Indigenous frameworks that emphasise a wholistic view of health and wellness align with the Capabilities framework. Both Indigenous worldviews and the Capabilities framework include mental, physical, emotional and spiritual health, in addition to connection to the environment, culture, social and economic facets of health and well-being.

An important and evolving area of research for strengthening the integration of PC and PH is the adoption of community-embedded, participatory approaches that emphasise relational and action-oriented processes, in which healthcare providers and researchers engage authentically and reciprocally with communities, empowering communities to mobilise collective strengths and resources to improve health outcomes. By positioning patients, communities and relationships at the centre of care, this perspective acknowledges the interdependencies among the broader social, cultural and structural factors that shape health. For example, recent work by Aggarwal et al[38] showed that COVID-19 vaccine distribution, particularly for equity-deserving groups, needs community-embedded approaches for implementation and delivery of proven treatments. Working in partnership with communities is not only critical for advancing integrated PC and PH initiatives but also essential for building resilience and preparedness to confront future health crises.

Community-engaged research that is in PC, PH, community or land-based requires weaving together knowledges. Settler researchers working alongside Indigenous communities, for example, need to privilege the perspective of community members, including Elders and Knowledge Keepers, and adapt healthcare innovations to prioritise community values and traditional healing practices alongside Western clinical care.[39] This braided approach will ensure that Indigenous and Western perspectives are equally valued and inform each stage of design, evaluation and knowledge mobilisation. Moreover, a community-embedded approach to research could better align with wise practices versus best practices,[40] where community-based knowledge is used to guide care, instead of always relying on best practices, which have been developed with a biomedical model in mind and are best fit for well-documented, comparatively static health concerns with clear boundary conditions.

12.4.2 Strengthening Data Systems for Use by Communities

PC and PH are recognised as having a significant role to play in recognising and decreasing institutional racism and other forms of discrimination that sustain health inequities.[12,34,41] An enduring structure that organisations can put in place is using digital health records. Good data lead to better outcomes, such as enabling personalised cancer medicines and treatments for rare diseases. Harnessing digital PC data—starting with electronic health records—for PH surveillance (eg syndromic surveillance), quality improvement and research is needed. Three areas are worth emphasising, with the acknowledgement that much research is needed in the area of digital health solutions.[8,10] First, data elements exist in electronic health records, but the codification of understanding by humans (experts) using standardised terminologies and ontologies and analysis is needed. Informaticians, data scientists, patients from diverse backgrounds and clinicians who work with them are all required to improve what is being collected digitally. Second, interprofessional thinking, paired with knowledge keepers and patients, is needed to critically analyse the algorithms that are being rapidly adopted by PC and PH. Artificial intelligence (AI) use is rapidly advancing, currently seen as an approach to decrease administrative burden by summarising patient encounters or to write medication prescriptions. With AI increasingly being used as decision support, more work is needed to understand the equity impacts of further reliance on these algorithms. Finally, using the FAIR (Findability, Accessibility, Interoperability and Reusability) principles is needed to examine further the ability to create connected, interoperable information systems and their impact on deployment for real-world issues. The technological solutions to linking data from different sources (eg PC charts, PH registries, administrative billing data, hospitalisations, wearables) are abundant, and challenges can be overcome.

Integrating these data across systems and organisations, understanding what data to use and when, and overcoming the regulatory, privacy and interoperability issues remain challenging.[42] Because data collection and the analyses of these data have big advantages for PC and PH systems, we also acknowledge that knowledge without the wisdom to apply it correctly could be useless, if not dangerous. An established framework in Canada is OCAP (ownership, control, access and possession), which provides guidance on how First Nations data and information should be collected, protected, used and shared.[43] Data sovereignty, especially in Indigenous communities, is a critical element of a common understanding of how and under what circumstances researchers can use data for good.[44,45] In strengthening data systems for use by communities, relationships and processes can help guard against the exploitation of their data.

Innovations in research that develop the science of comprehensive measurement and reporting across jurisdictions and communities are needed. Population health and integrated healthcare systems require the collection of real-world data from multiple sources, including patients, healthcare practices and broader systems of care within the community. Public reporting can be used for change, although there is potential for negative, unintended consequences, such as gaming or a preoccupation with a small number of published, often easily measurable, indicators.[46] However, public reporting of health system performance at all levels can promote accountability, highlight variation, identify areas for improvement, and support change.[47] Regional case studies of performance reporting[48] indicate that public reporting can influence decision makers' and clinicians' quality-improvement agendas. Public reporting may improve performance[49] because it has the potential to 'facilitate public participation and increase accountability in healthcare, impact societal and professional values and direct attention to issues not currently on the policy agenda'.[50,51] Therefore, data from multiple sources can be used to create a portrait of whether PC and PH are meeting stated objectives and identify opportunities for improvement. For example, research in three Canadian provinces showed low performance in both care integration and accessibility across all regions,[54] which led to renewed improvement work.[52] Reporting on PC and PH performance remains nascent, but it is needed to focus individual, organisational and systems efforts to strengthen our healthcare systems.

12.5 Approaches to Research: Implementation Science, Learning Health Systems and Complexity

The interaction between PH and PC is inherently complex, shaped by overlapping mandates, shared goals and distinct accountabilities. Some functions sit squarely within one domain, but many occupy the interface between the two. PC, for example, routinely undertakes activities that are traditionally PH functions—such as immunisation, screening and interventions to support healthier lifestyles. Conversely, PH enhances the effectiveness of PC by generating population-level surveillance data, informing planning and priority setting and contributing to evaluation and quality improvement. Greater integration between these domains is widely seen as desirable, but the evidence base for integration remains limited and uneven.[53–55]

At the same time, integration is not without risks: aligning functions may create additional burdens on already stretched financial, human and organisational resources, and may introduce unintended consequences if implementation is poorly designed. This is precisely where implementation science plays a critical role. By systematically studying how integration efforts unfold in diverse contexts, implementation science provides the tools to identify facilitators and barriers, adapt interventions to local needs and generate evidence on the effectiveness, efficiency and equity of the innovation.[56] In doing so, it can help policymakers and health system leaders move beyond aspirational calls for integration toward practical, evidence-informed strategies that strengthen both PH and PC in ways that are sustainable and responsive to communities.

Additionally, a Learning Health System (LHS) approach builds on this foundation by providing a framework for advancing equity-driven improvement across PC and PH. LHSs embed iterative cycles of data collection, reflection and action into everyday practice, creating the conditions for systems that can learn and adapt in real time. They also provide the infrastructure to scale and spread promising innovations—such as Advanced Access scheduling and case management models—that have the potential to improve equitable access and strengthen the delivery of PC at scale.[56,57] At their core, LHSs empower individuals and communities to articulate and pursue their own health priorities. Achieving this vision requires sustained investment in the health workforce, including expanding team-based models that bring together diverse professionals, community partners and sectors.

Finally, acknowledging the complexity of PC and PH work, and the interplay between them, necessitates the use of a complexity framework that can help us understand complex systems, guide analysis and establish a common language and logic for dialogue, discussion and learning. Frameworks used to understand complexity often describe differences between simple, complicated, complex and chaotic systems. One example is the Cynefin framework developed by Snowden,[58] which is used to aid decision-making by focusing on cause and effect within different contexts. For complex issues, such as integration of PC and PH, innovations and emergent learnings are discovered through trial and error. Existing practice-based research and learning networks could serve as an environment where novel approaches to implementation, scale and spread of innovations are tested and refined.

12.6 Conclusion

The COVID-19 pandemic may seem long past, but we know that future pandemics, syndemics and poly-crises will occur. Evidence-based science and research can strengthen PC and PH alongside these workforces that protect and improve the health of all. Although many areas of future research are needed, we discussed three in this chapter. First, engaging communities to strengthen PC and PH in their areas fosters trust, relationship-based care delivery and their collective strengths and resources to improve health outcomes. Second, developing and using data generated by PC and PH for good and learning is foundational for building scientific evidence. Finally, this chapter suggests improving the science of implementation and learning in order to help guide PC and PH to apply, spread and scale innovations that serve to maintain or improve the health of all.

References

1. Rabeneck L, McCabe C, Dobrow M, et al. Strengthening health care in Canada post-COVID-19 pandemic. *Facets*. 2023;8:1–10. https://doi.org/10.1139/facets-2022-0225
2. Mashford-Pringle A, Skura C, Stutz S, et al. What we heard: Indigenous peoples and COVID–19. Ottawa: Public Health Agency of Canada; 2021. [Available from: https://nccdh.ca/resources/entry/what-we-heard-indigenous-peoples-and-covid-19]
3. Druedahl LC, Minssen T, Price WN. Collaboration in times of crisis: A study on COVID-19 vaccine R&D partnerships. *Vaccine*. 2021;39(42):6291–5. https://doi.org/10.1016/j.vaccine.2021.08.101
4. Lee BE, Sikora C, Faulder D, et al. Early warning and rapid public health response to prevent COVID-19 outbreaks in long-term care facilities (LTCF) by monitoring SARS-CoV-2 RNA in LTCF site-specific sewage samples and assessment of antibodies response in this population: Prospective study protocol. *BMJ Open*. 2021;11:e052282. https://doi.org/10.1136/bmjopen-2021-052282
5. Campbell-Scherer D, Chiu Y, Ofosu NN, et al. Illuminating and mitigating the evolving impacts of COVID-19 on ethnocultural communities: A participatory action mixed-methods study. *CMAJ*. 2021;193:E1203–12. https://doi.org/10.1503/cmaj.210131
6. Salvalaggio G, Hyshka E, Brown C, et al. A comparison of the COVID-19 response for urban underserved patients experiencing healthcare transitions in three Canadian cities. *Can J Public Health*. 2022;113:846–66. https://doi.org/10.17269/s41997-022-00651-7
7. Glegg S, McCrae K, Kolla G, et al. "COVID just kind of opened a can of whoop-ass": The rapid growth of safer supply prescribing during the pandemic documented through an environmental scan of addiction and harm reduction services in Canada. *Int J Drug Policy*. 2022;106. https://doi.org/10.1016/j.drugpo.2022.103742
8. National Academies of Sciences, Engineering, and Medicine, Health and Medicine Division, McCauley L, Phillips RL, Meisnere M, et al. Implementing high-quality primary care: Rebuilding the foundation of health care. Washington: National Academies Press; 2021.
9. Khatri RB, Hill PS, Wolka E, et al. Beyond astana: Configuring the world health organization collaborating centres for primary health care. *PLoS Glob Public Health*. 2023;3(7):e0002204. https://doi.org/10.1371/journal.pgph.0002204
10. Aggarwal M, Hutchison B, Abdelhalim R, et al. Building high-performing primary care systems: After a decade of policy change, is Canada "Walking the Talk?" *Milbank Q*. 2023;101(4):1139–1190. https://doi.org/10.1111/1468-0009.12674
11. Lavoie JG, Wong ST, Ibrahim N, et al. Underutilized and undertheorized: The use of hospitalization for ambulatory care sensitive conditions for assessing the extent to which primary

healthcare services are meeting needs in British Columbia First Nation communities. *BMC Health Serv Res.* 2019;19:50. https://doi.org/10.1186/s12913-018-3850-y

12. Browne AJ, Varcoe CM, Wong ST, et al. Closing the health equity gap: Evidence-based strategies for primary health care organizations. *Int J Equity Health.* 2012;11:59. https://doi.org/10.1186/1475-9276-11-59
13. Phillips RL. Implementing high-quality primary care: To what end? *Ann Fam Med.* 2022;20:107–8. https://doi.org/10.1370/afm.2802
14. Sparer MS, Brown LD. Politics and the public health workforce: Lessons suggested from a five-state study. *Milbank Q.* 2023;101(3):815–40. https://doi.org/10.1111/1468-0009.12657
15. Valiavska A, Smith-Frigerio S. Politics over public health: Analysis of Twitter and reddit posts concerning the role of politics in the public health response to COVID–19. *Health Commun.* 2023;38(11):2271–80. https://doi.org/10.1080/10410236.2022.2063497
16. Adams J, Carmona R, Elders J, et al. Six surgeons general: It's our duty to warn the nation about RFK Jr. *Washington Post.* 2025.
17. Harris M. The interface between primary health care and population health: Challenges and opportunities for prevention. *Public Health Res Pract.* 2016;26(1): e2611601. doi.org/10.17061/phrp2611601
18. Banarsee R, Kelly C, El-Osta A, et al. Towards a strategic alignment of public health and primary care practices at local levels—the case of severe and enduring mental illness. *Lon J Prim Care.* 2018;10(2):19–23. https://doi.org/10.1080/17571472.2018.1437070
19. World Health Organization. World Health Assembly endorses resolution on social participation. 2024. [cited 11 Oct 2025; Available from: https://www.who.int/news/item/29-05-2024-world-health-assembly-endorses-resolution-on-social-participation]
20. Straus SE, Beckett R, Fahim C, Pak N, Kasperavicius D, Clifford T, et al. Health research system recovery: Strengthening Canada's health research system after the COVID-19 pandemic. *Facets.* 2024 Sep;9. [cited 9 Oct 2025; Available from: https://www.facetsjournal.com/doi/full/10.1139/facets-2023-0233]
21. Canadian Primary Care Research Network Website. University of British Columbia. 2025. [cited 9 Oct 2025; Available from: https://cpcrn-rcrsp.ca/]
22. Crowshoe L, Sehgal A, Montesanti S, et al. The Indigenous primary health care and policy research network: Guiding innovation within primary health care with Indigenous peoples in Alberta. *Health Policy.* 2021;125(6):725–31. https://doi.org/10.1016/j.healthpol.2021.02.007
23. Ermine W. The ethical space of engagement. *Indig Law J.* 2007;6.
24. Magesh S, John D, Li WT, et al. Disparities in COVID-19 outcomes by race, ethnicity, and socioeconomic status: A systematic-review and meta-analysis. *JAMA Netw Open.* 2021;4(11):e2134147. https://doi.org/10.1001/jamanetworkopen.2021.34147
25. Parolin Z, Lee EK. The role of poverty and racial discrimination in exacerbating the health consequences of COVID–19. *Lancet Reg Health Am.* 2022;7:100178. https://doi.org/10.1016/j.lana.2021.100178
26. Thakur N, Lovinsky-Desir S, Bime C, et al. The structural and social determinants of the racial/ethnic disparities in the U.S. COVID-19 pandemic: What's our role? *Am J Respir Crit Care Med.* 2020;202(7):943–9. https://doi.org/10.1164/rccm.202005-1523PP
27. Paremoer L, Nandi S, Serag H, et al. Covid-19 pandemic and the social determinants of health. *BMJ.* 2021;372:n129. https://doi.org/10.1136/bmj.n129
28. Khedmati Morasae E, Derbyshire DW, Amini P, et al. Social determinants of spatial inequalities in COVID-19 outcomes across England: A multiscale geographically weighted regression analysis. *SSM Popul Health.* 2024;25. https://doi.org/10.1016/j.ssmph.2024.101621
29. Browne AJ, Varcoe C, Ford-Gilboe M, et al. EQUIP healthcare: An overview of a multi-component intervention to enhance equity-oriented care in primary health care settings. *Int J Equity Health.* 2015;14:152. https://doi.org/10.1186/s12939-015-0271-y

30. Vanden Bossche D, Zhao QJ, Ares-Blanco S, et al. Addressing health inequity during the COVID-19 pandemic through primary health care and public health collaboration: A multiple case study analysis in eight high-income countries. *Int J Equity Health.* 2023;22:171. https://doi.org/10.1186/s12939-023-01968-6
31. Wong ST, MacDonald M, Martin-Misener R, et al. What systemic factors contribute to collaboration between primary care and public health sectors? An interpretive descriptive study. *BMC Health Serv Res.* 2017;17:796. https://doi.org/10.1186/s12913-017-2730-1
32. Valaitis RK, Wong ST, MacDonald M, et al. Addressing quadruple aims through primary care and public health collaboration: Ten Canadian case studies. *BMC Public Health.* 2020;20:507. https://doi.org/10.1186/s12889-020-08610-y
33. Richard L, Furler J, Densley K, et al. Equity of access to primary healthcare for vulnerable populations: The IMPACT international online survey of innovations. *Int J Equity Health.* 2016;15:64. https://doi.org/10.1186/s12939-016-0351-7
34. Ford-Gilboe M, Wathen CN, Varcoe C, et al. How equity-oriented health care affects health: Key mechanisms and implications for primary health care practice and policy. *Milbank Q.* 2018;96(4):635–71. https://doi.org/10.1111/1468-0009.12349
35. Timmins N, Baird B. The Covid-19 vaccination programme trials, tribulations and successes. London, England: The King's Fund; 2022. [cited 21 Dec 2025; Available from: https://www.kingsfund.org.uk/insight-and-analysis/reports/covid-19-vaccination-programme]
36. Sen A. Development as freedom. New York: Anchor Books; 1999.
37. Claassen R, Düwell M. The foundations of capability theory: Comparing nussbaum and gewirth. *Ethical Theory Moral Pract.* 2013;16:493–510. https://doi.org/10.1007/s10677-012-9361-8
38. Aggarwal M, Katz A, Kokorelias KM, et al. What are effective vaccine distribution approaches for equity-deserving and high-risk populations during COVID-19? Exploring best practices and recommendations in Canada: Protocol for a mixed-methods multiple case codesign study. *BMJ Open.* 2023;13:e072238. https://doi.org/10.1136/bmjopen-2023-072238
39. Melro CM, MacDonald K, Cowan T, et al. Integrating Indigenous ways of knowing into learning health systems: Moving from learning health systems to learning communities. *Can J Psychiatry.* 2025;10:1–6. https://doi.org/10.1177/07067437251380734
40. Calliou B, Wesley-Esquimaux C. A wise practices approach to Indigenous community development in Canada. In: Voyageur C, Calliou B, Brearley L, eds. Restorying Indigenous leadership: Wise practices in community development. Banff, Alberta: Banff Centre Press; 2015.
41. Allan B, Smylie first peoples, second class treatment: The role of racism in the health and well-being of Indigenous peoples in Canada. Toronto: The Wellesley Institute; 2015. [Available from: https://www.wellesleyinstitute.com/wp-content/uploads/2015/02/Summary-First-Peoples-Second-Class-Treatment-Final.pdf]
42. Health Data Research Network Canada. Indigenous data sovereignty. 2025. [cited 9 Oct 2025; Available from: https://www.hdrn.ca/en/dash/resources/indigenous-data-sovereignty/]
43. First Nations Information Governance Centre. The first nations principles of OCAP. 2025. [cited 9 Oct 2025; Available from: https://fnigc.ca/ocap-training/]
44. Black Health Equity Working Group. Engagement, governance, access, and protection (EGAP): A data governance framework for health data collected from Black communities. 2021. [cited 9 Oct 2025; Available from: https://blackhealthequity.ca/wp-content/uploads/2021/03/Report_EGAP_framework.pdf]
45. Animikii. Niiwin is your Indigenous data sovereignty platform. 2025. [cited 9 Oct 2025; Available from: https://animikii.com/]

46. Salvalaggio G, Brooks H, Caine V, et al. Flawed reports can harm: The case of supervised consumption services in Alberta. *Can J Public Health.* 2023;114:928–33. https://doi.org/10.17269/s41997-023-00825-x
47. Levesque JF, Sutherland K. Combining patient, clinical and system perspectives in assessing performance in healthcare: An integrated measurement framework. *BMC Health Serv Res.* 2020;20:23. https://doi.org/10.1186/s12913-019-4807-5
48. Martin-Misener R, Wong ST, Johnston S, et al. Regional variation in primary care improvement strategies and policy: Case studies that consider qualitative contextual data for performance measurement in three Canadian provinces. *BMJ Open.* 2019;9:e029622. https://doi.org/10.1136/bmjopen-2019-029622
49. Schneider EC, Shah A, Doty MM, et al. Mirror, mirror 2021: Reflecting poorly. New York: The Commonwealth Fund. [Available from: www.commonwealthfund.org/sites/default/files/2021-08/Schneider_Mirror_Mirror_2021.pdf]
50. Slater M, Abelson J, Wong ST, et al. Priority measures for publicly reporting primary care performance: Results of public engagement through deliberative dialogues in 3 Canadian provinces. *Health Expect.* 2020;23:1213–23. https://doi.org/10.1111/hex.13100
51. Johnston S, Abelson J, Wong ST, et al. Citizen perspectives on the use of publicly reported primary care performance information: Results from citizen-patient dialogues in three Canadian provinces. *Health Expect.* 2019;22:974–82. https://doi.org/10.1111/hex.12902
52. Ellins, J; McIver S. Supporting patients to make informed choices in PC: What works? 2009 May;2011:12. [Available from: http://www.birmingham.ac.uk/Documents/college-social-sciences/social-policy/HSMC/publications/PolicyPapers/Policy-paper-4.pdf]
53. Oxman AD, Lavis JN, Lewin S, Fretheim A. Support tools for evidence-informed health policymaking (STP) 1: What is evidence-informed policymaking? *Health Res Policy Syst.* 2009;7(Suppl 1):S1. https://doi.org/10.1186/1478-4505-7-S1-S1
54. Wong ST, Johnston S, Burge F, et al. Comparing the attainment of the patient's medical home model across regions in three Canadian provinces: A cross-sectional study. *Healthcare Policy.* 2021;17(2):19–37. https://doi.org/10.12927/HCPOL.2021.26659
55. Montesanti S, Robinson-Vollman A, Green LA. Designing a framework for primary health care research in Canada: A scoping literature review. *BMC Fam Pract.* 2018;19(144). https://doi.org/10.1186/s12875-018-0839-x
56. Nilsen P, Bernhardsson S. Context matters in implementation science: A scoping review of determinant frameworks that describe contextual determinants for implementation outcomes. *BMC Health Serv Res.* 2019;19(189). https://doi.org/10.1186/s12913-019-4015-3
57. Finegood D, Bradd S, Yakimov C. Simon Fraser university faculty of science. *Complex Systems Frameworks Collection.* 2025. [cited 9 Oct 2025; Available from: https://www.complexsystemsframeworks.ca/]
58. Snowden D. The Cynefin framework. 2025. [cited 9 Oct 2025; Available from: https://thecynefin.co/about-us/about-cynefin-framework/]

CHAPTER

13

Interprofessional, Interdisciplinary and Transdisciplinary Collaboration in Primary Care Research

Ülkü Sur Ünal and Maria van den Muijsenbergh

13.1 Introduction

13.1.1 Collaboration in Primary Care

Primary care addresses a wide array of health issues influenced by biological, psychological, social and environmental factors. No single profession can fully understand or resolve these multifaceted problems; therefore, professionals from different disciplines have to work together in primary care. There are different levels of collaboration: professionals may work alongside doing their own jobs and referring the patient to other professionals also doing their own jobs (multiprofessional collaboration), or they may set goals together and work in a team, called interprofessional collaboration:[1–3]

> members of different professional groups with different specialties, a different sense of self-perception and ways of being perceived by others, different areas of expertise and work, and a different level of status all work directly together to provide high-quality, patient-oriented care, so that the patient benefits from the specific skills of each individual profession.[4,5]

Interprofessional collaboration in primary care practice can lead to better outcomes, including the development of community-centred services and improved alignment between health and social care systems.[6–8] There will be improved healthcare quality and safety as well as better patient outcomes in chronic care.[9–11] Recent systematic reviews highlight that interprofessional training initiatives further enhance team effectiveness and patient outcomes.[12,13]

DOI: 10.1201/9781003652106-16

13.1.2 Collaboration in Primary Care Research

Incorporating diverse professional perspectives, such as medicine, nursing, social work and public health, also enables researchers to examine health phenomena holistically, capturing the full scope of patient needs and systemic challenges.[14,15] The holistic approach specified in the WONCA tree[16] should therefore be implemented not only in primary care practice but also in research, thus ensuring that research topics are evaluated from multiple perspectives.

There are different types of collaboration. Interprofessional research involves collaboration among professionals from different fields within health practice settings, e.g., doctors, nurses, pharmacists. Early interprofessional training and ongoing teamwork foster a culture that supports the implementation of research into routine care.[10] It promotes mutual understanding and respect, which are essential for effective teamwork and patient-centred care and drive innovation in research and practice.[9,17] Primary care providers involved in interprofessional research initiatives can become more familiar with each other's roles and expertise, which benefits interprofessional collaboration in practice.

In interdisciplinary research, there is collaboration beyond other health academic disciplines to non-health academic disciplines, such as sociology, bioengineering, environmental science and law. Combining different scientific disciplines in the research team has its merits, as it brings together unique frameworks, research approaches and analytical techniques. It encourages innovative methodologies such as mixed-methods and participatory research, which significantly enhance the validity and applicability of findings. Research involving multiple professions and disciplines tends to produce findings that are more directly translatable into practice, ensuring interventions are feasible, culturally appropriate and aligned with clinical workflows,[1,17] which helps bridge the research-to-practice gap.[18,19] This is even more so the case when not only different academic and professional disciplines are involved, but also community members, policymakers, etc participate as equal partners in research—see Chapter 21 on community engagement and co-design. Collaborative efforts help identify pressing issues and develop community-relevant interventions, promoting more effective policy and system changes, supporting the development of integrated, patient-centred healthcare systems that are more effective, equitable and resilient.[9,19–21]

However, these collaborations need to be learned and acquired; they do not arise out of thin air. Interdisciplinarity requires high competence in one's own discipline. It does not mean that one should become a bit of a specialist in another area; rather, it means that one is open-minded and poses new questions to another field of study.[18]

In this chapter, we describe facilitators and barriers to perform interprofessional, interdisciplinary and transdisciplinary primary care research and provide some practical guidance on how to build a collaborative research team.

13.2 Barriers and Facilitators in Primary Care Research Collaborations

Research on interprofessional collaboration in primary care more often describes the implementation and evaluation of integrated healthcare services than the actual collaboration dynamics and skills. However, various barriers and facilitators to implementation of interprofessional collaboration in practice and research have been identified, and teaching programmes have been described, as well as systemic policies that can support interprofessional collaboration.[22–29]

13.2.1 Barriers to Collaborative Primary Care Research

The main barriers relate to differences in culture and language, and lack of acknowledgement of one another's roles and competencies.[30,31] There can be a lack of understanding and respect. Each discipline and profession has its own values, beliefs, norms, activities and practices. Differences in ways of describing a research problem, in research methods, or in vocabulary can act as a barrier for collaboration when not recognised, acknowledged and discussed.[34] This is especially challenging when some team members deem their own profession or discipline superior to others, without being aware of this view. Medical doctors often see their view on medical issues as the only one, and they think quantitative research is what is usually done in medicine, with the double-blind randomised controlled trial as the gold standard, is the best scientific approach. When professionals see each other as rivals or want to keep their own ideas to themselves, this can block teamwork.

Trust is another issue. If there is rivalry or bad past experiences, people may not want to work closely together.[13,14,36,37] In these circumstances, misunderstandings or confusion about exactly who will do what can easily arise. Frequent and extensive communication is therefore necessary to become aware of and bridge differences in views, in scientific approaches, and in vocabulary.

Good collaboration often takes a long time; hence, collaborative research may be considered less productive. Journals accepting interdisciplinary papers may also be lower impact, a further barrier. Organisations and departments may not be able to or do not want to make time, provide support or be flexible in their structures to enable this time-consuming, boundary-crossing teamwork. When professionals are not recognised or rewarded for teamwork, they might not want to do it.

13.2.2 Facilitators to Collaborative Primary Care Research

There are, however, a number of ways by which collaborative research can be facilitated. One principle of this is common interest: the different actors' common interest in collaboration, perceiving opportunities to improve quality of care.[30] People often do not know the skills and competencies of other professionals and disciplines. Only when they trust each other are they able to hand over responsibility.[31,32] Roles and responsibilities need to be discussed and explicitly articulated and written down to avoid confusion, differences in understanding, or thinking that others will do the job.[30–32]

Excellent and frequent communication is required, to establish trust, define common goals, roles and responsibilities.[31,32] Frequent formal as well as informal communications, in person and written down, are a prerequisite.[18] Informal rules should be developed and conditions set in place to engage researchers across disciplines, which may be challenging due to vast differences between disciplinary and professional jargon. In this area, special care has to be taken to develop a common/shared understanding of terms. A joint glossary can be helpful. Core to a constructive dialogue is also fostering shared empathy and respect. Sharing the different professional perspectives and being explicit about the assumptions helps overcome misunderstandings due to different jargon or paradigms.[34] In addition to these general facilitators of interprofessional collaboration, Brown's principles for interdisciplinary research[21,33] have proven to be helpful.

A shared mission needs to be forged, developing a collective, compelling overall goal for the project, including impact as a necessary outcome, with meaningful roles across the different disciplines. Reaching a shared understanding of the purpose and goals of the research amongst the team is a first priority.[18] This makes it easier for different professionals to work together. Participatory processes are important to co-design goals, mission, aims and approach, and to develop a shared understanding.

'T-shaped' researchers need to be developed, who can possess strong disciplinary expertise while fostering the ability to look beyond their own discipline and appreciate the norms, theories, approaches and breakthroughs of other disciplines.

Collaborative research requires more time and organisational flexibility, which can only be realised with the support of the research leaders and the heads of departments in charge. Collaboration is easier when leaders and organisations support teamwork. There has to be a fair division of labour; not every team member needs to contribute equally, but they must be able to contribute appropriately and accountably.[18]

Creating enduring connections among researchers, policymakers and practitioners is necessary for the adoption of interdisciplinary research outputs in practice, to ensure that there is active work towards real-world impact. Different types of training may help develop the skills and attitude necessary for interdisciplinary research.[19,35]

13.3 Practical Tips for Building a Research Collaboration

We present some recommendations for building research collaborations at each step in a research process, with a focus on international research projects, as they contain an additional layer of complexity due to different mother tongues and differences in national regulations and healthcare organisation—see Box 13.1 and Table 13.1.

BOX 13.1 PRACTICAL TIPS FOR BUILDING AN INTERPROFESSIONAL, INTERDISCIPLINARY RESEARCH TEAM

Research proposal

Involve all from the start
Strong project leader and support organisation
Online meetings
Budget for extra time
Conduct preliminary studies
Have common goals

Start of the project

Get to know each other:

- Define clear roles
- Define outputs
- Define desired outcomes

Joint training
Joint glossary

During the project

Sufficient rewards
Regular meetings
Personal contacts
Check expectations

Dissemination of results

Discuss the number and order of authors at the start
Give back to communities involved
Provide clear recommendations for practice and policies

TABLE 13.1 Examples from International Research Projects

Project name	RESTORE project[38–42] 2010–2015 https://restoreeuproject.eu/	RAPIDE project Started in 2024 https://www.rapideproject.eu/	PRIMORE project Started in 2018 https://euprimarycare.org/portfolio-items/primore/
Professionals involved	General practices, social workers, psychologists, professional interpreters, migrant service users, anthropologists	Community nurses, social workers, general practitioners, public health doctors, medical specialists, mathematicians, engineers	Family doctors, community nurses, occupational therapists, physiotherapists, social workers, psychologists, public health professionals
Scientific disciplines involved	Medicine, social sciences (anthropology, sociology, psychology)	Medicine, social sciences, linguistics, mathematics, information specialists	Medicine, social sciences
Aim	To improve cross-cultural communication in primary care	To develop, validate and demonstrate a portfolio of powerful tools that enable healthcare systems to embed robustness of decisions, resilience of the healthcare professionals and patients and flexibility in the modalities of care delivery to maintain access to regular care during cross-border health emergencies	Encourage development and exchange of interprofessional research in primary care in Europe with a focus on young researchers from CEE countries and developing evidence on primary care, resulting in EFPC position papers
Countries involved	Ireland, UK, Austria, Greece, The Netherlands	Ireland, Malta, Italy, Slovenia, Norway, Lithuania, The Netherlands	Norway, Turkey, Greece, Germany, Slovenia, The Netherlands, Ukraine, Belgium, UK, Spain, Portugal, Italy, Austria
Facilitators	Using networks (WONCA and NAPCRG) Extensive joint training on normalisation process theory and participatory learning and action research methods	Good existing contacts from previous research collaborations Joint modelling and scenario enacting Joint glossary after professional differences were revealed in thinking about patient care pathways and patient journeys and on primary care definition	Good personal and professional contacts between European Forum for Primary Care member organisations Regular online and personal meetings Involvement in professional masterclasses in interprofessional collaboration for young researchers

13.3.1 Building Trust, Mutual Understanding and Respect

This is something to work on from the start of the writing of your research proposal. Involve different professions and disciplines from different countries from the start, and preferably also patient representatives. It helps when you can draw from existing networks. Organise online meetings to get to know each other, explore common goals, discuss research methods, and determine division of roles and tasks.

This process can be facilitated with a strong project leader, who has the ability to listen well, to recognise and acknowledge the different strengths of participating researchers, and is familiar with a broad range of research methods. She or he should be able to establish trust and confidence also from participants with different professional or scientific backgrounds. Also very important is the involvement from the start of a strong project support organisation, which is familiar with these processes as well as with all procedures in grant-making. The budget should provide for sufficient time and financial rewards for all participants, including time for joint training and meetings. Planning should consider that procedures such as ethical permission can take a considerably longer time in some disciplines and countries than in others. During the project, frequent contact is necessary to ensure mutual understanding of goals, tasks, roles and research methods. Besides sufficient financial rewards, it is important to acknowledge openly each one's contribution.

13.3.2 Communication

Start with extensive getting-acquainted sessions and training, taking time to learn about each profession and discipline, teaching interprofessional collaboration, understanding that these research methods might be new to some. Setting ground rules and using participatory methods can help ensure equal participation of all professionals and disciplines. Defining clear roles and discussing expectations will be one of the topics to discuss at the start. Research rules may vary across disciplines. For instance, social sciences often have fewer authors per article compared to clinical fields. Clearly defining roles and setting expectations early can help manage these differences and facilitate smoother collaboration.

Developing a joint glossary of terms is important to reach terminological consistency and to ensure that all participants understand and use the same language. Definitions can differ considerably among professions and disciplines. During the project, frequent meetings (online, webinars, but also in-person meetings) and open channels for feedback can help identify misunderstandings early and keep all team members aligned throughout the research process. Time and space for personal contact about non-research-related topics can add to building trust and mutual understanding. An attitude of flexibility and adaptability is required; being open to adjusting plans or methods as the project develops is important, especially when working with diverse disciplines that may have different approaches or expectations.

13.3.3 Embracing New Research Methods

One of the strengths of interprofessional and interdisciplinary research is the wealth of different research approaches. However, these have to be appreciated and understood by all participants. Conducting preliminary research can be beneficial due to varying opinions on clinical outcomes and research priorities, particularly in qualitative studies, where analytical approaches may vary. Training can be necessary when all participants have to apply the same techniques. Software compatibility is important. Computer programs or platforms have to be carefully chosen, taking into account differences in commonly used software.

13.4 Conclusion and Future Perspectives

In 2024–25, the PRImary care Multi-prOfessional REsearcher network PRIMORE—a multidisciplinary group of young researchers within the European Forum for Primary Care—performed a systematic review of the existing research on interprofessional collaboration in primary care (will be published). This revealed the growing interest in this topic, with 125 papers on the subject since 2020 compared to 30 between 2004–09. It also showed that most studies were carried out in the US, Canada and the Netherlands, mainly by academic researchers in collaboration with primary care practitioners. Although many different primary care professionals were involved in the projects described, the vast majority included general practitioners and nurses (see Figure 13.1).

This review showed a gap in mixed-methods and process evaluations, which are crucial for understanding implementation in complex, real-world primary care. Research on collaborative primary care research primarily appears to focus on treatment and system/organisational aspects, while prevention and rehabilitation remain relatively underrepresented. System-level results, such as improved

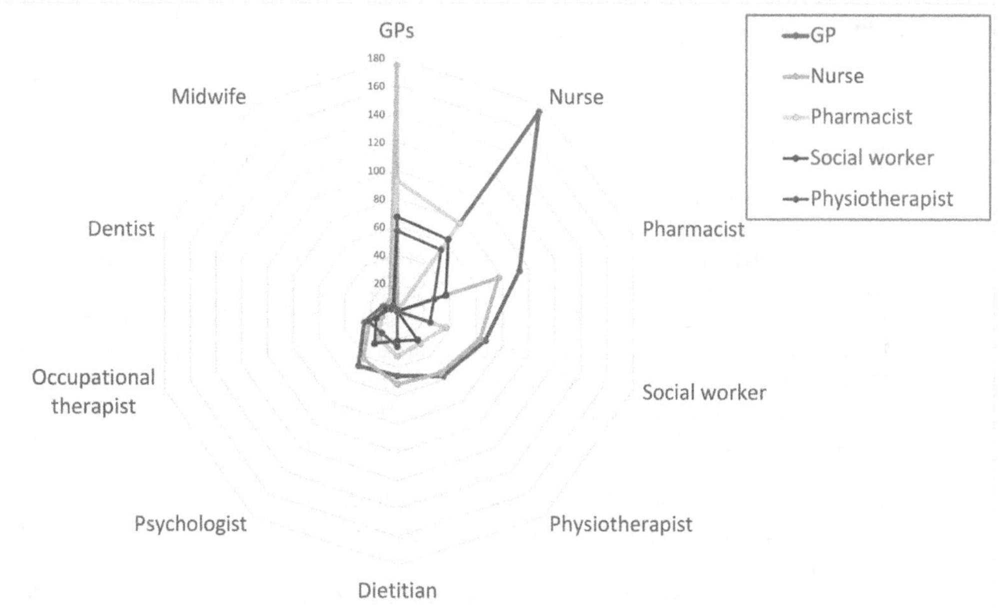

FIGURE 13.1 Professionals involved in the PRIMORE project collaboration

coordination of care, service redesign and cost efficiency, dominated the field. In contrast, fewer studies explicitly focussed on patient-reported outcomes or provider well-being.

The importance and relevance of interprofessional collaboration in primary care research and practice is increasingly acknowledged as essential for robust primary care that can address the future challenges of growing healthcare needs, due to ageing and global crises, despite a decrease in available labour and financial funds. To implement this, more interdisciplinary mixed-methods research is warranted on interprofessional collaboration in primary care in different countries, with an increased range of healthcare professionals and a focus on patient-reported outcomes and provider well-being.

This can be extended to create interdisciplinary research networks that include different professionals and different disciplines, such as medicine, healthcare, social sciences and economics, of which the PRIMORE network is an example. Forging strong relations from the start of a research proposal, setting common goals and a clear task division, and maintaining frequent communication are the essential elements for successful interdisciplinary and interprofessional collaboration in research. Interprofessional education could enhance later interprofessional collaboration. Transdisciplinary research that includes end-users means that solutions will be acceptable and implementable.

As the future of primary care depends heavily on continued interprofessional collaboration, it will be important to focus on integrating the expertise of all primary care professionals. Ultimately, interprofessional collaboration is more than a tool of clinical practice: it is the foundation of resilient, patient-centred and sustainable primary care systems.

References

1. Zwarenstein M, Goldman J, Reeves S. Interprofessional collaboration: Effects of practice-based interventions on professional practice and healthcare outcomes. *Cochrane Database Syst Rev.* 2009;(3).
2. Reeves S, Xyrichis A, Zwarenstein M. Teamwork, collaboration, coordination, and networking: Why we need to distinguish between different types of interprofessional practice. *J Interprof Care.* 2018 Jan 2;32(1):1–3.
3. Gilbert JHYJHS. A WHO report: Framework for action on interprofessional education and collaborative practice. *J Allied Health.* 2010;39(Suppl 1):196–7.
4. Kälble K. Berufsgruppen- und fachübergreifende Zusammenarbeit—Terminologische Klärung. In: Kaba-Schönstein L, Kälble K, eds. Interdisziplinäre Kooperation im Gesundheitswesen: Eine Herausforderung für die Ausbildung in der Medizin, der Sozialen Arbeit und der Pflege; Ergebnisse des Forschungsprojektes MESOP. Frankfurt am Main: Mabuse-Verl; 2004. p. 29–41.
5. Mahler C, Gutmann T, Karstens S, Joos S. Terminology for interprofessional collaboration: Definition and current practice. *GMS Z Med Ausbild.* 2014;31(4):1–10.
6. Thomas P, Burch T, Ferlie E, Jenkins R, Wright F, Sachar A, et al. Community-oriented integrated care and health promotion—views from the street. *London J Prim Care.* 2015 Nov 1;7(5):83–8.
7. Jacobsen FF, Akman M, Aarendonk D. The establishment and functioning of the PRIMORE (European Primary care Multiprofessional Researcher network) project. *Prim Health Care Res Dev.* 2019;20:e114.

8. Rawlinson C, Carron T, Cohidon C, Arditi C, Hong QN, Pluye P, et al. An overview of reviews on interprofessional collaboration in primary care: Barriers and facilitators. *Int J Integr Care*. 2021;21(2).
9. Reeves S, Pelone F, Harrison R, Goldman J, Zwarenstein M. Interprofessional collaboration to improve professional practice and healthcare outcomes. *Cochrane Database Syst Rev*. 2017 Jun 22;2017(6).
10. Reeves S, Perrier L, Goldman J, Freeth D, Zwarenstein M. Interprofessional education: Effects on professional practice and healthcare outcomes (update). *Cochrane Database Syst Rev*. 2013 Mar 28;2013(3).
11. Bouton C, Journeaux M, Jourdain M, Angibaud M, Huon JF, Rat C. Interprofessional collaboration in primary care: What effect on patient health? A systematic literature review. *BMC Prim Care*. 2023 Dec 1;24(1).
12. Weinstein AR, Dolce MC, Koster M, Parikh R, Hamlyn E, McNamara EA, et al. Integration of systematic clinical interprofessional training in a student-faculty collaborative primary care practice. *J Interprof Care*. 2018 Jan 2;32(1):104–7.
13. Thistlethwaite J. Interprofessional education: A review of context, learning and the research agenda. *Med Educ*. 2012 Jan 1;46(1):58–70.
14. D'Amour D, Ferrada-Videla M, San Martin Rodriguez L, Beaulieu MD. The conceptual basis for interprofessional collaboration: Core concepts and theoretical frameworks. *J Interprof Care*. 2005 May;19(Suppl. 1):116–31.
15. Kivits J, Ricci L, Minary L. Interdisciplinary research in public health: The 'why' and the 'how'. *J Epidemiol Community Health*. 2019 Dec 1;73(12):1061.
16. Windak A, Rochfort A, Jacquet J. The revised European definition of general practice/family medicine. A pivotal role of One Health, planetary health and Sustainable Development Goals. *Eur J Gen Pract*. 2024 Dec 31;30(1):2306936.
17. Green BN, Johnson CD. Interprofessional collaboration in research, education, and clinical practice: Working together for a better future. *J Chiropr Educ*. 2015 Mar 1;29(1):1–10.
18. Barkovic D. Challenges of interdisciplinary research. *Interdiscip Manag Res*. 2010;6:951–60.
19. Terry AL, Stewart M, Ashcroft R, Brown JB, Burge F, Haggerty J, et al. Complex skills are required for new primary health care researchers: A training program responds. *BMC Med Educ*. 2022 Dec 1;22(1):1–8.
20. Apramian T, Karim A, Parker K, Sinclair L, Ladak Z, Ku C, et al. How national healthcare change initiatives balance emergent and deliberate change: A principles-focused evaluation. *Healthc Manag Forum*. 2025;38(1):52–7.
21. Brown R, Werbeloff L, Raven R. Interdisciplinary research and impact (Global challenges 4/2019). *Glob Challenges*. 2019 Apr;3(4).
22. Ndibu Muntu Keba Kebe N, Chiocchio F, Bamvita JM, Fleury MJ. Variables associated with interprofessional collaboration: A comparison between primary healthcare and specialized mental health teams. *BMC Fam Pract*. 2020 Jan 8;21(1):1–11.
23. Angeles RN, Cuenter D, McCarthy L, Bauer M, Wolfson M, Chacon M, et al. Group interprofessional chronic pain management in the primary care setting: A pilot study of feasibility and effectiveness in a family health team in Ontario. *Pain Res Manag*. 2013 Jan 1;18(5):237–42.
24. Markle-Reid MF, McAiney C, Forbes D, Thabane L, Gibson M, Hoch JS, et al. Reducing depression in older home care clients: Design of a prospective study of a nurse-led interprofessional mental health promotion intervention. *BMC Geriatr*. 2011 Aug 25;11(1):1–21.
25. Janson SL, Cooke M, McGrath KW, Kroon LA, Robinson S, Baron RB. Improving chronic care of type 2 diabetes using teams of interprofessional learners. *Acad Med*. 2009;84(11):1540–8.
26. Müller CA, Fleischmann N, Cavazzini C, Heim S, Seide S, Geister C, et al. Interprofessional collaboration in nursing homes (interprof): Development and piloting of measures to improve interprofessional collaboration and communication: A qualitative multicentre study. *BMC Fam Pract*. 2018 Jan 11;19(1):1–11.

27. Ashcroft R, Feryn N, Lam S, Hussain A, Donnelly C, Mehta K, et al. Social workers' formal and informal leadership in interprofessional primary care teams in Ontario, Canada. *Healthc Manag Forum*. 2023 Sep 1;36(5):304–10.
28. Khan AI, Barnsley J, Harris JK, Wodchis WP. Examining the extent and factors associated with interprofessional teamwork in primary care settings. *J Interprof Care*. 2022 Jan 2; 36(1):52–63.
29. Laatikainen T, Dumcheva A, Kiriazova T, Zeziulin O, Inglin L, Collins D, et al. Capacity building of health care professionals to perform interprofessional management of non-communicable diseases in primary care—experiences from Ukraine. *BMC Health Serv Res*. 2021 Dec 1;21(1):1–15.
30. Supper I, Catala O, Lustman M, Chemla C, Bourgueil Y, Letrilliart L. Interprofessional collaboration in primary health care: A review of facilitators and barriers perceived by involved actors. *J Public Health*. 2015;37(4):716–27.
31. Schot E, Tummers L, Noordegraaf M. Working on working together: A systematic review on how healthcare professionals contribute to interprofessional collaboration. *J Interprof Care*. 2020 May 3;34(3):332–42.
32. Morgan S, Pullon S, McKinlay E. Observation of interprofessional collaborative practice in primary care teams: An integrative literature review. *Int J Nurs Stud*. 2015 Jul 1;52(7):1217–30.
33. Brown RR, Deletic A, Wong THF. Interdisciplinarity: How to catalyse collaboration. *Nature*. 2015 Sep 16;525(7569):315–7.
34. Daniel KL, McConnell M, Schuchardt A, Peffer ME. Challenges facing interdisciplinary researchers: Findings from a professional development workshop. *PLoS One*. 2022 Apr 1;17(4).
35. Stewart M, Wuite S, Ramsden V, Burge F, Beaulieu MD, Fortin M, Godwin M, Harris S, Reid G, Haggerty J, Brown JB, Thomas R, Wong S. Transdisciplinary understandings and training on research: Successfully building research capacity in primary health care. *Can Fam Physician*. 2014 Jun;60(6):581–2.
36. El-Awaisi A, Yakti OH, Elboshra AM, Jasim KH, AboAlward AF, Shalfawi RW, et al. Facilitators and barriers to interprofessional collaboration among health professionals in primary healthcare centers in Qatar: A qualitative exploration using the "Gears" model. *BMC Prim Care*. 2024 Dec 1;25(1):1–14.
37. Lee CS, Poon Z, He JCE, Goh BQ, Poh CXY, Paulpandi M, et al. Qualitative study on the perceived enablers and barriers to interprofessional education in primary care in Singapore. *BMC Prim Care*. 2025 Dec 1;26(1):1–12.
38. MacFarlane A, O'Donnell C, Mair F, O'Reilly-de Brún M, de Brún T, Spiegel W, et al. REsearch into implementation STrategies to support patients of different origins and language background in a variety of European primary care settings (RESTORE): Study protocol. *Implement Sci*. 2012 Nov 20;7(1).
39. O'Donnell CA, Mair FS, Dowrick C, O'Reilly-De Brún M, De Brún T, Burns N, et al. Supporting the use of theory in cross-country health services research: A participatory qualitative approach using normalisation process theory as an example. *BMJ Open*. 2017 Aug 1;7(8):e014289.
40. O'Reilly-de Brún M, de Brún T, O'Donnell CA, Papadakaki M, Saridaki A, Lionis C, et al. Material practices for meaningful engagement: An analysis of participatory learning and action research techniques for data generation and analysis in a health research partnership. *Health Expect*. 2018 Feb 1;21(1):159–70.
41. de Brún T, O'Reilly-De Brún M, Van Weel-Baumgarten E, Burns N, Dowrick C, Lionis C, et al. Using participatory learning & action (PLA) research techniques for inter-stakeholder dialogue in primary healthcare: An analysis of stakeholders' experiences. *Res Involv Engagem*. 2017 Dec 6;3(1):1–25.
42. van den Muijsenbergh METC, LeMaster JW, Shahiri P, Brouwer M, Hussain M, Dowrick C, et al. Participatory implementation research in the field of migrant health: Sustainable changes and ripple effects over time. *Health Expect*. 2020 Apr 1;23(2):306–17.

CHAPTER

14

Primary Care Performance Measurement and Management for Improvement

Óscar Brito Fernandes, Erica Barbazza and Dionne Kringos

14.1 Introduction

Healthcare performance measurement is a helpful tool for evaluating the work of healthcare professionals, organisations and systems. It provides performance information (intelligence) for governance, management and clinical decision-making.[1] Over time, the focus of performance measurement has shifted from volume-based to outcome-based and then, more recently, to value-based measurement.[2–4] Implementing learning health systems is now seen as a key pathway towards value-based healthcare.[5] This approach requires a fundamental change in how we measure, report and use performance data as intelligence for decision-making.

In primary care, the adoption of routine performance measurement for continuous learning and improvement has followed a unique path. Although it has been slower and more fragmented compared to specialised hospital settings, performance measurement in primary care is becoming increasingly common. In general, the difference in its trajectory can be said to stem largely from primary care's distinctive structure—characterised by small, independent, and often private practices—which creates challenges for standardised measurement.[6–8] Primary care also faces unique obstacles, including ambiguous data ownership, hybrid data structures (combining structured, semi-structured and unstructured elements), quality concerns and resource limitations.[9,10]

Primary care information systems have also in large part been developed incrementally, through piecemeal policies and innovations,[7,11] with generally slow adoption of digital solutions.[8,10] Without robust data infrastructure, many countries have relied on periodic assessments rather than integrated health information systems for performance measurement. The complexity of measuring the primary healthcare approach and the heterogeneity in how primary care is organised across contexts has typically led to a focus on "what" to measure rather than "how" to use measurement effectively. Consequently, primary care–focused measurement initiatives often remain disconnected from governance and management cycles.[12]

DOI: 10.1201/9781003652106-17

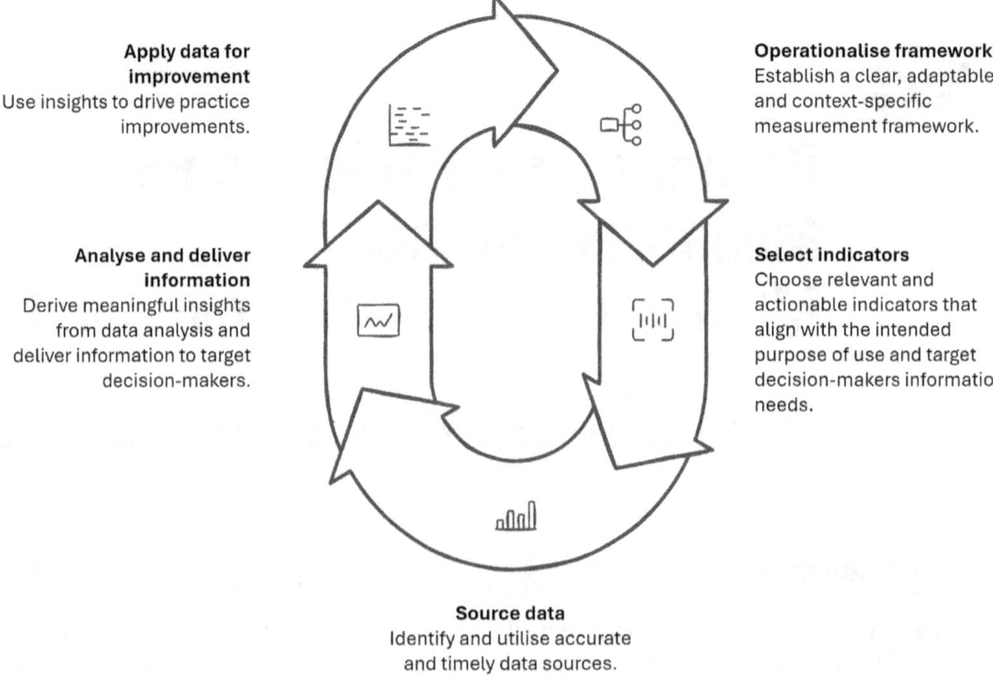

FIGURE 14.1 Iterative cycle of primary care performance measurement and management for improvement

This chapter aims to support primary care practitioners and researchers in developing a systematic approach to primary care performance measurement that leverages continuous data collection, analysis, and iterative feedback loops to support data-driven decision-making that contributes to a learning healthcare system. We guide readers through five inter-related considerations for performance measurement in primary care (Figure 14.1):

1. Operationalising a framework for performance measurement
2. Selecting indicators that are fit for purpose
3. Sourcing appropriate data
4. Analysing and delivering information that is fit for use
5. Applying data for performance management

By addressing these key areas, we can create a more effective and actionable approach to primary care performance measurement and management, ultimately leading to better health outcomes and more efficient use of resources. To conclude, we adopt a future-oriented perspective and consider areas for further development and exploration to advance primary care performance measurement.

14.2 Operationalising a Framework for Performance Measurement

Integrating performance data into decision-making requires a structured approach, beginning with defining improvement objectives and ensuring that performance indicators align with a stated goal. The success of measurement efforts depends on the clarity of this direction of change.[13] This means that performance indicators should not only track past achievements but also guide future actions, helping decision-makers at any level in focus—from policymakers to frontline providers—to steer healthcare systems toward better outcomes.

With a clear strategic direction set, operationalising primary care performance measurement involves defining which components should be measured, including both traditional (eg quality, accessibility) and emerging dimensions (eg resilience, environmental sustainability, digital integration) of care. To effectively assess these areas, selecting an appropriate measurement framework and the measures therein is essential for guiding the interpretation of data and informing action for improvement.

This task can present several challenges. Primary care is inherently context-specific, and consequently no one framework will be a fit for all. Additionally, variations in how primary care is defined and scoped across different countries and even sub-nationally make knowledge transfer and learning between and within countries more difficult. The complexity of primary care services, such as task-sharing and shifting of roles, coupled with the coexistence of multiple, often overlapping definitions, adds to the theoretical ambiguity surrounding primary care and hinders consistent measurement and improvement efforts.

Selecting a robust framework to support primary care performance measurement and management is therefore crucial. Box 14.1 outlines guiding principles to inform framework selection. Established frameworks, such as the WHO Primary Health Care Operational Framework,[14,15] offer structured methodologies that systematically capture policy levers, key performance dimensions and metrics. Their strength lies in their alignment with existing national and subnational plans and priorities, as well as with performance tools such as Health System Performance Assessment (HSPA) frameworks. This alignment ensures consistency, comparability and relevance in policymaking and service delivery. When an HSPA framework is already in place, integrating these tools can reinforce continuous improvement and evidence-based decision-making across, and beyond, primary care. This approach not only fosters accountability and transparency but also enhances learning and adaptation across various contexts[16], ultimately contributing to improved primary care outcomes.

This is not a comprehensive list, but by adhering to these guiding principles, the selection of a primary care performance measurement framework can be a more robust and effective process, leading to more meaningful and actionable insights for improving primary care.

BOX 14.1 GUIDING PRINCIPLES TO INFORM FRAMEWORK SELECTION

- **Alignment with purpose and context:** The framework should align with its intended purpose (eg quality improvement, accountability) and the core goals and functions of primary care.
- **Stakeholder relevance and engagement:** The framework should be meaningful and understandable to all relevant stakeholders (patients, providers, policymakers) and, ideally, engage them in its design to enhance its relevance and acceptance.

- **Prioritise outcomes and care experiences**: The framework should consider the impact of primary care on intended health outcomes and care experiences, fostering accountability and monitoring responsiveness of primary care to individuals' and communities' needs, preferences and expectations.
- **Emphasise actionability and improvement**: The framework should provide actionable insights across essential domains of primary care that can inform decision-making and support quality improvement at practice, organisational and policy levels.
- **Consider context and promote adaptability**: The framework should be flexible and adaptable to various contexts, recognising diverse populations, settings and health needs while remaining sensitive to local and regional variations. It should also account for the broader social, economic, cultural and political factors that influence primary care performance.
- **Consider feasibility and burden**: The framework should be practical and feasible to implement, minimising administrative burdens while ensuring effective data collection and reporting, underpinned by robust methodological considerations.
- **Continuous review and updating**: The framework, including its domains and measures, should be considered a living document, subject to ongoing review and revision to ensure adaptability. It should balance core domains of primary care performance with emerging evidence, such as policy priorities, new data sources (eg people-reported metrics) and evolving information needs (eg environmental sustainability).

14.3 Selecting Indicators That Are Fit for Purpose

The past two decades have seen substantial improvements in the scientific rigour of healthcare performance indicators, particularly related to their validity and reliability criteria.[17] Guidelines have emerged for developing streamlined indicator sets,[18,19] along with methodologies such as the Delphi technique and RAND appropriateness index to support processes for their selection.[20–23] Despite this progress, an indicator's 'usefulness' ultimately goes beyond its statistical quality. Even the most robust, statistically sound indicator that meets established criteria may still fall short in supporting decision-making. Primary care physicians and researchers now face a different challenge: not "is there an indicator?" for their area of interest but rather "which one should I choose?"

To address this selection challenge, focus has shifted toward an indicator's *actionability*, beginning with its fitness for purpose.[13] An indicator's fitness for purpose depends largely on its alignment with strategic priorities. For true utility, an indicator must deliver information relevant to its intended user—the decision-maker. This relevance varies based on several factors, including whether decisions are intended to occur at the micro (clinical), meso (organisational) or macro (policy) level of healthcare systems. The specific decision-maker's role and how they will apply the information further influences this relevance.

Consider the example of improving antibiotic prescribing: at the micro-level, a primary care clinician might track new and repeat antibiotic prescriptions quarterly within their practice; at the meso-level, an insurer might annually review practices' adherence to prescribing guidelines for payment incentive decisions; and at the macro-level, a policymaker might analyse antibiotic volumes per 100,000 population regionally, nationally and internationally to inform policy cycles.[24]

As Table 14.1 demonstrates, different intended uses and users create cascading effects on what constitutes a 'good' indicator. It will also influence what are the ideal data sources, precision requirements, timeliness needs and relevant comparisons. The varied uses of indicators across micro-meso-macro contexts highlight the importance of clearly defining an indicator's intended purpose. When selecting indicators for measurement frameworks and creating indicator sets that span multiple health system levels, primary care physicians and researchers must consider these diverse uses, as different decision-making functions often need to work in concert.

Box 14.2 outlines key considerations to help readers systematically evaluate and balance various actionability factors when selecting fit-for-purpose indicators.

TABLE 14.1 Illustrative Example of Different Uses, Users and Information Needs Related to Antibiotic Prescribing in Primary Care

Context	Purpose of Use	User	Information Need	Possible Data Source
Macro (policy)	System performance monitoring	Ministry of Health	Total volume of antibiotics prescribed, per 100,000 population per region, nationally	Administrative/claims data
Meso (organisational)	Quality-based financing	Insurer	Adherence of practices to prescribing guidelines for benchmarking performance across practices annually	Electronic medical records; administrative/claims data
Micro (clinical)	Individual performance improvement	Primary care physician	New and re-prescribing of antibiotics in practice annually	Electronic medical record

Source: Adapted from[13,24]

BOX 14.2 KEY CONSIDERATIONS FOR AN INDICATOR'S FITNESS FOR PURPOSE

Purpose of Use Considerations

- What is the intended use of the indicator?
- Which context of decision-making will it inform? (micro/clinical-level; meso/organisational-level; macro/policy-level)
- Who are the intended users (decision-makers) of the analysed data?

Other Methodological Considerations

- Is the indicator sufficiently sensitive to change?
- Are the entry points for acting feasible?
- Does the indicator signal a clear direction?
- Is the indicator a reflection of the system?

Source: Adapted from[13,25]

14.4 Sourcing Appropriate Data

The landscape of data sourcing for primary care performance measurement has undergone a major change over the past decades, rendering concerns over data scarcity increasingly obsolete. Previously constrained by limited availability, researchers and practitioners now navigate an unprecedented volume of data from different sources. Electronic Health Records (EHRs) remain a cornerstone of clinical data collection, capturing comprehensive information on medical history, diagnoses, medications and treatment plans. These records support the tracking of patient outcomes, care processes and guideline adherence while enhancing care coordination through seamless information sharing. However, challenges persist, including the burden of data entry and the difficulty of automated aggregation and analysis. Similarly, administrative data offers insights into staffing levels, patient flow and healthcare expenditures. When integrated with other datasets, these records enable in-depth assessments of primary care performance and resource allocation. Beyond clinical and administrative data, disease-specific registers, such as cancer registries, also play a crucial role in quality measurement.

Surveys targeting both patients and healthcare providers provide additional insights, particularly in measuring patient-reported outcomes (PROMs) and experiences (PREMs). These measures offer a nuanced understanding of primary care responsiveness to individual and community needs. The OECD's PaRIS (Patient-Reported Indicators Survey) initiative exemplifies ongoing efforts to standardise these measures internationally, facilitating cross-country comparability.[26]

Geospatial and social media data have also emerged as valuable sources. A geographic information system (GIS) is a technology that is used to create, manage, analyse and map all types of data, connecting data to a map, integrating location data. GIS enables sophisticated spatial analyses of healthcare access and utilisation patterns, which proved critical during the COVID-19 pandemic for tracking service disruptions and vaccination efforts.[27,28] Social media platforms, meanwhile, provide real-time surveillance of patient sentiment and emerging health trends, allowing for early detection of public health concerns.[29] The proliferation of innovative data sources further expands the scope of performance measurement. Mobile health applications and wearable devices generate continuous health-related data, including physical activity and cardiovascular metrics.[30] Additionally, the Internet of Things (IoT) facilitates real-time patient monitoring through interconnected devices and smart sensors, supporting proactive and responsive healthcare interventions.[31]

Despite the vast array of available data, significant challenges remain in sourcing and utilising these data effectively. Issues such as data fragmentation, gaps in service delivery data and difficulties in evaluating both patient and provider experiences pose barriers to comprehensive performance assessment. Moreover, privacy concerns, security risks and ethical considerations must be addressed, particularly when incorporating novel data sources. Ensuring robust data governance, standardisation and interoperability is essential to optimising the use of both traditional and innovative datasets. Furthermore, investment in workforce training and the development of secure data environments can enhance data accessibility while safeguarding patient privacy.

With the appropriate integration of diverse data sources and advanced analytical methodologies, primary care leaders and researchers can refine data-driven decision-making, fostering continuous improvement in primary care delivery. The shift from overcoming data scarcity to strategically curating and applying high-quality data underscores the evolving nature of primary care performance measurement. By translating these rich data into actionable intelligence, health systems can drive meaningful, evidence-based improvements that enhance patient outcomes and optimise primary care service delivery.

14.5 Analysing and Delivering Information That Is Fit for Use

Beyond selecting purpose-driven indicators and sourcing relevant data, two additional critical steps in an indicator's use cycle determine its fitness for use: applying appropriate analysis techniques to produce values that are meaningful and delivering the information in an effective modality that clearly communicates the findings to the target decision-makers.[13] Both processes require careful consideration across multiple dimensions.

First, when selecting the appropriate analysis for indicators, several key decisions must be made. The most suitable analytical approach—whether benchmarking, time trend analysis, case mix correction or other methods—should align with the intended purpose. Reference groups and data breakdowns should also be tailored accordingly. For instance, a physician analysing their practice might examine data by postal code, while a regional health authority might utilise broader geographic boundaries such as districts or provinces. The time intervals selected for analysis should also directly serve the intended user's needs and decision-making timeline.

Second, how data are returned to decision-makers also impacts their ability to act.[13] Key considerations include determining the appropriate degree of 'storytelling' to accompany the results and support their interpretation of the findings.[32,33] Equally important are decisions about dissemination frequency, the medium of reporting (eg reports, newsletters, dashboards) and channels for delivering information.[34]

The medium for reporting performance information has evolved dramatically over the past decade, accelerated in large part by the COVID-19 pandemic. Dashboards emerged as the standard for both public and internal reporting. Early examples, such as the Johns Hopkins Coronavirus Resource Center dashboard,[35] established a global standard for pandemic information delivery. The widespread adoption of dashboards that followed can be attributed to varied factors, including the availability of software solutions, accessible data sources and increasing digital literacy among users. Their permanence reflects the effectiveness of dashboards to meet decision-makers' information needs during crises by providing interactive, geographically oriented information in a concise, visual format.[36] Their dynamic displays adapt to changing information priorities and deliver near real-time data updates.

Prior to the pandemic, public-facing uses of dashboards were relatively limited, mainly appearing in hospital management,[37,38] clinical decision support,[39] and international benchmarking.[40,41] Although dashboards were occasionally used during previous disease outbreaks,[42,43] the scale and speed of their development during COVID-19 was unprecedented.

Dashboard-style displays for primary care data are already operational in several regions in Canada, including initiatives in British Columbia[44] and Ontario.[45] The expansion of dashboards for delivering primary care information merits further prioritisation, guided by a strong audience segmentation based on clearly defined purposes and user needs.[46] Importantly, dashboards should be complemented by other communication and engagement strategies, like those used in pandemic reporting.[47]

Key considerations outlined in Box 14.3 can inform decisions related to determining the appropriate analytical approaches and delivery formats to ensure that healthcare performance information effectively supports the intended users and aligns with decision-making objectives.

BOX 14.3 KEY CONSIDERATIONS FOR REFLECTING ON ANALYSIS AND DELIVERY OF DATA

- How will the data be analysed? (eg benchmarking, time trend, case mix correction)
- How can composites/indices be used to simplify data?
- Who is the reference group?
- How will the data be disaggregated? (eg age, sex, ethnicity, geographically)
- How will values be calculated? (eg means, median, SD, top 10% mean)
- Should a time trend be reported and at what interval?
- How will risk adjustments be applied? (eg variable specification, source, weighting scheme)
- How will missing data points be handled?
- What other data are needed to give the indicator meaning?
- How will the data be visualised? (eg chart, map, table)
- What techniques to simplify the meaning can be applied? (eg colour, size variation, icons)
- How can users customise the data? (eg change of display, change of information)
- How can the quality and the meaning of data be narrated?
- How will it be reported? (eg print, mobile, web-based)
- What is the relevant reporting cycle? (eg real time, quarterly, annually, biennially)
- How will users be reached? (eg mail, email, champions)
- How can users be supported to make use of findings?

Source: Adapted from[13,25]

14.6 Applying Data for Performance Management

14.6.1 From Measurement to Management

The ultimate goal of performance measurement in primary care is not merely to collect data but to use it effectively to drive meaningful improvements in health outcomes, system efficiency and patient experience. Achieving this goal requires moving beyond measurement towards management, where data informs decision-making, supports continuous learning cycles and fosters a culture of improvement. Despite the increasing availability of data in primary care, many healthcare systems struggle to transition from passive reporting to active use of performance intelligence. The challenge often lies in ensuring that measurement is embedded within governance structures and quality improvement processes, rather than existing as a disconnected reporting exercise.[12]

14.6.2 Strategies for Driving Improvement

Evidence suggests that when primary care measurement is linked to concrete improvement mechanisms, such as quality assurance initiatives or financial incentives, it is more likely to drive meaningful change.[48] Pay-for-performance schemes, for example, have been widely implemented to align financial incentives with quality goals. These schemes can encourage providers to focus on specific health outcomes, but their effectiveness depends on careful design to prevent unintended consequences.[49,50] Similarly, public reporting of performance metrics can promote transparency and accountability, but its impact varies depending on how data are presented and the extent to which it is used to support improvement rather than punitive measures.[51]

14.6.3 Overcoming Behavioural and Systemic Barriers

One of the key challenges in applying data for improvement lies in influencing behaviour at multiple levels—among healthcare providers, managers, policymakers and patients. The Behaviour Change Wheel model[52] offers a useful framework for understanding how different factors interact to drive change. Research has shown that external motivators, such as financial incentives or public recognition, must be balanced with intrinsic motivators, including professional autonomy and a sense of purpose. In primary care, where professional discretion is often a defining characteristic, improvement strategies should foster engagement rather than impose rigid compliance measures.[53]

Measurement has the potential to drive improvement, but it can also produce unintended consequences. Some of the most common pitfalls include the "spotlight effect," where easily measurable indicators receive disproportionate attention, while more complex aspects of care remain unmeasured and undervalued. Another risk is gaming, where providers adjust behaviour to meet performance targets without making meaningful improvements in care quality. These risks highlight the importance of designing measurement strategies with input from stakeholders, ensuring that indicators reflect real-world priorities and do not distort clinical practice.[1]

14.6.4 Evaluating Impact and Scaling Up What Works

A key step in ensuring that performance measurement translates into tangible improvements is the evaluation of impact. This involves moving beyond simple outcome tracking to deeper assessments of what works, for whom, and under what conditions. Realist evaluation approaches, which consider the context in which interventions operate, have been particularly useful in understanding why some performance initiatives succeed where others fail.[54] For instance, a performance dashboard that successfully drives change in one setting may not be as effective in another if local governance structures and data literacy levels differ significantly.

To maximise the potential of performance measurement for driving improvement, health systems need to establish feedback loops that enable real-time learning. This means continuously refining indicators based on emerging evidence, updating targets to reflect shifting priorities and creating spaces for primary care providers to engage with data in meaningful ways. Dashboards, interactive data platforms and AI-driven analytics are increasingly being used to support decision-making at the point of care, but their success depends on how well they integrate with existing clinical workflows.[55]

14.6.5 Embedding Measurement Into Primary Care Governance

Ultimately, applying data for improvement requires an iterative, learning-based approach that transcends simple benchmarking (see Box 14.4). Performance measurement should not be an end in itself, but rather a tool that enables continuous reflection and adaptation. By embedding measurement within governance structures, aligning incentives and fostering a culture of continuous improvement, primary care can ensure that data becomes a catalyst for better patient outcomes and a more efficient healthcare system.

BOX 14.4 KEY CONSIDERATIONS FOR REFLECTING ON STRATEGIES TO TURN PERFORMANCE DATA INTO ACTION

- Is the goal to ensure minimum standards or stimulate excellence?
- At what level will change occur (system, organisation, provider or patient)?
- What structural, regulatory or cultural factors shape feasibility?
- Are governance and leadership structures supportive of change?
- Are you addressing known gaps in care or variation in performance?
- Have you engaged stakeholders to validate these priorities?
- Can combining strategies (e.g., audit and feedback, public reporting and pay-for-performance) reinforce impact?
- What is known about the strategy's effectiveness and cost-effectiveness?
- Are data availability and infrastructure sufficient to support it?
- Does your approach allow feedback loops for adjustment and scaling?
- Is it embedded in a broader quality governance framework?
- How might indicators be gamed or distract from holistic care?
- Is professional engagement strong enough to support intrinsic motivation?

Source: adapted from[56]

14.7 Future Perspectives on Primary Care Performance Measurement

Primary care performance measurement has advanced significantly in the past decade. Many of these developments have been highlighted in this chapter, including globally aligned indicator frameworks, the expansion of digital health data sources and a growing emphasis on people-centred and equity-sensitive indicators. These advances reflect an important shift from narrow technical monitoring to a broader understanding of how primary care contributes to resilient and high-performing health systems.

Nonetheless, significant challenges remain. Many systems continue to suffer from fragmented health information infrastructure, with major data gaps in community-based care, patient experience, care coordination and environmental sustainability. Opportunities offered by electronic health records and real-world data are not yet fully realised, owing to limited interoperability, weak governance and insufficient analytical capacity. Moreover, many indicators still lack actionability, often failing to inform or influence decision-making across micro, meso and macro levels. A myriad of factors contributes to this situation, including limited time and technical capacity to use the available information for improvement, as well as challenges to fully embed measurement within managerial cycles.

Looking ahead, performance measurement should be more explicitly designed for action. This means prioritising indicators that are co-developed with users, adapted to local contexts and embedded in decision-making cycles. Performance intelligence—transforming (health) data into timely, fit-for-purpose and useful insights—is central to this vision. To fully harness this potential, countries must invest in data governance, capacity building and interoperable infrastructure that facilitates appropriate and efficient use of diverse data sources.

Finally, future research should go beyond indicator development to evaluate how performance data is used to influence practice and policy. It should examine the enabling conditions by varied purposes of use under which measurement leads to improvement, and how to embed indicators within learning systems. Ultimately, the goal is not just to produce better indicators but to contribute to better health outcomes, fairer systems and stronger primary care as the foundation for resilient and sustainable health systems.

14.8 Key Takeaways

- Primary care performance measurement has transitioned from volume-based to outcome- and value-based models. This underscores a shift towards measuring what matters, notably system efficiency and patient health outcomes and experiences. Learning health systems have become integral to this transition, serving as catalysts for embedding outcome-based and value-based strategies into everyday clinical and managerial practices, and thus supporting better governance and decision-making.

- Embedding performance data into decision-making requires a clear, structured approach. Defining improvement objectives, aligning performance indicators with strategic priorities, and facilitating timely information-sharing among relevant stakeholders are essential for transforming data into knowledge that supports more effective decision-making processes.

- Managing primary care performance for improvement requires addressing unique challenges such as siloed information systems, ambiguous data ownership and resource constraints. Effective management entails fostering a culture of continuous improvement, linking measurement to tangible incentives, and ensuring that data use drives engagement and informed decision-making at all levels.

Future research should not only continue to refine the technical quality of primary care performance indicators but also explore how measurement contributes to system learning, policy change and improved outcomes. This includes understanding the contextual factors that enable data to be used effectively, ensuring indicators support equity and sustainability, and embedding performance intelligence in everyday decision-making.

References

1. Smith P, Mossialos E, Papanicolas I, et al. Part 1: Principles of performance measurement. In: Smith P, Mossialos E, Papanicolas I, et al., eds. Performance measurement for health system improvement: Experiences, challenges and prospects. Copenhagen: WHO Regional Office for Europe; 2008.
2. Cassel CK, Conway PH, Delbanco SF, et al. Getting more performance from performance measurement. *N Engl J Med.* 2014;371(23):2145–7. https://doi.org/10.1056/NEJMp1408345
3. Berwick DM, Nolan TW, Whittington J. The triple aim: Care, health, and cost. *Health Aff (Millwood).* 2008;27(3):759–69. https://doi.org/10.1377/hlthaff.27.3.759
4. Porter ME. What is value in health care? *N Engl J Med.* 2010;363(26):2477–81. https://doi.org/10.1056/NEJMp1011024
5. Friedman C, Rubin J, Brown J, et al. Toward a science of learning systems: A research agenda for the high-functioning learning health system. *J Am Med Inform Assoc.* 2015;22(1):43–50. https://doi.org/10.1136/amiajnl-2014-002977
6. OECD. Realising the potential of primary health care. Paris: OECD Health Policy Studies; 2020.
7. Bogaert P, Verschuuren M, Van Oyen H, et al. Identifying common enablers and barriers in European health information systems. *Health Policy.* 2021;125(12):1517–26. https://doi.org/10.1016/j.healthpol.2021.09.006
8. Doty MM, Tikkanen R, Shah A, et al. Primary care physicians' role in coordinating medical and health-related social needs in Eleven countries. *Health Aff (Millwood).* 2020;39(1):115–23. https://doi.org/10.1377/hlthaff.2019.01088
9. OECD. Health in the 21st century: Putting data to work for stronger health systems. Paris: OECD Health Policy Studies; 2019.
10. Oderkirk J. Readiness of electronic health record systems to contribute to national health information and research. Paris: OECD Health Working Papers; 2017.
11. Chang F, Gupta N. Progress in electronic medical record adoption in Canada. *Can Fam Physician.* 2015;61(12):1076–84.
12. Young RA, Roberts RG, Holden RJ. The challenges of measuring, improving, and reporting quality in primary care. *Ann Fam Med.* 2017;15(2):175–82. https://doi.org/10.1370/afm.2014
13. Barbazza E, Klazinga NS, Kringos DS. Exploring the actionability of healthcare performance indicators for quality of care: A qualitative analysis of the literature, expert opinion and user experience. *BMJ Qual Saf.* 2021;30(12):1010–20. https://doi.org/10.1136/bmjqs-2020-011247
14. World Health Organization, (UNICEF). Operational framework for primary health care: Transforming vision into action. Geneva: WHO; 2020.
15. World Health Organization, United Nations Children's Fund (UNICEF). Primary health care measurement framework and indicators: Monitoring health systems through a primary health care lens. Geneva: WHO; 2022.

16. Brito Fernandes O. Citizen-driven health care system performance: Studies on care experiences and engagement. University of Amsterdam; 2022.
17. Loeb JM. The current state of performance measurement in health care. *Int J Qual Health Care*. 2004;16 Suppl 1:i5–9. https://doi.org/10.1093/intqhc/mzh007
18. Schang L, Blotenberg I, Boywitt D. What makes a good quality indicator set? A systematic review of criteria. *Int J Qual Health Care*. 2021;33(3). https://doi.org/10.1093/intqhc/mzab107
19. Kara P, Valentin JB, Mainz J, et al. Composite measures of quality of health care: Evidence mapping of methodology and reporting. *PLoS One*. 2022;17(5):e0268320. https://doi.org/10.1371/journal.pone.0268320
20. Damberg CL, Sorbero ME, Lovejoy SL, et al. An evaluation of the use of performance measures in health care. *Rand Health Q*. 2012;1(4):3.
21. Fink A, Kosecoff J, Chassin M, et al. Consensus methods: Characteristics and guidelines for use. *Am J Public Health*. 1984;74(9):979–83. https://doi.org/10.2105/ajph.74.9.979
22. Linstone H, Turoff M. Delphi method: Techniques and applications. Reading: Addison-Wesley; 1975.
23. de Koning JS, Kallewaard M, Klazinga NS. Prestatie-indicatoren langs de meetlat—het AIRE instrument. *TSG*. 2007;85(5):261–4. https://doi.org/10.1007/BF03078683
24. Barbazza E, Verheij RA, Ramerman L, et al. Optimising the secondary use of primary care prescribing data to improve quality of care: A qualitative analysis. *BMJ Open* 2022;12(7):e062349. https://doi.org/10.1136/bmjopen-2022-062349
25. HealthPros. A practical guide towards actionable healthcare performance indicators: Selecting healthcare performance indicators that are fit for purpose and use for various stakeholders. Healthcare Performance Intelligence; 2022.
26. OECD. Does healthcare deliver? Results from the patient-reported indicator surveys (PaRIS). Paris: WHO; 2025.
27. Ahasan R, Alam MS, Chakraborty T, et al. Applications of GIS and geospatial analyses in COVID-19 research: A systematic review. *F1000Res*. 2020;9:1379. https://doi.org/10.12688/f1000research.27544.2
28. Ozdenerol E. The role of GIS in COVID-19 management and control. Boca Raton: CRC Press; 2023.
29. Charles-Smith LE, Reynolds TL, Cameron MA, et al. Using social media for actionable disease surveillance and outbreak management: A systematic literature review. *PLoS One*. 2015;10(10):e0139701. https://doi.org/10.1371/journal.pone.0139701
30. Seshadri DR, Davies EV, Harlow ER, et al. Wearable sensors for COVID-19: A call to action to harness our digital infrastructure for remote patient monitoring and virtual assessments. *Front Digit Health*. 2020;2:8. https://doi.org/10.3389/fdgth.2020.00008
31. Dang LM, Piran MJ, Han D, et al. A survey on internet of things and cloud computing for healthcare. *Electronics*. 2019;8(7):768.
32. Raleigh VS, Foot C. Getting the measure of quality: Opportunities and challenges. London: The King's Fund; 2010.
33. Robicsek A. Six modest proposals for health care measurement. *Catalyst Carryover*. 2019;5(3). https://doi.org/10.1056/CAT.19.0658
34. Brehaut JC, Colquhoun HL, Eva KW, et al. Practice feedback interventions: 15 suggestions for optimizing effectiveness. *Ann Intern Med*. 2016;164(6):435–41. https://doi.org/10.7326/M15-2248
35. Johns Hopkins University. COVID-19 dashboard by the Center for Systems Science and Engineering (CSSE) at Johns Hopkins University. 2020. [cited 3 Oct 2023; Available from: https://coronavirus.jhu.edu/map.html accessed 24 March 2025].
36. Ivankovic D, Barbazza E, Bos V, et al. Features constituting actionable COVID-19 dashboards: Descriptive assessment and expert appraisal of 158 public web-based COVID-19 dashboards. *J Med Internet Res*. 2021;23(2):e25682. https://doi.org/10.2196/25682

37. Weggelaar-Jansen A, Broekharst DSE, de Bruijne M. Developing a hospital-wide quality and safety dashboard: A qualitative research study. *BMJ Qual Saf.* 2018;27(12):1000–7. https://doi.org/10.1136/bmjqs-2018-007784
38. Lee K, Jung SY, Hwang H, et al. A novel concept for integrating and delivering health information using a comprehensive digital dashboard: An analysis of healthcare professionals' intention to adopt a new system and the trend of its real usage. *Int J Med Inform.* 2017;97:98–108. https://doi.org/10.1016/j.ijmedinf.2016.10.001
39. Dowding D, Randell R, Gardner P, et al. Dashboards for improving patient care: Review of the literature. *Int J Med Inform.* 2015;84(2):87–100. https://doi.org/10.1016/j.ijmedinf.2014.10.001
40. Ghazisaeidi M, Safdari R, Torabi M, et al. Development of performance dashboards in healthcare sector: Key practical issues. *Acta Inform Med.* 2015;23(5):317–21. https://doi.org/10.5455/aim.2015.23.317-321
41. Damman OC, van den Hengel YK, van Loon AJ, et al. An international comparison of web-based reporting about health care quality: Content analysis. *J Med Internet Res.* 2010;12(2):e8. https://doi.org/10.2196/jmir.1191
42. Kamadjeu R, Gathenji C. Designing and implementing an electronic dashboard for disease outbreaks response: Case study of the 2013–2014 Somalia Polio outbreak response dashboard. *Pan Afr Med J.* 2017;27(Suppl 3):22. https://doi.org/10.11604/pamj.supp.2017.27.3.11062
43. Meng Y, Zhang Y, Wang S, et al. Lessons learned in the development of a web-based surveillance reporting system and dashboard to monitor acute febrile illnesses in Guangdong and Yunnan provinces, China, 2017–2019. *Health Secur.* 2020;18(S1):S14–S22. https://doi.org/10.1089/hs.2019.0079
44. Health Data Coallition. Welcome to the Health Data Coalition. 2025. [cited 25 Mar 2025; Available from: https://hdcbc.ca]
45. Ontario MD. EMR quality dashboard completes successful proof of concept. Ontario MD. 2019. [cited 15 Apr 2019; Available from: https://www.ontariomd.ca/emr-quality-dashboard-poc-complete]
46. Dasgupta N, Kapadia F. The future of the public health data dashboard. *Am J Public Health.* 2022;112(6):886–8. https://doi.org/10.2105/AJPH.2022.306871
47. Thorpe LE, Gourevitch MN. Data dashboards for advancing health and equity: Proving their promise? *Am J Public Health.* 2022;112(6):889–92. https://doi.org/10.2105/AJPH.2022.306847
48. Berenson RA, Pronovost PJ, Krumholz HMM. Achieving the potential of health care performance measures. Robert Wood Johnson Foundation and Urban Institute. 2013. [cited May 2013; Available from: https://www.urban.org/sites/default/files/publication/23636/412823-achieving-the-potential-of-health-care-performance-measures.pdf]
49. Gosden T, Forland F, Kristiansen IS, et al. Capitation, salary, fee-for-service and mixed systems of payment: Effects on the behaviour of primary care physicians. *Cochrane Database Syst Rev.* 2000;2000(3):CD002215. https://doi.org/10.1002/14651858.CD002215
50. Petersen LA, Woodard LD, Urech T, et al. Does pay-for-performance improve the quality of health care? *Ann Intern Med.* 2006;145(4):265–72. https://doi.org/10.7326/0003-4819-145-4-200608150-00006
51. Campbell SM, Kontopantelis E, Reeves D, et al. Changes in patient experiences of primary care during health service reforms in England between 2003 and 2007. *Ann Fam Med.* 2010;8(6):499–506. https://doi.org/10.1370/afm.1145
52. Michie S, van Stralen MM, West R. The behaviour change wheel: A new method for characterising and designing behaviour change interventions. *Implement Sci.* 2011;6:42. https://doi.org/10.1186/1748-5908-6-42 [published Online First: 26 Apr 2011]
53. Doran T, Maurer KA, Ryan AM. Impact of provider incentives on quality and value of health care. *Annu Rev Public Health.* 2017;38:449–65. https://doi.org/10.1146/annurev-publhealth-032315-021457

54. Pawson R, Tilley N. Realistic evaluation. London: Sage; 1997.
55. Kvedar J, Coye MJ, Everett W. Connected health: A review of technologies and strategies to improve patient care with telemedicine and telehealth. *Health Aff (Millwood).* 2014;33(2):194–9. https://doi.org/10.1377/hlthaff.2013.0992
56. OECD/WHO. Improving healthcare quality in Europe: Characteristics, effectiveness and implementation of different strategies. Paris/Geneva: WHO; 2019.

CHAPTER

15

New Approaches to Evaluating the Climate Resilience of Primary Care Facilities and Services

Robert Mash, Kiran Jobanputra and Patricia Nayna Schwerdtle

15.1 Introduction

The resilience of health facilities and services is becoming an important issue for health systems.[1] Following the Astana Declaration,[2] the World Health Organization (WHO) published a framework to measure the performance of health systems from a primary healthcare (PHC) lens.[3] There were three important service delivery processes: the model of care; systems for improving quality and patient safety; and evaluating the resilience of facilities and services. Resilience was also seen as a key cross-cutting dimension alongside quality and equity.

The WHO broadly defined *resilience* as "the capacity of health actors, institutions and populations to prepare for and effectively respond to crises; maintain core functions when a crisis hits; and, informed by lessons learned during the crisis, reorganize if conditions require it".[4] Resilience is needed in the face of many challenges, such as pandemics, financial crises and climate change. Infectious disease outbreaks and pandemics from agents such as COVID-19, Ebola, West Nile Virus and Severe Acute Respiratory Syndrome (SARS) have all tested the resilience of health systems.[3] Austerity economics can undermine and challenge health systems as budgets and resources are severely cut.[5]

When resilience is seen as a cross-cutting dimension in the WHO framework, then the whole measurement framework becomes relevant.[3] Resilience of PHC will be related to all the components of PHC: multisectoral policy and action, empowered people and communities, as well as integrated health services.[6] All the health system building blocks can be related to resilience.[7] Strong governance, policy, stakeholder and community engagement, financing and priority setting will lay a foundation of resilience. Ensuring that all the health system inputs are on track will also build resilience. For example, strong infrastructure, competent and complete primary care

DOI: 10.1201/9781003652106-18

teams, reliable medicine and other supplies, and a functional health information system supported by digital technology. Exploring new approaches to the evaluation of resilience in all these dimensions is clearly beyond the scope of this chapter.

Climate change is an ubiquitous and growing challenge to health facilities and services in all countries. It should also be noted that the ecological planetary crisis is more than just climate change and includes increasing pollution of the oceans, air and land, loss of species and biodiversity, changes in land use and altered biogeochemical cycles.[8] In this chapter however we primarily consider the challenges of climate change.

Many health systems are still waking up to the need to incorporate the challenges of climate change into their policy and plans. Previous guidance on resilience has focused more on pandemics, conflicts and disasters and has not fully considered climate hazards. Climate change amplifies the risks associated with these other challenges, so improving all-hazards resilience must include climate resilience.[7]

We are also cognisant that this book is intended for primary care providers and researchers who are concerned with service delivery at the coalface of the health system. We therefore focus on climate resilience and examine new approaches to evaluating resilience at the level of primary care facilities and services.

15.2 Climate Resilience

Climate change has three important relationships to health: the health and social effects, the impact on health facilities and services, and the contribution of health systems to greenhouse gas emissions.

15.2.1 Impact of Health

Firstly, a changing climate affects air quality, food production, infectious disease exposures, access to adequate clean water and many weather-related hazards.[8] These impacts can influence the whole burden of disease, including infectious disease, non-communicable diseases and psychosocial issues. Health-related social effects include displacement, migration and conflict. The resilience of societies to these challenges is related to many factors, such as government performance, wealth, available technology, culture and belief systems, and of course the strength of the health system.[8]

15.2.2 Impact on Health Facilities and Services

Secondly, the same factors that impact people's health also impact the health facilities and services trying to help the population.[1] The WHO states that

> climate resilient health care facilities are those that are capable to anticipate, respond to, cope with, recover from and adapt to climate-related shocks and stress, so as to bring ongoing and sustained healthcare to their target populations, despite an unstable climate.[1]

Climate shocks include extreme weather events such as cyclones, hurricanes, storm surges and extreme temperatures that occur suddenly, while stressors may take time to develop and have an impact, such as drought.

Over time, a primary care facility has different opportunities to prepare for climate hazards (shocks and stressors), to respond adequately and to recover as part of a learning health system. The ability to respond and recover will partly depend on the baseline level of capacity. We know, for example, that many primary facilities in low- and middle-income countries have a low baseline capacity due to issues such as poor infrastructure, inadequate workforce and limited access.[9] Following a challenge, a primary care facility may collapse, recover to the same level as baseline or even transform to be more resilient. In low- and middle-income countries such as Malawi and Mozambique, the climate shocks may destroy primary care facilities.[10,11] Recurrent and frequent shocks may also impede the ability to fully recover between challenges.

15.2.3 Contribution to Greenhouse Gas Emissions

The third important relationship is the significant carbon footprint of health systems.[12] Approximately 5% of all carbon emissions globally come from the health sector. Reducing the carbon footprint, particularly in high-income countries, is therefore also a priority. Ensuring that health systems develop with a low-carbon trajectory is also important, even when the priority in low- and middle-income countries may be resilience. Many interventions to improve resilience can also improve environmental sustainability, so it can be helpful for evaluations to consider both.[1] For example, solar energy can improve resilience by reducing reliance on the national grid, while also reducing the carbon footprint of the facility.

The risks faced by a primary care facility can be considered as an equation that includes exposure to the climate hazards expected in that community, the adaptive capacity of the facility and its vulnerabilities. This is illustrated in Figure 15.1, and Table 15.1 defines some of the key terms used in the framework.[13] This implies that not all hazards result in risks, where there are significant capacities present to attenuate the impact of that hazard.

15.3 Approaches to Measuring the Climate Resilience of Health Facilities

Measuring the climate resilience of health facilities produces insights into their capacity to maintain function during and after climate-related disruptions. Although the assessment of climate-specific resilience is a relatively recent area of focus, it is grounded in a longer tradition of evaluating the overall resilience of health facilities within the field of disaster risk reduction.

The WHO has developed guidance for assessing climate risks and identifying solutions to build resilient health facilities, focusing on four key areas: (1) the health workforce; (2) water, sanitation and healthcare waste; (3) energy; (4) and infrastructure, technologies and products. This facility-level guidance is intended to be used alongside the WHO's broader health system resilience framework, which includes ten modules based on the building blocks of health systems.

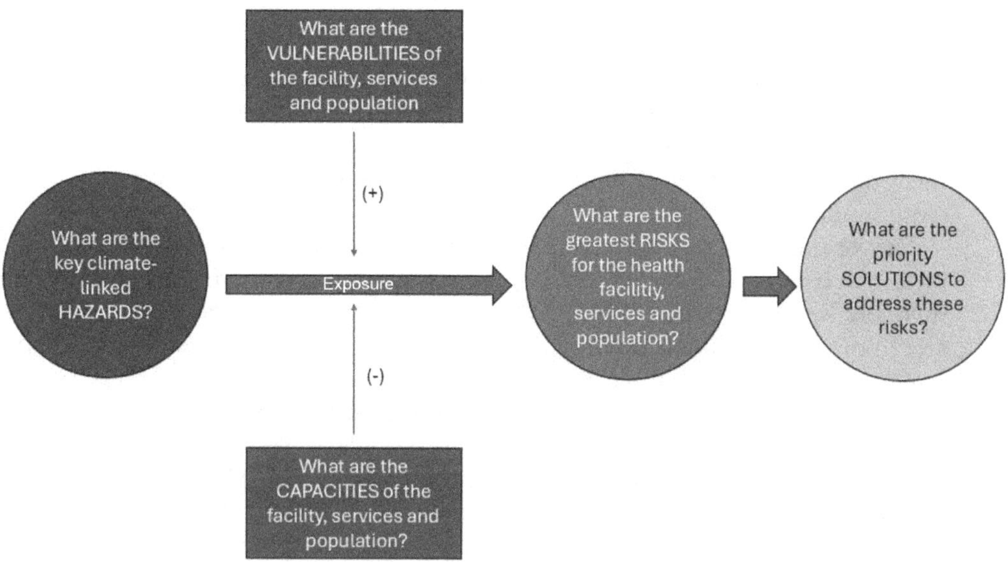

FIGURE 15.1 Conceptual framework for evaluating climate resilience of facilities and services

TABLE 15.1 Definitions of Key Concepts[13,14]

Concept	Definition
Climate hazard	A climate-related shock (sudden onset) or stress (slow onset) that causes damage to health, health facilities or services
Vulnerability	The likelihood of facilities and services to be negatively affected by climate hazards and the specific characteristics that make them vulnerable
Capacity	The ability of facilities and services to adapt or respond to climate hazards and the specific characteristics that give them capacity
Risk	The probability of particular harmful or negative consequences to facilities and services resulting from interactions between hazards, vulnerabilities, exposures and adaptive capacities that need to be addressed.

Although a growing number of global tools and frameworks exist to support climate resilience and sustainability in health systems, most are designed for system-wide or national-level application and are not tailored to the unique vulnerabilities or capacities of individual facilities.[15] Many tools use checklists, stress tests or readiness diagnostics, and these are valuable for assessing risks or identifying gaps but fall short in producing a context-specific, actionable list of feasible solutions to strengthen facility-level resilience in a low-carbon and sustainable manner.[15] These approaches often use hazard-specific granularity, or focus only on one type of hazard, limiting their relevance in settings where multiple, compounding climate threats occur or where there is a high level of uncertainty, which calls for a multi-hazard approach.[15]

In contrast, our participatory, mixed-methods approach to measuring climate vulnerability and adaptive capacity at the facility level can fill these gaps. It enables the integration of local knowledge, facility-specific data and stakeholder perspectives to identify which climate risks are most likely to impact the facility now and in the future. Also, by involving frontline health workers, managers and communities, our Climate Action Accelerator (CAA) Health Facility Climate Vulnerability and Capacity Assessment (VCA) approach enhances the relevance and acceptability of resilience-building strategies and also produces grounded, implementable solutions. This makes them more operationally useful than the multitude of top-down tools that are currently available.

One of the key requirements of any approach to measurement is that it should inform decision-makers on how to improve climate resilience. Measurement should therefore be incorporated into a process of identifying and prioritising solutions and finding ways of implementing these in the context. Measurement is also important for demonstrating which interventions bring value and how much they cost; this is provided through a monitoring framework at the implementation phase, not addressed in this chapter.

Both sets of WHO guidance emphasise the links between climate resilience and environmental sustainability. To support implementation, the WHO also provides a checklist of issues for health facilities and services to consider.[16] Drawing on these WHO resources, the CAA developed the Climate Resilience and Environmental Sustainability of Health Facilities (CRESH) process—an integrated, mixed-methods participatory approach for evaluating resilience and sustainability.[13]

This health service–level VCA method was initially piloted at N'gouri Hospital in Chad, a low-income country setting that had substantial conflict and security issues,[17] and then in primary care facilities within the Cederberg subdistrict of South Africa. We outline this new approach to assessing climate resilience as a case study example.

15.4 A Practical Approach to Evaluating Climate Resilience and Identifying Interventions to Mitigate Climate Risks

15.4.1 Preparation for the Climate VCA

The local research team in Cederberg consisted of a family physician, a researcher in planetary health and primary healthcare, an emergency medicine specialist, a public health specialist and a psychologist with a special interest in public health. The CAA team consisted of a global health researcher and two other experts who had developed the VCA process and piloted it in Chad.

The research team also partnered with the local Department of Health and Wellness. The need for this research study was suggested by the Chief Director, who also led the Department's Climate Change Forum. In addition, the research team engaged with the public health specialist for the rural health services and the provincial head of disaster management.

Once the Cederberg subdistrict was identified, a workshop was held with the district manager, subdistrict manager, facility-level operational managers and provincial-level experts. The research team and one member of CAA outlined the five stages in the VCA process (Figure 15.2). The purpose of this workshop was to ensure that the health services were willing to adopt and engage with the VCA process.

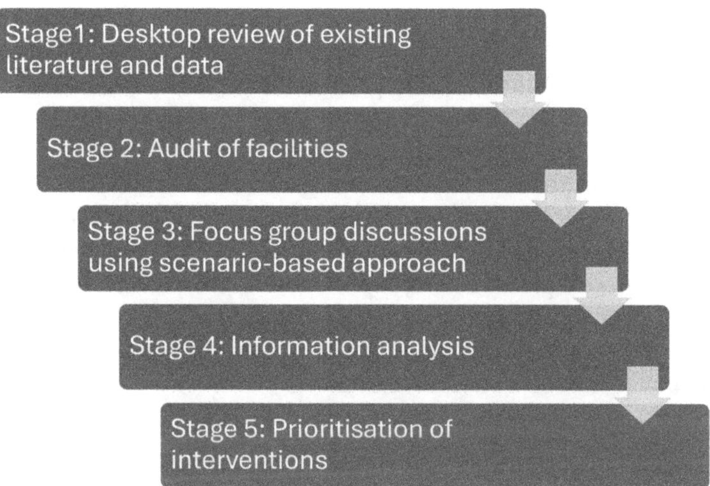

FIGURE 15.2 Five stages of the VCA process

15.4.2 Stage 1: Desk Review

The purpose of the desk review is to produce a preliminary list of hazards, potential vulnerabilities and capacities based on existing literature and data. The research team gathered existing data on the local climate hazards, population demographics, disease burden and health facilities. The information was collated in a short review document. The review identified the key current and future climate hazards facing this population and pointed towards key health and facility-level vulnerabilities. This rapid desk review helped to define the information and adapt the tools needed to collect data in stages 2 and 3.

The desk review took four weeks to complete. Sources of information were the Department of Environmental Affairs and Development,[18] the District Health Barometer (district health information system indicators)[19] and internal reports from the subdistrict on infection prevention and control. The subdistrict manager also created a useful presentation on the subdistrict as part of the preparation step.

15.4.3 Stage 2: Audit of the Facilities

The facility audit enables a detailed elaboration of the facility vulnerabilities and capacities with regard to climate-related hazards, enabling a preliminary identification of the most important climate risks for that facility. The original audit tool that had been piloted in the hospital in Chad required substantial customisation for the South African context. The research team went back to the WHO guidance on facility-level resilience and their checklist of issues to validate the content of the tool for the context.[16] The draft audit tool was content validated by all members of the research team and the subdistrict manager. They assessed whether the relevant items were included and reviewed the response options (usually yes, no or not applicable). Some items were based on environmental sustainability initiatives taken by the Department of Health and Wellness elsewhere in the province. Space was also given for explanatory field notes to elaborate on the responses. The final tool had the following sections: (1) workforce; (2) service delivery and emergency preparedness; (3) water, waste and sanitation; (4) energy; and (5) infrastructure, which covered all six domains of the CAA Climate VCA approach.

The audit tool was completed by a 60-minute interview with the operational manager at each of the six facilities and a tour of the facility to observe and verify key issues. Photographs of infrastructure, equipment and relevant standard operating procedures also taken. The audit took three days to complete.

The tool was completed for each facility and the answers captured in an Excel spreadsheet. Some of the questions were deferred for an answer at the subdistrict level, when they could not be answered at the facility level. The findings were then summarised for the subdistrict as a whole.

15.4.4 Step 3: Focus Group (Scenario-Based) Discussions

The focus group discussions enrich the lists of vulnerabilities and capacities, and the ensuing risks, as well as providing an initial list of solutions that are generated by the participants. A week after the audit, the research team returned to conduct focus group discussions at three of the six primary care facilities. Facilities were purposefully selected based on the results of the audit in step 2. The audit helped identify which facilities had substantial prior experience of climate hazards and were large enough to participate in a group discussion. Three interviews were thought to give sufficient 'information power',[20] but if data saturation was not obtained, further focus groups were possible.

The focus group discussions were based on the two most common climate hazard scenarios that were identified in step 1 and confirmed in step 2. The one was extreme summer temperatures and the other was winter flooding and high episodic rainfall. Participants included members of the facility-based primary care team (eg nurses, pharmacy assistant, receptionists), as well as community health workers and their nurse coordinators from the community-based services. Groups comprised eight to ten people in total and brought together perspectives from the facility and community.

Each focus group was facilitated by two people using a scenario-based tabletop approach. One person facilitated the group discussion in a stepwise manner (Figure 15.3). Each discussion started by creating a visual prop to help people recall their experience and engage them in the discussion. Usually this involved drawing a picture on newsprint of the facility and surrounding community on the tabletop. The facilitator then orientated the group to the climate scenario and encouraged them to elaborate on what happened and what were the strengths (capacities) and vulnerabilities (weaknesses) of the facility and services in this situation. Then people were encouraged to reflect on their experience and possible solutions to improve coping strategies. All members of the group were encouraged to participate.

Although formal qualitative data analysis was not conducted, a structured approach was used to capture key insights from the focus group discussions. The second person in the group served as an observer, using a prepared template to systematically document the group's discussion, including key vulnerabilities, capacities and solutions. Key quotes that highlighted these points were also recorded

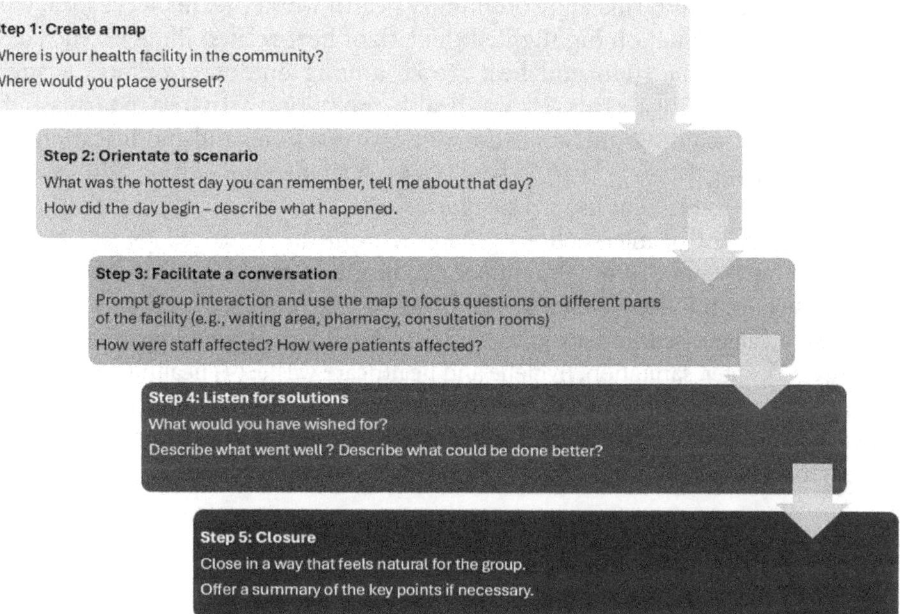

FIGURE 15.3 Steps in focus group discussion

verbatim. Additionally, the discussions were audio-recorded. Following each session, the note taker compiled a two- to three-page summary, outlining the main themes identified during the discussion, drawing on both their notes and the audio-recordings to ensure accuracy and completeness.

15.4.5 Step 4: Information Analysis

The information analysis step involves triangulating the information from the previous steps to produce a final list of the most important climate risks for the target facilities, as well as a list of potential interventions to mitigate those risks. The research team integrated the information from steps 1, 2 and 3 into a 'Risk and Intervention' matrix on a spreadsheet. The matrix included the following columns:

1. Climate hazards and sustainability challenges
2. Vulnerabilities
3. Capabilities
4. Risks
5. Potential interventions

The matrix had horizontal logic, linking climate hazards to vulnerabilities, capacities, risks and potential interventions. For example, under the broad climate hazard category of extreme heat and drought, one identified vulnerability was that farm and manual labourers work in extreme heat. The corresponding capacity was that mobile clinics visit farms and community health worker teams serve local communities. The combination highlighted the risk of heat-related illnesses such as dehydration, heat exhaustion and heat stroke among outdoor workers. A suggested intervention to mitigate this risk was health-promotion activities in farms and other workplaces, including guidelines for protective actions and modification of work patterns during extreme heat. In some cases, a single intervention addressed multiple risks across different hazard categories.

The initial list of interventions generated from the focus groups was enriched by potential interventions from the climate and health literature,[21,22] as well as the CAA climate resilience solution inventory.[13] Once all the potential interventions were identified, they were categorised into six groups: (1) infrastructure, technology and products; (2) energy; (3) water, sanitation, hygiene and healthcare waste; (4) health workforce; (5) service delivery; and (6) governance and financing. At this stage, the matrix underwent review by technical experts from the CAA to identify any inappropriate or obsolete interventions, as well as any key interventions that had been missed.

15.4.6 Step 5: Prioritisation and Planning

The final step in the process involved an assessment and prioritisation of the identified interventions and a collective decision on the final intervention list that can form the basis for a facility or district-level climate action plan. Two members of the research team presented the potential interventions to the subdistrict management team—the subdistrict manager, PHC manager and community-based services manager. Each category of potential interventions was presented in turn and discussed with the management team. Several factors were also considered to help prioritise the interventions:

- The likely cost of the intervention
- The expected impact on climate resilience
- The expected impact on the carbon footprint
- The expected impact on other environmental parameters

Some of the interventions were immediately discarded as not within the control of the Department of Health and Wellness but could be considered by local government or other sectors. Some of the proposed interventions were already being implemented, and some were modified considering feedback from the managers. For each of the remaining factors, the cost or impact was assessed as low, moderate or high. A final list of feasible and prioritised interventions was entered into an action plan and divided into short-term and longer-term actions that the subdistrict could take forward.

15.5 Discussion

This five-step process took five months to complete and resulted in a list of actions that the subdistrict could take to improve climate resilience and/or environmental sustainability. This included six days of field trips to the subdistrict (steps 2, 3 and 5) and approximately two weeks full-time equivalent (steps 1 and 4).

Given the current austerity measures in place in the health system of South Africa, the subdistrict will need support from the provincial government and university to identify potential sources of funding to implement and evaluate the prioritised interventions to build climate resilience. The process therefore is not complete at the end of step 5.

Although the team retained the essence of the methodology and five steps that had been applied in the original pilot in Chad, the content of the process was substantially customised to the context. The time and skills required to customise the method to the context should be anticipated for future applications of the methodology.

This facility-level climate VCA stands out from other health sector climate assessments, as most VCAs are typically conducted at the national level to inform national adaptation plans or at the health system level to guide system-wide adaptation strategies.[23] Few documented examples of primary-level climate VCAs exist.[24] Additionally, there are very few studies evaluating the implementation of a holistic package of solutions to build climate resilience and environmental sustainability—as this climate VCA process enables. Of the examples that do exist, they mostly comprise checklist-based approaches and sometimes single-hazard analysis (as opposed to multi-hazard analysis). Although there are several examples of assessments focused on the general resilience of primary care facilities, assessments specifically addressing climate resilience (and integrating sustainability considerations) at the facility level remain scarce. This approach is also unique because of its mixed-methods, participatory and transdisciplinary nature, which involved diverse stakeholders.

References

1. World Health Organization. WHO guidance for climate-resilient and environmentally sustainable health care facilities. Geneva: WHO; 2020.
2. World Health Organization. Astana declaration on primary health care [Internet]. 2018. [cited 18 Dec 2018; Available from: https://www.who.int/primary-health/conference-phc/declaration]
3. World Health Organization (WHO). Primary health care measurement framework and indicators: Monitoring health systems through a primary health care lens. Geneva; 2022. [cited 13 Mar 2022; Available from: https://www.who.int/publications/i/item/9789240044210]
4. Kruk M, Myers M, Tornorlah-Varpilah S, Dahn B. What is a resilient health system? Lessons from Ebola. *Lancet*. 2015;385(9980):1910–2.
5. Mash B. World Health Day: SA's public health sector facing crisis amid budget cuts. *Mail and Guardian*. 2024 Apr 7. [Available from: https://mg.co.za/thought-leader/opinion/2024-04-07-world-health-day-sas-public-health-sector-facing-crisis-amid-budget-cuts]
6. World Health Organization. Operational framework for primary health care: Transforming vision into action. Geneva: World Health Organization; 2020.
7. World Health Organization. Operational framework for building climate resilient and low carbon health systems. Geneva; 2023. [Available from: https://www.who.int/publications/i/item/9789240081888]

8. Myers S, Frumkin H. Planetary health: Protecting nature to protect ourselves. Washington: Island Press; 2020.
9. Mash R, Howe A, Olayemi O, Makwero M, Ray S, Zerihun M, et al. Primary health care and family medicine in sub-Saharan Africa. *BMJ Glob Health*. 2018;3:e000662.
10. Mailosi A, Mwalwanda S, Hassan C, Zinkanda S, Matanje B, Munyaneza F, et al. Experiences from Cyclone Anna and Cyclone Dumako: A short report. *Afr J Prm Heal Care Fam Med*. 2022;14(1):a3761.
11. Lokotola CL, Uyttersprot T, Felimone P, Scheerens C. How did primary health care in Beira experience Cyclone Idai? *African J Prim Heal Care Fam Med*. 2022 Nov 1;14(1).
12. Lenzen M, Malik A, Li M, Fry J, Weisz H, Pichler P, et al. The environmental footprint of health care: A global assessment. *Lancet Planet Health*. 2020;4(7):e271–9.
13. Climate Action Accelerator. Health facility level climate Vulnerability and Capacity Assessment (VCA). 2024. [cited 18 Oct 2024; Available from: https://climateactionaccelerator.org/climate-vca/]
14. Matthews J. Global warming of 1.5°C: An IPCC special report on the impacts of global warming of 1.5°C above pre-industrial levels and related global greenhouse gas emission pathways, in the context of strengthening the global response to the threat of climate change. Cambridge: Cambridge University Press; 2018. p. 541–562.
15. Haider Z, Rocklov J, Berry P, Jobanputra K, Ebi K, Ngo T, et al. Towards resilience: Investigating resources for enhancing climate resilience in health care facilities in low and middle-income countries: A scoping review. *BMC Health Serv Res*. 2025;In Press.
16. World Health Organization. Checklists to assess vulnerabilities in health care facilities in the context of climate change. Geneva; 2021. [Available from: https://www.who.int/publications/i/item/9789240022904]
17. Schwerdtle N. Building climate resilience: A climate change vulnerability and capacity assessment in Chad. *Glob Heal Sci Pract*. 2024;Under revi.
18. van Weele G, Nakase Z. Environmental risk & vulnerability: Understanding the biophysical risks of the Western Cape. 2023. [Available from: https://resource.capetown.gov.za/documentcentre/Documents/City%20research%20reports%20and%20review/Vulnerability_and_Hazard_Assessment_Report.pdf]
19. Ndlovu N, Padarath A, editors. District health barometer 2022/23. Durban: Health Systems Trust; 2024.
20. Malterud K, Siersma V, Guassora A. Sample size in qualitative interview studies: Guided by information power. *Qual Heal Res*. 2016;26(13):1753–60.
21. Pan American Health Organization. Smart hospitals toolkit. 2017. [cited 16 Jun 2025; Available from: https://www.paho.org/en/health-emergencies/smart-hospitals/smart-hospitals-toolkit]
22. Climate ADAPT. Practical guide for building climate-resilient health systems. 2024. [cited 16 Jun 2025; Available from: https://climate-adapt.eea.europa.eu/en/metadata/publications/practical-guide-for-building-climate-resilient-health-systems]
23. Schwerdtle P, Ngo T, Hasch F, Phan T, Quitmann C, Montenegro-Quiñonez C. Climate change resilient health facilities: A scoping review of case studies in low and middle-income countries. *Environ Res Lett*. 2024;19(7):074041.
24. Mash R, Blows S, Lahri S, McRae M, Lokotola C, Jobanputra K, Nayna Schwerdtle P. Building climate-resilient primary care: A convergent mixed-methods climate vulnerability and capacity assessment in the Cederberg subdistrict, South Africa. *Public Health*. 2026 Mar;252:106106. doi: 10.1016/j.puhe.2025.106106. Epub 2026 Jan 16. PMID: 41546982.

CHAPTER

16

Planetary Health and Primary Care Research

Özden Gökdemir, Dilge Kocabaş, Amber Wheatley Buckell, Nathaly Karina Velásquez Ipanaqué, Sankha Randenikumara and Enrique Falceto de Barros

16.1 The Need to Incorporate Planetary Health Research Into Primary Care

Planetary health can be defined as the health of human civilisation and the state of the natural systems on which it depends.[1] It promotes a systems-oriented approach to health, moving beyond individual biology to include ecological, societal and environmental determinants. The concept of planetary health acknowledges the connection between the condition of Earth's natural systems and human health. Primary care is in a unique position to address the health effects of environmental change and to advance sustainable healthcare practices because of its comprehensive, community-based approach. There is broad agreement that in order to guarantee robust, just and sustainable health systems, planetary health integration into primary care is both vital and urgent.[2–5]

Health effects due to climate change, such as heat stress, vector-borne diseases and mental health issues, are initially evident locally and first observed by primary care physicians.[6] Nevertheless, research in primary care has not yet consistently incorporated planetary health concepts.

16.2 Core Concepts and Importance of Research in Planetary Health

Many core principles of primary care have a deep correlation with the principles of planetary health. Holistic care, equity, continuity of care, collaboration and community orientation are some of the values that could be easily shared by both domains.

According to the theory of planetary health, maintaining natural systems is essential to ensuring human well-being because human health is closely related to their proper operation. With at least six of the nine boundaries—climate change, freshwater, novel entities, biosphere integrity, land-use and biogeochemical flows—having already been crossed, this viewpoint recognises that human activity has driven Earth's natural systems beyond safe and just planetary boundaries.[7]

DOI: 10.1201/9781003652106-19

There are a number of areas where research is vital. Understanding complex interactions can help identify how environmental factors such as air pollution and extreme weather lead to chronic diseases, worsen mental health and disrupt healthcare.[8] Scientific evidence is crucial for creating effective climate adaptation strategies and informing decisions on public health policies, such as the World Health Organization (WHO) air quality guidelines, and practical interventions such as sustainable urban planning. Research is important in evaluating co-benefits and trade-offs, for example, to assess how climate actions can also improve health (eg through cleaner air) while identifying potential negative side effects.[9–12]

16.3 Areas of Research in Planetary Health That Are Already Implemented

Addressing the health impacts of climate change demands a comprehensive and interconnected research strategy that operates on multiple levels. Globally, initiatives are tracking health indicators to monitor the crisis, while locally, the focus is shifting to actionable solutions.[13–15] This includes redesigning urban environments with green infrastructure to save lives,[16] empowering communities through citizen science, and making the healthcare sector itself more sustainable and climate-resilient.[17] These diverse efforts—from educating health professionals to developing integrated data models—are converging to prepare primary care for a new reality, enabling it to tackle the environmental roots of disease and build health systems ready for a changing planet.

16.4 Emerging Research Areas

16.4.1 Resilient Health Systems

Developing the resilience of primary care systems is crucial, so they can withstand climate-related disruptions such as floods, wildfires and heatwaves. Research into strategies to improve primary care infrastructure and services is quickly becoming an urgent need. Current active areas include research into the use of telehealth technologies, alternative models of care and mobile clinics in areas affected by climate-related events to ensure continuity of care during crises.[18,19] In addition to developing resilient infrastructure, the healthcare workforce will also need to be able to adapt to changes caused by climate events. This includes flexible training and support mechanisms.[20–22]

Healthcare has been shown to have a significant contribution to greenhouse gases, resulting in research on strategies to reduce the carbon footprint of clinics. This has led to strategies such as low-carbon prescription, reuse and recycle models in primary care and research into understanding the environmental, as well as health and economic, implications of greener healthcare practices.[23]

16.4.2 Planetary Health in Medical Education and Clinical Practice

As planetary health becomes more prominent, there is an increasing need to integrate planetary health topics and climate science into primary care training and education. In order for planetary health education in primary care to be effective, research into what knowledge, skills and attitudes are required to address the impacts of climate change on health is needed. Healthcare professionals also need to have sound educational strategies for counselling patients on climate-sensitive topics such as sustainable healthy diets, exercising safely and environmentally friendly transport.[24]

16.4.3 Surveillance of Diseases Affected by Climate Change

Due to ongoing ecological changes, new vector-borne, zoonotic and respiratory diseases are expected to emerge. To address these diseases, research is needed to create effective predictive models and real-time surveillance systems that can link local climate data directly with health outcomes tracked in primary care.[25]

16.4.4 Healthcare Technology Innovation and Integration

As healthcare becomes increasingly digitised, it is anticipated that climate risk alerts and weather warnings such as air quality indices or heatwave warnings will be integrated into electronic health record systems. There is increasing research into the utilisation of wearable technologies and mobile applications to track vital signs, as well as climate events. This can be particularly useful for populations who are sensitive to climate events, such as the elderly, and those in rural and remote areas. Primary care services may also begin using artificial intelligence or geographic information systems to identify and manage high-risk patient groups who may be most affected by environmental exposures.[26]

16.4.5 Social Prescribing and Community-Led Initiatives

To build resilience, communities who are most vulnerable to climate impacts can engage in community-based research to develop culturally appropriate strategies. These may include nature-based initiatives such as 'green prescribing' and urban greening, which can also serve as a form of advocacy to address health inequities from an environmental justice perspective.[26]

16.5 Evaluation Tools and Planetary Health Metrics

The development of new metrics and indicators is a core need for planetary health strategies. This includes creating specific measures to assess the impact of climate events on patient and population health,[27] as well as 'planetary health quality indicators' that link healthcare outcomes to environmental sustainability goals such as the United Nations Sustainable Development Goals.[28] Achieving this will likely require integrated evaluation models that combine data from multiple sectors, including healthcare, environment and equity.[1,6]

16.6 Policy and Governance

Finally, to implement new planetary health research, policy and governance structures must adapt to facilitate the transition from evidence to practice. This includes creating policies that enable multisectoral collaboration and data sharing among areas such as urban planning, transport and healthcare. Consequently, the influence of primary care advocacy on shaping local and national climate adaptation policies will become an important area of investigation.[29,30]

16.7 Future Directions for Research

Despite progress, significant challenges remain in planetary health research and its implementation. To address planetary health challenges effectively, a transformative and multi-faceted research approach is urgently needed. This involves bridging knowledge gaps by simplifying complex information for broader communication and strengthening local evidence in under-resourced regions. It is critical to overcome siloed disciplines by fostering cross-disciplinary collaboration and to develop innovative, adaptive study designs that are scalable and community-engaged. Furthermore, research must actively integrate Indigenous knowledge, standardise evaluation methods and explicitly address underlying power dynamics and inequities to ensure that solutions are equitable and effective. Ultimately, achieving a healthier global population requires concerted effort, urgent investment and widespread education to embed planetary health as a core value across all sectors.

We recommend that local evidence is strengthened, with a focus on low- and middle-income countries' planetary health knowledge translated into actionable, context-specific tools. Use participatory approaches to include Indigenous and community knowledge, ensuring equitable, culturally relevant solutions. Addressing power dynamics and ensuring that research benefits vulnerable populations will help prioritise equity. Collaboration should be promoted to foster interdisciplinary and cross-sector research, bridging academic and healthcare silos.

Climate change is a dynamic and evolving phenomenon, requiring adaptive and scalable research methods. Innovative study designs and implementation research need to be applied. Adaptive trial designs enable testing of interventions under changing environmental conditions, while community-based participatory research ensures local ownership and contextual relevance, particularly in resource-limited settings. Implementation science helps translate and scale sustainable, evidence-based climate–health interventions into real-world practice. Clear metrics and reporting frameworks for interventions linking health and environment need to be developed for standardised evaluation.

Planetary health should be integrated into workforce training and support to embed sustainability into healthcare practice. Investment in long-term, transformative research with a focus on implementation, resilience and cross-national collaboration is needed to tackle our current Anthropocene-period challenges.

16.8 Equity and Planetary Health

A central, urgent theme in planetary health is the pursuit of equity. This perspective asserts that a healthy environment is a universal human right, and it directly confronts the stark reality that the burdens of climate change and environmental degradation are not borne equally. Marginalised groups—including low-income communities, Indigenous populations, and those living in high-risk areas such as coastlines and floodplains—are disproportionately vulnerable. Therefore, research in primary care must extend beyond purely clinical outcomes to actively address issues of access, resilience and justice. This equity-focused approach demands that interventions are not only effective but are also prioritised to protect those most at risk, ensuring that the movement for planetary health is intrinsically a movement for social justice.[31]

The planetary health crisis demands we expand our ethical vision beyond individual professional conduct to embrace a broader social ethics. This perspective requires a collective commitment to the common good, where we reflect on how our actions impact global society and the planet itself.

At the heart of this ethical challenge is a profound injustice: the health burdens of climate change—from extreme heat to infectious diseases—disproportionately fall on populations who have contributed the least to the problem. This inequity creates a clear moral obligation to protect the most at-risk communities. It compels us to prioritise their well-being and ensure that policies and the allocation of limited resources are guided by justice, aiming to build a more equitable and sustainable society for all.[32]

16.9 Occupational Health in the Era of Climate Change and the Green Transition

Occupational health is changing as a result of climate change and the world's transition to a green economy. Both direct climate impacts (such as heat and extreme weather) and the introduction of new materials, technologies and work processes in green jobs present workers with new and changing risks. In order to safeguard worker health and guarantee a fair transition, literature emphasises the urgent need for research.

Climate change is triggering a multifaceted health crisis, impacting society from specific workplaces to the general population. Direct dangers include increasing heat stress and extreme weather, causing more illnesses and reducing productivity, especially for high-risk outdoor workers. Meanwhile, the essential shift to a green economy brings its own novel occupational hazards, demanding new safety measures. On a broader scale, the warming planet is worsening respiratory and cardiovascular diseases, facilitating the spread of infectious diseases, and escalating mental health issues and mortality, revealing the pervasive and complex nature of climate change's threat to health.[33–35]

Another crucial problem is not only for employees and citizens of our global village; as employees, society and all living things, we still bear the consequences of policies that take advantage of nature and disregard living things in order to increase profits. On 13 February 2024, tonnes of cyanide, sulphuric acid and heavy metals mixed into the Euphrates basin at a gold mine in the Çöpler village area of the İliç district in Erzincan, trapping nine workers beneath debris in a landslide in the heap leach area. This collapse was one of the most significant environmental catastrophes seen in Turkey's mining industry.[36] Research finding out root reasons, needs, burdens and planning for similar areas would be helpful for those who are living or working in this region.

Other examples are disasters following an earthquake. If there is any suspicion that asbestos or asbestos-containing materials are present in any structure or environment where the employer is working, hasty removal of debris and dumping it in wetlands or agricultural land must be avoided. The employer shall ensure that the removal, demolition, repair, maintenance and disposal of materials that may contain asbestos are carried out under supervision, and research to assess this will also need to be undertaken.[37,38]

16.10 Conclusion

Climate change and the green transition are fundamentally reshaping occupational health, introducing risks from extreme heat, new technologies and socioeconomic shifts. To safeguard workers, a critical need exists for expanded research and targeted policy action. Table 16.1 provides a checklist to incorporate climate change into primary care research. Key priorities include filling knowledge gaps on understudied areas such as air pollution and industrial transitions, as well as understanding how climate effects worsen health inequities and mental well-being. Addressing this evolving landscape proactively requires enhanced surveillance systems, region-specific adaptation strategies and specialised training for health professionals.

TABLE 16.1 Checklist: Incorporating Climate Change Into Primary Care Research

Understanding Context and Risks	• Have you identified local climate-related health risks (eg, heat stress, air pollution, vector-borne diseases)? • Have you assessed how environmental and social determinants interact to affect health in your population?
Community and Collaboration	• Are community voices included in framing research questions and interpreting findings? • Have you established partnerships with local authorities, environmental agencies or non-government organisations (NGOs) to strengthen data and impact?
Study Design and Systems Thinking	• Does your study design account for system complexity (eg interactions between health, environment and socioeconomic factors)? • Does it include adaptive methods suitable for rapidly changing climate conditions?
Monitoring and Data Collection	• Are you integrating environmental indicators (such as temperature, humidity or air quality) into routine health data? • Can digital tools or open datasets enhance your analysis or improve real-time monitoring? • Have you considered setting up early warning systems or surveillance for climate-sensitive diseases?

(Continued)

TABLE 16.1 Checklist: Incorporating Climate Change Into Primary Care Research (Continued)

Mitigation and Adaptation Strategies	• Have you considered both mitigation (reducing healthcare's carbon footprint) and adaptation (supporting resilience) strategies? • Does your research explore ways to strengthen primary care infrastructure and workforce adaptability to climate-related disruptions?
Equity and Sustainability	• Does your study promote equitable and inclusive approaches that protect vulnerable groups? • Are your recommendations aligned with sustainable healthcare practices and planetary health goals (eg UN SDGs)?

References

1. Whitmee S, et al. Safeguarding human health in the Anthropocene epoch: Report of the Rockefeller Foundation-Lancet Commission on planetary health. *Lancet.* 2015;386:1973–2028.
2. Xie E, de Barros EF, Abelsohn A, Stein AT, Haines A. Challenges and opportunities in planetary health for primary care providers. *Lancet Planet Heal.* 2018;2:e185–e7.
3. Lauriola P, et al. Family doctors to connect global concerns due to climate change with local actions: State-of-the art and some proposals. *World Med Health Policy.* 2021;13:199–223.
4. Gonzalez-Holguera J, et al. Translating planetary health principles into sustainable primary care services. *Fron Public Health.* 2022;10:1–10.
5. Hale I, Green S, Davis M, Nowlan, J. Planetary health lens for primary care. *Can Fam Physician.* 2024;70:224–7.
6. Baumgartner J. Planetary health: Protecting nature to protect ourselves. Samuel Myers and Howard Frumkin (eds). *Int J Epidemiol.* 2021;50:697–8.
7. Richardson K, et al. Earth beyond six of nine planetary boundaries. *Sci Adv.* 2023;9:1–16.
8. Andalib E, et al. The interplay between the built environment, health, and well-being: A scoping review. *Urban Sci.* 2024;8.
9. Mahajan SL, et al. Accelerating evidence-informed decision-making in conservation implementing agencies through effective monitoring, evaluation, and learning. *Biol Conserv.* 2023;286.
10. Brennan M, O'Shea PM, Mulkerrin EC. Preventative strategies and interventions to improve outcomes during heatwaves. *Age Ageing.* 2020;49:729–32.
11. Dewi SP, Kasim R, Sutarsa IN, Dykgraaf SH. A scoping review of the impact of extreme weather events on health outcomes and healthcare utilization in rural and remote areas. *BMC Health Serv Res.* 2024;24:486–97.
12. Lokotola CL. Towards a climate-resilient primary health care service. *South African Fam Pract.* 2023;65:1–6.
13. Bichueti RS, et al. Climate change and urban resilience in smart cities: Adaptation and mitigation strategies in Brazil and Germany. *Urban Sci.* 2025;9:1–24.
14. Akras Z, Dresser C, Ashworth H. Integration of environmental data into electronic health records for clinical and public health decision making: A viewpoint on expanding development in the United States. *J Med Internet Res.* 2025;27.
15. Matsumoto T, Bohorquez M. OECD regional development papers building systemic climate resilience in cities. OECD Regional Development Papers. OECD; 2023. p. 37. [Available from: https://www.oecd.org/content/dam/oecd/en/publications/reports/2023/10/building-systemic-climate-resilience-in-cities_a040ad72/f2f020b9-en.pdf]
16. Filonchyk M, Peterson MP, Zhang L, Hurynovich V, He Y. Greenhouse gases emissions and global climate change: Examining the influence of CO2, CH4, and N2O. *Sci Total Environ.* 2024;935.

17. World Health Organization. WHO global air quality guidelines. Particulate matter (PM2.5 and PM10), ozone, nitrogen dioxide, sulfur dioxide and carbon monoxide. WHO. 2021. [cited Sep 2021; Available from: https://www.who.int/publications/i/item/9789240034228]
18. Mathew S, et al. Telehealth for primary healthcare delivery in rural and remote contexts in high-income countries: A scoping review. *mHealth*. 2025;11.
19. Herrera CA, et al. No time to wait: Resilience as a cornerstone for primary health care across Latin America and the Caribbean, a World Bank-PAHO Lancet Regional Health Americas Commission. *Lancet Reg Health—Am*. 2025;50:101240.
20. Kemple T. Planetary health and primary care. *Br J Gen Pract*. 2019;69:536–7.
21. Mosadeghrad AM, Isfahani P, Eslambolchi L, Zahmatkesh M, Afshari M. Strategies to strengthen a climate-resilient health system: A scoping review. *Global Health*. 2023;19:1–11.
22. Strus JA, et al. Adaptation and mitigation for the planetary health crisis: A scoping review from the perspective of primary health care providers. *J Clim Chang Health*. 2025;22:100440.
23. Malani K, et al. Student challenges and successes in integration of planetary health in medical education: A mixed methods analysis. *Front Public Health*. 2025;13:1–10.
24. Walker R, et al. Health promotion interventions to address climate change using a primary health care approach: A literature review. *Health Promot J Austr*. 2011;22 Spec No, 6–12.
25. Mulligan C, Kumar SG, Berti G. Community-based resilience: Digital technologies for living within planetary boundaries. *Technol Soc*. 2025;82:102915.
26. Braithwaite J, Zurynski Y, Smith CK. *Routledge handbook of climate change and health system sustainability*. 2024. https://doi.org/10.4324/9781032701196.
27. Redvers N, Wright K, Hartmann-Boyce J, Tonkin-Crine S. Physicians' views of patient–planetary health co-benefit prescribing: A mixed methods systematic review. *Lancet Planet Health*. 2023;7:e407–e17.
28. Walsh SJ, et al. Primary healthcare's carbon footprint and sustainable strategies to mitigate its contribution: A scoping review. *BMC Health Serv Res*. 2024;24.
29. MacNeill AJ, McGain F, Sherman JD. Planetary health care: A framework for sustainable health systems. *Lancet Planet Heal*. 2021;5:e66–e8.
30. Martens P. *Planetary health: The recipe for a sustainable future*. 2023. https://doi.org/10.26481/spe.20230421pm
31. Haines A, Ebi K. The imperative for climate action to protect health. *N Engl J Med*. 2019;380:263–73.
32. US Global Change Research Program. The impacts of climate change on human health in the United States. *Fresenius' Zeitschrift für Analytische Chemie*. 2016;311.
33. Schulte PA, et al. Updated assessment of occupational safety and health hazards of climate change. *J Occup Environ Hyg*. 2023;20:183–206.
34. Vitale E, Salvago P, Campanella AF, Cirrincione L. A protocol of prevention and protection measures on new occupational risk factors in green jobs in Italian workplaces. *Sustain*. 2024;16:1–20.
35. Jia JA, Jia NI. Impacts of climate change on occupational health and safety: A comprehensive review. *Asian J Ad Res Reports*. 2024;18:136–54.
36. Soysal A. Altın Madenlerinin Denetimi Sorunsalı. *Yesil Gazette*. 2024. p. 1–4. [cited 21 Jul 2024; Available from: https://yesilgazete.org/altin-madenlerinin-denetimi-sorunsali/]
37. United Nations Environment Programme. Asbestos health and safety requirements. *UN*. 2021. [cited 27 Jan 2021; Available from: https://www.unep.org/resources/toolkits-manuals-and-guides/asbestos-health-and-safety-requirements]
38. Yavuz CI. The additional burden of earthquakes: Asbestos risks rising in Türkiye. *Thorac Res Pract*. 2024;25:100–1.

SECTION

4

Innovations in Research Methodologies

CHAPTER

17

New Approaches to Clinical Trials in Family Medicine and Primary Health Care Research

Christopher C Butler and Max O Bachmann

17.1 Introduction

Primary health care (PHC) is a system-wide approach that includes 'first contact' primary care but is multi-agency and includes activities across areas that impact broadly upon health and well-being.[1] PHC is mission critical to achieving universal health coverage, improving equity and delivering efficient, person-centred care.[2] Much innovation in healthcare in the past seemed like a fantastic idea at the time and was introduced without being evaluated, so we do not know if the innovations brought the benefits we hoped for. Whenever we spend more time or money on something new, it generally means that there's less of these precious resources available for other things.

For PHC to deliver most cost-effectively on its promises and potential, it must be underpinned by rigorous evidence that shows what works. Many kinds of evidence can be used to help us figure out if interventions are beneficial and, if so, who do they benefit most and who might they harm? Analysing routinely collected data—either looking back on data already collected or looking forward using new data—is common, and people call this 'real-world evidence' in one form or another. Observational studies, whether they include an intervention, such as a before and after study, or case control studies, but without randomisation, are very helpful. But getting comparison groups that are similar in just about every way, apart from whether they have been exposed to an intervention or not, is very difficult or impossible with these non-randomised research designs. Randomised controlled clinical trials (RCTs) ensure that comparison groups are similar to start with, and are therefore the best way of ensuring that comparisons between groups give unbiased answers about the effect of interventions.[3] RCTs are ideal not only for testing new drugs but also for testing complex interventions such as care pathways and other health services interventions. Most clinical trials are conducted in hospital or specialist settings and often focus on narrow, pharmacologically driven questions. Sometimes, different, better ways of delivering care, so-called health services interventions, can save numerous lives and improve healthcare and quality of life.[4]

DOI: 10.1201/9781003652106-21

There is an urgent need to strengthen PHC trial research that covers a wider range of interventions, not only drug treatments, but also complex care pathways, behaviour change interventions, and different ways of delivering care.[4] This is especially true in low- and middle-income countries (LMICs), where the disease burden is high but research infrastructure is often underdeveloped.[5] The World Health Assembly recently passed Resolution 75.8 on strengthening clinical trials, calling for bigger and better trials that include more diverse people, to ensure that those for whom interventions are intended are included in the trials.[6] This chapter provides a practical guide to approaches in clinical trials that may be better suited to PHC and LMIC contexts, including adaptive and pragmatic designs, cluster randomised stepped-wedge decentralised 'democratic' trial delivery, and embedded research infrastructure.

17.2 The Limits of Traditional Trial Designs in PHC

New approaches are emerging to attempt to generate comparative effectiveness data using statistical manipulation of routinely collected data. Trial simulations, for example, are becoming increasingly popular. However, no amount of 'statistical magic' can eliminate the influence of unknown or unmeasured confounders that might affect outcomes. Many of the potential important confounders, or features of patients and their settings that may influence outcomes, are not captured in routinely collected data and so cannot be considered in the analysis. The risk is always there that differences between groups are not the result of the intervention, but rather are caused by differences that existed already and that influence outcomes. Typical examples would be baseline differences in health literacy between groups, or in access to healthier food, which really cause differences in obesity, rather than the introduction of a new drug treatment being evaluated. Prospective randomisation thus remains the most robust way to reduce the risk of bias when comparing interventions.

Traditionally, we think of RCTs as one group being randomised to receive an active treatment and the other group receiving a dummy version of that treatment. Traditional RCTs often face significant limitations, particularly in PHC settings and in LMICs:

- Rigid inclusion criteria that exclude people with comorbidities or features common in PHC populations may make it hard to apply trial findings to a particular individual receiving care.[7] Small, selected trial populations that often are not diverse or large, making it hard to know whether the treatment is likely to benefit patients with specific characteristics.[8]
- They typically test single interventions, reducing efficiency.[9]
- Most are conducted in hospital settings, not community-based or primary care environments.
- They frequently aim to support drug licensing rather than integration into routine care pathways.[10]
- Cost-effectiveness is often not evaluated or a secondary outcome.

- Participation is frequently limited to those living near, or receiving care from, the sites that are contracted and set up for trials.[4]
- Implementation is usually slow, resource-intensive and often impractical in LMIC contexts.[11]

17.3 Adaptive Trials

Changing aspects of a clinical trial once it has started may be considered bad practice that introduces risk of error and bias. However, some trial protocols are intentionally designed to include flexibility to respond to changing circumstances and emerging data. Adaptive clinical trials thus 'use accumulating data to decide on how to modify aspects of the study as it continues, without undermining the validity and integrity of the trial.'[12]

Possible study design modifications can include changes to:

- Eligibility criteria
- Randomisation procedure
- Treatment regimens
- Total sample size of the study
- Concomitant treatments used
- Follow-up time
- Primary endpoint
- Secondary endpoints
- Statistical analysis methods
- Study end date

There are many adaptive trial design features, for example:

- Adaptive randomisation
- Adaptive group sequential design
- N-adjustable design
- Drop-the-loser design
- Adaptive dose-escalation design
- Biomarker-adaptive design
- Adaptive treatment-switching design
- Adaptive-hypothesis design
- Adaptive seamless Phase II/III trial design
- Multiple adaptive design

However, we will consider mainly adaptive platform trial designs.

17.4 Adaptive Platform Trials

In contrast to a traditional placebo-controlled single-question trial, platform trials are ongoing research infrastructures designed to answer multiple clinical questions about a single disease area.[13] Instead of focusing on only one intervention, platform trials use a master protocol to evaluate several treatment arms, which may enter or leave the trial over time.[14] These designs are especially well established in oncology and are now being adapted to PHC. Patients are randomised to a shared control or to any one of multiple arms. Frequent interim analyses allow ineffective treatments to be dropped and promising ones to be added.

This adaptability increases efficiency and ensures sustained relevance over time. Information from the trial itself can help determine the right sample size for evaluations within the trial. Sometimes, sample size calculations are based on information from trials done elsewhere and at a different time, and the estimated effect sizes and therefore sample numbers may not apply to a new trial. Frequent interim analyses overcomes this problem, because as soon as there is enough information in the trial to show that an intervention stands very little chance of being successful, or that it is indeed clearly beneficial, then that intervention can be removed from the trial and new participants will contribute to evaluating the next interventions.[11] Bayesian statistical methods can enable data to be leveraged from those who have already been in the trial to add power to comparisons of future interventions, and can take into account the changing nature of the illness or natural history overtime.[15]

A master protocol governs how treatments are added or removed, typically based on interim analyses.[16] These decisions about dropping arms for futility, or declaring an intervention to be successful, at an interim analysis are based on pre-specified thresholds of probability for futility and success. As treatments are dropped or new ones are added, the trial platform continues. When a new arm is added, the master protocol is amended, with a new intervention specific appendix (ISA) outlining the rationale, and any additional relevant eligibility criteria and safety monitoring.

Platform trials can include multiple arms with stratification by subgroup (eg age, comorbidity), allowing for fine-grained information about which interventions work or do not work so well for which subgroups, tailoring evaluation across heterogeneous populations. Their statistical efficiency, flexibility and ability to produce policy-relevant results make them particularly attractive for LMICs, where infrastructure may be limited, but the need for real-world, adaptable evidence is high. This 'trial without end' infrastructure allows the trial infrastructure to be embedded into routine care, for research expertise to be retained and developed in an ongoing way (rather than disappearing when a single-question trial comes to an end), and for emerging findings from the trial to be implemented straightaway. If the comparison is usual care and the trial shows that an intervention is better than usual care, then that intervention can be incorporated into a new version of best usual care, and future interventions can be compared to that. In this way, we end up with an ever-learning, ever-evolving and ever-improving healthcare system (Box 17.1).

BOX 17.1 PRINCIPLE AND PANORAMIC TRIALS—THERAPEUTICS FOR COVID-19 IN THE COMMUNITY

The PRINCIPLE and PANORAMIC individually randomised adaptive platform controlled trials enrolled more than 40,000 participants to evaluate nine treatments over time for COVID-19 in the community.[21,23] They pioneered adaptive platform designs and decentralised methods, allowing rapid participation without the need to always attend clinical sites. The PRINCIPLE trial started by testing one drug, but by the time it closed, it had tested seven different treatments for COVID-19. The PANORAMIC trial focused on novel treatments, starting out with one drug and ending up by evaluating two agents. These trials addressed the 'inverse research participation law' by enabling inclusion of participants across diverse geographies and socioeconomic backgrounds. Their results informed national and global guidelines, supporting both treatment decisions and antimicrobial stewardship.[24,25]

Key enablers included prior experience with adaptive trials, rapid funding mechanisms and prioritisation by national research networks. A 'hub and spoke' recruitment model enabled more than 4,500 general practices to refer patients to 65 research hubs. Regulatory innovations permitted electronic eligibility checks, remote consent, home delivery of study medication and digital follow-up, even during lockdowns.

17.5 Basket and Umbrella Platform Trials

Basket trials evaluate a single intervention across different diseases or populations sharing a characteristic (eg a genetic marker). Umbrella trials, conversely, evaluate several interventions across subgroups within a single condition. Both trial designs offer efficiency and are valuable in LMICs, where resources for multiple separate trials may be limited. The beauty of the platform trial, however, is that within a single trial, the basket and umbrella approaches can be integrated so that the trial can simultaneously give answers about several interventions and different subgroups and patient characteristics.

17.6 Pragmatic, Cluster and Stepped-Wedge Designs

17.6.1 Pragmatic Trials

Pragmatic trials assess interventions under real world conditions, in settings like those in which the interventions would be implemented.[7,17] They typically include diverse populations, allow flexibility in delivery, and often use routine data for follow-up and outcome ascertainment.[18] The comparison group should be as close to real-world usual practice as possible, because often the question is whether there is benefit to adding in something new or in addition to current best practice, rather than whether something works better than its dummy version. The intervention can be applied flexibly; for example, different individuals might get different treatments.

Outcome measures should be those that matter to healthcare professionals, the healthcare system, and, most importantly, to the people for whom the intervention is intended for. Pragmatism in trials is particularly useful for evaluating cost-effectiveness, as costs of the new way of doing things or the new intervention can be compared directly with existing care. Usual care—the comparator group in pragmatic trials—does not include the use of placebos, which can alter help-seeking behaviour, thus impacting on costs. Not using placebos also avoids nocebo effects, which means that some people feel worse or get so-called adverse effects from taking an inert version of medicine. In such cases, outcomes in the control group will be worse than if there had been no placebo, so the effect of an intervention might be exaggerated.

17.6.2 Cluster Randomised Trials

Cluster randomised trials (CRTs) allocate groups—such as groups of patients attending clinics or living in communities—to trial arms rather than individuals. This is particularly appropriate when interventions are delivered at the organisational or population level, or where individual randomisation risks contamination.[19] CRTs are well suited to PHC settings, where team-based or system-wide changes (eg new models of care, triage protocols or point-of-care testing) are often evaluated. These designs can often make it unnecessary to obtain individual consent from participants, given that reasonable alternative approaches to system-wide care are being compared, so that there is real equipoise and risks to individuals are very low. Furthermore, whether patients give their consent or not would not affect the care they receive. CRTs usually need larger numbers of participants than individually randomised trials because, although there might be large numbers of individuals in each cluster, the most important contribution to the power of these trials is the number of clusters randomised rather than the total number of individuals in the trial. The reason for this need for large sample size is that individuals attending the same clinic, for example, are likely to be more like each other than they are to individuals attending facilities elsewhere, and thus may respond not as independent individual observations, but are more likely to respond in the same way as other members of that cluster (Box 17.2).

17.6.3 Stepped-Wedge Cluster Randomised Trials

Stepped-wedge cluster randomised trials are a subtype of CRT in which the intervention is rolled out sequentially across clusters over time, with all eventually receiving the intervention. Typically, groups of clusters (eg clinics and their patients) are randomised so that one group begins with the intervention while the other groups initially serve as controls. After a defined period, some of the control clusters then receive the intervention. This is repeated in steps over time, providing pre- and post-intervention data across all clusters. The effect of the intervention is estimated by comparing all outcomes measured while clusters are exposed to the intervention (the 'wedge') with all outcomes measured while clusters have not yet been exposed to the intervention. This approach enhances statistical power, as each cluster serves as its own control, but requires outcomes to be measured repeatedly at each step.

BOX 17.2 STRETCH TRIAL—INNOVATION IN HIV CARE DELIVERY

The STRETCH trial addressed delays in HIV treatment initiation in South Africa by enabling nurse-led ART (NIMART).[26] The trial was built on response to community concern and public engagement was central throughout. This pragmatic cluster randomised trial included all 31 PHC clinics in one province, with 16 randomised to the intervention. It leveraged electronic records for participant identification and follow-up, enrolling more than 15,000 participants. Individual consent was not required as a new, plausible way of delivering treatment was to be compared to existing practice. Everyone attending a particular clinic was managed according to the same care pathway. Although large numbers of participants contributed data, the trial took into account clustering, which means that power is reduced compared to a trial in which 15,000 individuals were randomised, rather than 31 clinics. Despite real-world challenges—including staff shortages and a moratorium on ART initiation due to funding cuts—the trial showed at least equivalent clinical and ART programme outcomes from NIMART compared to when doctors initiated treatment.

The trial coincided with a national policy shift to NIMART, supporting rapid scale-up of ART delivery. Sustained engagement with national and provincial health authorities, including their representation on the trial steering committee, ensured policy relevance and impact. This trial illustrates a pragmatic cluster design with appropriate ethical oversight and real-world applicability through its influence of national policy. It showed how the way we deliver care and medicines can have massive impact on policy and lives saved.

This design is especially valuable when the intervention is expected to do more good than harm, so that all participants will eventually receive it, and may be continued beyond the life of the trial. It ensures ethical equity, as no group is permanently denied access. In LMICs, stepped-wedge designs are particularly practical: they allow for phased roll-out of limited resources, accommodate local adaptations and facilitate comparisons both within and between clusters over time.

17.6.4 Trials That 'Take Research to the People': So-Called Decentralised Trials

Decentralised methods improve inclusivity and reduce participation barriers.[20] Key features include remote eligibility screening, consent and data collection and follow-up using mobile devices. Community health workers may support engagement and sample collection. Integrated digital platforms enable eligibility checks, consent, randomisation, data capture and long-term follow-up.[4]

These designs, proven during COVID-19, are ideal for evaluating low-cost, low-risk interventions and for maintaining trial continuity during disruptions. Using visiting healthcare workers or remote enabling technologies, such as phones, text and e-mail, and taking treatments directly to people sick in bed at home can ensure that people can contribute to trial research without ever having to leave their sick bed. This minimises the burden on people as they participate in trials and, if it is an infectious condition, reduces the chance of spread.

17.7 Digital Enablement

Digital tools can facilitate real-time recruitment, adaptive randomisation, e-consent and linkage to electronic health records (EHRs). Routine care data can help ascertain outcomes such as hospitalisation or mortality, reducing the need for burdensome data collection. For example, participants may be identified through diagnostic codes, triaged through automated eligibility checkers and followed up through phone, text or app-based surveys. This approach proved critical during the COVID-19 pandemic, when traditional face-to-face research models became unfeasible.[21] In LMICs, the use of mobile phones and SMS for follow-up may be more feasible than computer-based platforms, and community health workers can serve as essential links between participants and digital systems.

17.8 Embedding Trials in PHC

Embedding research in PHC systems improves recruitment, implementation and long-term sustainability. Practice-based research networks and clinical trial networks provide shared infrastructure, community engagement and capacity building.[22] Informal networks including community health workers and non-government organisations are often central to research delivery and should be supported with training, mentorship and funding. Practice-based research networks often evolve from long-standing collaborations and provide infrastructure for continuous quality improvement and research translation. Engagement with civil society organisations and existing community networks (eg faith-based groups) can help bridge the gap between researchers and underserved populations.

Embedding trials in PHC also enables more sustainable implementation of trial findings, as providers are already familiar with the interventions and context. It also helps build trust in the research process, fostering participation and long-term partnerships. Incentivising PHC involvement in research—whether through protected time, training or accreditation—can support long-term engagement and capacity building (Box 17.3).

BOX 17.3 CHECKLIST FOR PLANNING A PHC TRIAL IN LMICS

- Align the research question with local health system priorities.
- Engage community stakeholders from the start.
- Consider a pragmatic or adaptive design suited to available infrastructure.
- Consider basket, umbrella, cluster or stepped-wedge cluster designs where appropriate.
- Use existing data systems for recruitment and outcome measurement where possible (eg electronic medical records and mobile phones).
- Plan for proportionate ethics and regulatory approvals.
- Include strategies to ensure equitable participation.
- Build local research capacity through training and mentorship.
- Budget for public engagement, dissemination and implementation.

17.9 Conclusion

Consider approaches that are broader than the traditional two-armed placebo control trials in family medicine and PHC, which are vital for ensuring evidence-based care, particularly in LMICs. Innovative trial designs—including adaptive platform, pragmatic, basket, umbrella and cluster and cluster stepped-wedge trials—can avoid some of the limitations of traditional RCTs. Digitally enabled, decentralised delivery and embedding trials within PHC systems are key strategies for inclusivity and sustainability. Strengthening local networks, building capacity and aligning with community needs will help democratise trials and ensure that those who are most in need are not left out of the evidence base.

References

1. World Health Organisation. Primary health care: WHO; 2023. [cited 10 Apr 2024; Available from: https://www.who.int/news-room/fact-sheets/detail/primary-health-care]
2. World Health Organization and the United Nations Children's Fund. A vision for primary health care in the 21st century: Towards universal health coverage and the Sustainable Development Goals. WHO and UNICEF. 2018. WHO/HIS/SDS/2018.X. Licence: CC BY-NC-SA 3.0 IGO.
3. World Health Organization. Guidance for best practices for clinical trials. Geneva: World Health Organization; 2024.
4. Butler CC, Mash R, Gobat N, et al. Democratising clinical trials research to strengthen primary health care. *Lancet Glob Health.* 2025;13(4):e749–e58. https://doi.org/10.1016/S2214-109X(24)00513-8
5. Crisp N. Global health capacity and workforce development: Turning the world upside down. *Infect Dis Clin North Am.* 2011;25(2):359–67. https://doi.org/10.1016/j.idc.2011.02.010
6. World Health Organization. Strengthening clinical trials to provide high-quality evidence on health interventions and to improve research quality and coordination. Seventy-Fifth World Health Assembly; 2022.
7. Ford I, Norrie J. Pragmatic trials. *N Engl J Med.* 2016;375(5):454–63. https://doi.org/10.1056/NEJMra1510059 [published Online First: 16 Aug 2016]
8. Jacobson LD, Edwards AG, Granier SK, Butler CC. Evidence-based medicine and general practice. *Br J Gen Pract.* 1997;47(420):449–52.
9. Butler CC, Coenen S, Saville BR, et al. A trial like ALIC(4)E: Why design a platform, response-adaptive, open, randomised controlled trial of antivirals for influenza-like illness? *ERJ Open Res.* 2018;4(2). https://doi.org/10.1183/23120541.00046-2018 [published Online First: 16 May 2018]
10. Kalkman S, van Thiel G, van der Graaf R, et al. The social value of pragmatic trials. *Bioethics.* 2017;31(2):136–43. https://doi.org/10.1111/bioe.12315 [published Online First: 7 Jan 2017]
11. Saville BR, Berry SM. Efficiencies of platform clinical trials: A vision of the future. *Clin Trials.* 2016;13(3):358–66. https://doi.org/10.1177/1740774515626362
12. Gallo P, Chuang-Stein C, Dragalin V, et al. Adaptive designs in clinical drug development: An executive summary of the PhRMA working group. *J Biopharm Stat.* 2006;16(3):275–83; discussion 85–91, 93–8, 311–2. https://doi.org/10.1080/10543400600614742
13. Butler CC, Connor JT, Lewis RJ, et al. Answering patient-centred questions efficiently: Response-adaptive platform trials in primary care. *Br J Gen Pract.* 2018;68(671):294–5. https://doi.org/10.3399/bjgp18X696569

14. Angus DC, Alexander BM, Berry S, et al. Adaptive platform trials: Definition, design, conduct and reporting considerations. *Nat Rev Drug Discov.* 2019;18(10):797–807. https://doi.org/10.1038/s41573-019-0034-3
15. Connor JT, Elm JJ, Broglio KR, et al. Bayesian adaptive trials offer advantages in comparative effectiveness trials: An example in status epilepticus. *J Clin Epidemiol.* 2013;66(8 Suppl):S130–7. https://doi.org/10.1016/j.jclinepi.2013.02.015 [published Online First: 17 Jul 2013]
16. Berry SM, Connor JT, Lewis RJ. The platform trial: An efficient strategy for evaluating multiple treatments. *JAMA.* 2015;313(16):1619–20. https://doi.org/10.1001/jama.2015.2316 [published Online First: 24 Mar 2015]
17. Zuidgeest MGP, Goetz I, Groenwold RHH, et al. Series: Pragmatic trials and real world evidence: Paper 1. Introduction. *J Clin Epidemiol.* 2017;88:7–13. https://doi.org/10.1016/j.jclinepi.2016.12.023 [published Online First: 28 May 2017]
18. Meinecke AK, Welsing P, Kafatos G, et al. Series: Pragmatic trials and real world evidence: Paper 8. Data collection and management. *J Clin Epidemiol.* 2017;91:13–22. https://doi.org/10.1016/j.jclinepi.2017.07.003 [published Online First: 19 Jul 2017]
19. Dron L, Taljaard M, Cheung YB, et al. The role and challenges of cluster randomised trials for global health. *Lancet Glob Health.* 2021;9(5):e701–e10. https://doi.org/10.1016/S2214-109X(20)30541-6
20. Butler CC. Democratising the design and delivery of large-scale randomised, controlled clinical trials in primary care: A personal view. *Eur J Gen Pract.* 2023; 30(1):2293702. https://doi.org/10.1080/13814788.2023.2293702
21. Gbinigie O, Ogburn E, Allen J, et al. Platform adaptive trial of novel antivirals for early treatment of COVID-19 in the community (PANORAMIC): Protocol for a randomised, controlled, open-label, adaptive platform trial of community novel antiviral treatment of COVID-19 in people at increased risk of more severe disease. *BMJ Open.* 2023;13(8):e069176. https://doi.org/10.1136/bmjopen-2022-069176 [published Online First: 7 Aug 2023]
22. Mash RJ, Von Pressentin K. Family practice research in the African region 2020–2022. *Afr J Prim Health Care Fam Med.* 2024;16(1):e1–e8. https://doi.org/10.4102/phcfm.v16i1.4329 [published Online First: 13 Feb 2024]
23. Hayward G, Butler CC, Yu LM, et al. Platform randomised trial of interventions against COVID-19 in older people (PRINCIPLE): Protocol for a randomised, controlled, open-label, adaptive platform, trial of community treatment of COVID-19 syndromic illness in people at higher risk. *BMJ Open.* 2021;11(6):e046799. https://doi.org/10.1136/bmjopen-2020-046799 [published Online First: 18 Jun 2021]
24. National Institute for Health and Care Excellence (NICE). Nirmatrelvir plus ritonavir, sotrovimab and tocilizumab for treating COVID-19: Technology appraisal guidance Reference number:TA878. 2025. [cited 1 May 2025; Available from: https://www.nice.org.uk/guidance/ta878/chapter/1-Recommendations accessed 8 Jun 2025].
25. World Health Organisation. Therapeutics and COVID-19: Living guideline. WHO; 2023. [cited 14 Jul 2023; Available from: https://www.who.int/publications/i/item/WHO-2019-nCoV-therapeutics-2022.4 accessed 6 Aug 2023].
26. Fairall L, Bachmann MO, Lombard C, et al. Task shifting of antiretroviral treatment from doctors to primary-care nurses in South Africa (STRETCH): A pragmatic, parallel, cluster-randomised trial. *Lancet.* 2012;380(9845):889–98. https://doi.org/10.1016/S0140-6736(12)60730-2 [published Online First: 15 Aug 2012]

CHAPTER

18

Mapping Exercises, Gap-Mapping and Scoping Reviews

Duygu Ayhan Başer and Mehmet Akman

18.1 Introduction

Primary care research is going through a vital change, broadening methodological horizons to respond to increasingly more complex questions regarding health systems, equity and pragmatic real-world interventions.[1] Scoping reviews, mapping exercises and gap-mapping are valuable tools in primary care research for synthesising evidence, identifying knowledge gaps and informing policy and practice. Scoping reviews are best suited for exploring broad or emerging topics, such as complex care models or social determinants of health. Mapping exercises help organise diverse evidence thematically or methodologically, providing a clear overview of research landscapes, often as a preparatory step before systematic reviews. Gap-mapping visually highlights areas where evidence is abundant and where critical gaps exist, supporting strategic research planning and funding decisions.[2,3] In a field such as primary care, which serves diverse populations and adapts to evolving health needs, these methods are essential for aligning research with real-world priorities. This chapter aims to describe and compare these approaches, drawing on recent methodological developments and global standards.

18.2 Mapping Exercises

Mapping exercises serve as a foundational step in understanding the scope, nature and characteristics of the available evidence on a specific healthcare topic and are intensive processes conducted to ascertain, organise and clarify the evidence base of a given topic as available in literature.[3] Mapping exercises are commonly undertaken as a first step prior to systematic reviews or to inform policy development and planning for research. Unlike systematic reviews, which focus on answering a narrowly defined research question, mapping reviews aim to provide a broad overview of existing studies, highlight key features and identify knowledge gaps.[4,5] They are

DOI: 10.1201/9781003652106-22

similar to scoping reviews in purpose, but they place greater emphasis on structure and categorisation.

18.2.1 Steps to Conduct Mapping Exercises

Follow these key steps when performing a mapping exercise:[3–5]

1. *Define the purpose and scope*: The initial step is to delineate the aim and scope of the mapping exercise precisely. This entails specifying the population of concern, the concept(s) under examination and the context under which the studies fall. The aim may range from establishing research gaps to gauging the diffusion of evidence over geographical or methodological fields.
2. *Develop a comprehensive search strategy*: A broad and in-depth search strategy is required to find the complete spectrum of accessible relevant literature. Most typically, this is a combination of defined terms (eg Medical Subject Headings, MeSH) and free-text keywords in more than one electronic database. The search should not be limited by language or publication date unless justified by research aims.
3. *Screen and select studies*: Once the literature is procured, two-stage study screening is done: title/abstract screening and full-text screening. Pre-decided inclusion and exclusion criteria should be consistently applied. It is preferable for two or more reviewers to screen to decrease selection bias, as well as make accurate judgments.
4. *Develop a framework of data classification*: A classification framework is built to group the included studies. This may involve coding by study design, population, intervention categories, outcomes measured, geographical location or other dimensions of interest. The framework is piloted with a subset of studies and, if necessary, adjusted for simplicity and comprehensiveness.
5. *Data extraction and chart data*: Data from all the studies are extracted on a standardised form. Key variables usually include publication details, study objectives, methods, characteristics of participants and key findings. The data are then graphed to facilitate descriptive analysis and visualisation.
6. *Summarise and visualise the evidence base*: The information retrieved is put into tables, matrices or visual evidence maps. Not only does this provide a descriptive overview of the literature, but it also reveals the density, diversity and distribution of evidence. Gaps and under-researched topics can be easily spotted using this process.
7. *Prioritise and refine areas for further review*: Based on the findings of the mapping, specific themes, groups or intervention types can be selected for further investigation in a subsequent systematic review or other form of synthesis. Stakeholder or advisory group feedback can be used to inform the prioritisation process.
8. *Report the mapping exercise*: The mapping exercise approach and outcomes should be documented in an open and structured format. The report should include rationale, methods, results, and, research, policy and practice implications.

Good reporting ensures replicability and the utility of the mapping exercise for additional research.

By visually and descriptively mapping the landscape of existing research, mapping exercises guide future investigations, inform practice guidelines and support healthcare planning. In primary care, such methods can be particularly valuable for exploring areas such as preventive interventions, health education strategies or integrated care models where diverse evidence types and outcomes are expected.[5]

18.3 Gap-Mapping

Gap-mapping is a systematic and formal method to identify areas where evidence is abundant, scarce or entirely lacking in a specific field of research. It is a helpful way of informing research agendas, funding and policy development in the future. Unlike traditional ways of evidence synthesis that merely state what is known, gap-mapping also shows what is not known.[6,7]

18.3.1 Steps to Conduct Gap-Mapping

The following provides the key steps involved in performing gap-mapping:[6–8]

1. *Build a conceptual framework*: The first step is to build a clear conceptual framework that outlines the relevant domains to map, for example, intervention types, target groups, outcomes and settings.
2. *Build mapping questions*: Specific mapping questions would have to be constructed to drive the scope and direction of the exercise. Normally, these would be on interactions between outcomes and interventions or to identify underrepresented groups or contexts discovered in the available evidence base.
3. *Conduct a systematic literature search*: A systematic and exhaustive search needs to be conducted in electronic databases, grey literature databases and institutional websites of significance. Predefined inclusion and exclusion criteria must be applied to maintain transparency and reproducibility.
4. *Screen and select eligible studies*: All the retrieved records should be screened at both the title/abstract and full-text levels. The selection process must conform to the predetermined criteria, and dual independent screening is recommended to minimise bias and enhance inter-rater reliability.
5. *Extract and code study data*: For each study included, the relevant data must be extracted, such as population information, intervention categories, measured outcomes, study design and location. The extracted data must then be coded according to the pre-set framework.
6. *Construct the mapping matrix*: Coded data must be reformatted into a two-dimensional matrix, where one dimension is intervention categories and the other is outcome types. Each cell of the matrix must be evidence at that specific intersection and can also contain metadata such as number of studies or quality ratings.

7. *Analyse gaps and clusters:* The completed matrix should be scanned for areas with a concentration of evidence (clusters) and areas with little or no data (gaps). Cross-cutting themes of study geographic distribution, equity considerations or study quality can be incorporated into this analysis as well.
8. *Report and disseminate findings:* The final step involves the presentation of the findings both in narrative and visual formats. The gap map needs to be shared through reports, scholarly articles, policy briefs or interactive websites.

Stakeholder participation at the stage of dissemination is highly recommended to achieve maximum impact and highest applicability of the findings.

18.4 Scoping Reviews

A scoping review is a form of evidence synthesis whereby existing or emerging literature on a specific topic is systematically and iteratively searched and summarised.[5] Scoping reviews are particularly useful for clarifying key concepts, summarising research findings for stakeholders and knowledge users, assessing the feasibility of conducting a full systematic review, and identifying gaps within the existing body of evidence.[9]

18.4.1 Steps to Conduct Scoping Studies

Prior to conducting a scoping review, significant consideration must go into choosing a sufficient research team, since the reviews are a group effort and not an individual one. Ideally, a subject specialist and an individual who has previously conducted scoping reviews should be included.[9–12] Arksey and O'Malley's 2025 framework provides six steps to conduct scoping studies:[10]

1. *Defining the research question*: Formulating a focused research question is the crucial initial step in a scoping review. A research question that is too broad will result in an uncontrollably large volume of studies to review, potentially rendering the project impossible to conduct. A question that is too narrow may unnecessarily limit the scope and depth of the review. A number of sub-questions can be developed.
2. *Identifying relevant studies*: Engaging a librarian early in the process is essential for developing a solid search strategy, including selecting appropriate keywords, MeSH terms and databases. As the search progresses, the strategy may need to be refined based on the types of results retrieved. In addition, it is important to clearly establish inclusion and exclusion criteria.
3. *Study selection*: Digital tools are valuable resources for streamlining the organisation and screening of studies. After gathering citations from a database search, these can be imported into platforms through reference managers. Once relevant studies are selected, their citations can be exported back into the reference manager for further use. Most reference management tools also

include features such as duplicate detection, abstract similarity comparison and inclusion/exclusion decision tracking. Having additional reviewers will speed up review time, but calibration is required to maintain consistency. During the screening stage, both the title and abstract should be read. If the abstract is not available, the entire article has to be read. Using only titles is not accurate as they might not reflect the article's content. Following this step, the full text should be read of all selected papers.

4. *Charting the data*: The data extraction form is collaboratively constructed by the research team. Although the specific data fields are at the discretion of the research question and the general purpose of the review, typical categories are the author's name, year of publication, site of study, study population details, key findings, limitations cited in the study and recommended future research areas. Depending on the topic, additional tailored categories may be required to gain more information. Before full data extraction begins, the form should be pilot tested.
5. *Collating, summarising and reporting results*: Once the data extraction process is complete, the next task is conducting the numerical and thematic analyses. Numerical data are either tabulated or put into a visual presentation, aiming to highlight the key findings and indicate how these align with the initial reasons behind the review.

   For thematic analysis, qualitative data (typically word snippets from studies) are coded with keywords that capture their meaning. After initial coding is complete, the research team as a whole revises and refines the codes collaboratively. Refined codes are then brought together based on similarity, patterns or conceptual relationships, forming higher-level themes. Each theme is a recurring pattern or problem that emerges in multiple different studies and is inextricably linked to the original research questions. A reflexive and iterative approach ensures that themes are inductively derived from the data and interpreted meaningfully in the evidence base.
6. *Stakeholder consultation (recommended)*: Stakeholder input may also be utilised to explain the results of the review and to determine areas that have not previously been touched on within the literature.

Table 18.1 presents a comparison between mapping exercises, gap-mapping and scoping reviews.

18.5 Conclusion

In primary care, where decisions must often be made in the face of complexity and resource limitation, evidence synthesis methods such as scoping reviews, mapping exercises and gap-mapping offer systematic tools for understanding, organising and prioritising knowledge. Each tool has a specific function, from scoping out broad topics to formally identifying evidence gaps. Collectively, they facilitate more informed, more equitable and more strategic research, policy and practice. Combining these strategies with primary care research reinforces the ability to respond to today's challenges and shape future trends with accuracy and certainty.

TABLE 18.1 Comparison of Mapping Exercises, Gap-Mapping and Scoping Reviews

Feature	Mapping Exercises	Gap-Mapping	Scoping Reviews
Goal	To organise and categorise studies descriptively	To identify where evidence exists and where gaps remain	To explore the breadth and depth of existing evidence
Output examples	Narrative synthesis, summary tables (e.g., by target, population, intervention type)	Descriptive tables, charts, 2D evidence matrices (e.g., intervention vs. outcome), heat maps showing geographic or topical gaps	Thematic narrative synthesis; charts showing study types, frequency or year of publication; tables
Visual presentation	Sometimes used (e.g., frequency bar charts, descriptive tables thematic maps)	Frequently included (e.g., interactive gap matrices, color-coded grids by intervention/outcome)	Optional, but may include graphs (e.g., bubble plots, maps of study settings)
Quality appraisal	Optional	Often included or at least noted	Rarely performed
Systematic method	Yes	Yes	Yes
Stakeholder Input	Optional	Optional	Recommended for relevance and framework development
Stakeholder input	Optional	Recommended for relevance and framework development	Optional
Best use	For preparing a systematic review or understanding research spread	For guiding research priorities and funding decisions	For clarifying concepts, identifying scope of evidence
Visual presentation	Sometimes used	Frequently included	Not required
Level of Detail	Moderate to high	High (structured by dimensions eg population, outcome)	Moderate
Framework use	Based on classification schemes	Requires predefined conceptual framework	PCC (Population–Concept–Context)
Integration with reviews	Often used as a preliminary step to review	Used to inform review scoping, commissioning or policy	Can inform or be a standalone product

References

1. Bierman AS, Tong ST, McNellis RJ. Realizing the dream: The future of primary care research. *Ann Fam Med.* 2022 Mar–Apr;20(2):170–4. https://doi.org/10.1370/afm.2788
2. Campbell F, Tricco AC, Munn Z, Pollock D, Saran A, Sutton A, et al. Mapping reviews, scoping reviews, and evidence and gap maps (EGMs): The same but different—the "Big Picture" review family. *Syst Rev.* 2023;12:45. https://doi.org/10.1186/s13643-023-02178-5
3. Frampton GK, Harris P, Cooper K, et al. Educational interventions for preventing vascular catheter bloodstream infections in critical care: Evidence map, systematic review and

economic evaluation. Southampton, UK: NIHR Journals Library; 2014 Feb. (Health Technology Assessment, No. 18.15. Chapter 2, Methods for the mapping exercise and systematic review of clinical effectiveness. [Available from: https://www.ncbi.nlm.nih.gov/books/NBK263094/]

4. Mapping exercise toolkit. [Available from: https://www.girlguiding.org.uk/globalassets/docs-and-resources/growing-and-promoting-guiding/mappingtoolkit_2013.pdf]
5. Sutton A, O'Keefe H, Johnson EE, Marshall C. A mapping exercise using automated techniques to develop a search strategy to identify systematic review tools. *Res Synth Methods.* 2023 Nov;14(6):874–81. https://doi.org/10.1002/jrsm.1665
6. Saran A, White H. Evidence and gap maps: A comparison of different approaches. *Campbell Syst Rev.* 2018;4(1):1–38. https://doi.org/10.4073/cmdp.2018.2
7. White H, Albers B, Gaarder M, Kornør H, Littell J, Marshall Z, Mathew C, Pigott T, Snilstveit B, Waddington H, Welch V. Guidance for producing a Campbell evidence and gap map. *Campbell Syst Rev.* 2020 Nov 19;16(4):e1125. https://doi.org/10.1002/cl2.1125
8. Saran A, White H. Evidence and gap maps: A comparison of different approaches. *Campbell Syst Rev.* 2018;14:1–38. https://doi.org/10.4073/cmdp.2018.2
9. Mak S, Thomas A. Steps for conducting a scoping review. *J Grad Med Educ.* 2022 Oct;14(5):565–7. https://doi.org/10.4300/JGME-D-22-00621.1
10. Arksey H, O'Malley L. Scoping studies: Towards a methodological framework. *Int J Soc Res Methodol.* 2005;8(1):19–32. https://doi.org/10.1080/1364557032000119616
11. Peters MDJ, Marnie C, Tricco AC, et al. Updated methodological guidance for the conduct of scoping reviews. *JBI Evid Synth.* 2020;18(10):2119–26. https://doi.org/10.11124/jbies-20-00167
12. Levac D, Colquhoun H, O'Brien KK. Scoping studies: Advancing the methodology. *Implement Sci.* 2010;5:69. https://doi.org/10.1186/1748-5908-5-69

CHAPTER

19

Implementation Research in Primary Care

Lisa R Hirschhorn, Joseph B Ross and Robert J Havey

19.1 Introduction

Improving health through primary care (PC) has always been a challenge, but this has been increasingly facilitated by the wealth of evidence-based interventions found to reduce preventable mortality and morbidity. Many of these clinical and technological innovations are measurably improving the access and quality of PC services in diverse contexts. These solutions have the potential to enhance the performance and operational efficiency of PC systems, driving progress toward more person-centred, effective and high-quality care. However, as more of these proven interventions have become available, it has become clear that implementing these potentially life-saving interventions presents its own set of challenges.

Effective implementation of evidence-based intervention in any PC system requires an understanding of the strengths and weaknesses, interdependencies and relationships of the system's policies, capacities and functions to support the planning and successful integration of the intervention through feasible and appropriate strategies. There have been considerable gaps in how these proven interventions are implemented, resulting in missed opportunities to reduce suffering and reduce deaths.[1,2] Implementation research emerged from the recognition of the long delay between research-identified evidence-based interventions (EBIs) found to improve health and their implementation into PC practice. In the last decade, implementation research has increasingly been used to select and measure the effectiveness of strategies chosen to strengthen the delivery of these EBIs through PC as well as to support their adaptation, scale and sustainability.[3] In this chapter, we provide a brief introduction to implementation research and then provide some examples of how it has been used to help improve the implementation of EBIs into PC.

DOI: 10.1201/9781003652106-23

19.2 What Is Implementation Research?

19.2.1 Implementation Research

Quality improvement work focuses on improving the quality of care through local change, but the field of implementation research is designed to understand the challenges of implementation and create generalisable knowledge needed to accelerate the spread of important EBIs. This knowledge includes understanding barriers and facilitators, and using these insights to guide the design of strategies needed to address the challenges and leverage opportunities. Implementation research also focuses on important outcomes beyond EBI effectiveness, including whether people are using the EBI, using it correctly, and reaching the right people. When done well, implementation research can help researchers and PC providers understand and address challenges to implementation while creating the broader knowledge needed to spread lessons learned and adapt to new settings.[4]

Implementation research is defined as the "study of the use of strategies to adopt and integrate evidence-based health interventions into clinical and community settings to improve individual outcomes and benefit population health".[5] More simply, Curran describes the components of implementation research as focusing on the "thing" (the EBI) that we want people and places to do, the strategies being the "stuff" we do to help them do the "thing". Implementation outcomes are how well and how much they deliver the "thing" (Box 19.1). Other authors have also written articles that can serve as an excellent introduction, as well as free online training such as the World Health Organization (WHO) Special Program for Research and Training in Tropical Diseases.[6–8]

The field of implementation research uses models, theories and frameworks to help guide the design and conduct of research. These can be roughly grouped into three types: determinants, process and evaluation (Table 19.1). Determinants frameworks such as the Consolidated Framework for Implementation Research (CFIR), as

BOX 19.1 IMPLEMENTATION SCIENCE DEMYSTIFIED

- **The intervention/practice/innovation** is THE THING.
- **Effectiveness research** looks at whether THE THING works.
- **Implementation research** looks at how best to help people/places DO THE THING.
- **Implementation strategies** are what we do to help people/places DO THE THING.
- **Implementation outcomes** are HOW MUCH and HOW WELL they DO THE THING and if it works in real life.
- **Contextual factors** are what helps or hinders the implementation strategies and outcomes to get people or places to do the thing.

Adapted from Curran, 2020, *Implementation science made too simple.*[27]

well as others such as the Practical, Robust Implementation and Sustainability Model (PRISM) help identify the contextual factors (barriers and facilitators) to understand why an EBI has or has not been put into practice and where change is needed.[9] Evaluative models and frameworks are used to measure success through implementation outcomes and include Reach, Effectiveness, Adoption, Implementation, Maintenance (RE-AIM) and Proctor's outcomes. Finally, process models and frameworks can help guide you through the decisions on which EBIs are needed, adapting as needed and testing. For example, the Assessment, Decision, Adaptation, Production, Topical experts, Integration, Training and Testing (ADAPT-ITT) model, originally designed for HIV, takes you through a series of eight phases from the initial decision of what is needed (your EBI, adaptation and strategies) through testing.[10]

19.2.2 What Do We Mean by Context?

Context is the setting in which you are planning to implement. These can present barriers and facilitators (also called determinants) at multiple levels, the individuals who are

TABLE 19.1 Selected Theories, Frameworks and Models Used in Implementation Science

Type	Use	Examples	Some Resources
Determinant	Provides guidance and definition for understanding and measuring factors that may hinder or facilitate implementation and moderate implementation outcomes	Consolidated Framework for Implementation Research (CFIR 2.0); Practical, Robust Implementation and Sustainability Model (PRISM); Promoting Action on Research Implementation in Health Services (PAHRIS); socioecological model	CFIR Research Team-Center for Clinical Management Research. 2025[28] Unversity of Colorado Denver. 2025. 4 steps to complete The iPRISM Webtool[29] Bergstrom et al[30]
Process	Used to guide the process from context assessment to implementation and sustainability	Exploration, Preparation, Implementation, Sustainment (EPIS). ADAPT-ITT*	EPIS FRAMEWORK[31] Wingood and DiClemente[10]
Evaluative	Used to identify outcomes and to measure or evaluate the success of the work	RE-AIM Proctor Implementation Outcomes (2011)	RE-AIM[32] Proctor et al[33]

Adapted from L Damschroder, 2019, *Clarity out of chaos: Use of theory in implementation research*[34]
*ADAPT-ITT steps include:

- Assessment—identify barriers, facilitators and causes for the health outcome challenges
- Decision—select EBIs and whether to adopt or adapt
- Adaptation—adapt the EBI if needed based on contextual factors
- Production—create your plan for adaptation of EBI and strategies
- Topical experts—identify and provide needed mechanical assistance and expert inputs
- Integration—integrate the decisions and information
- Training—train all relevant implementers and stakeholders
- Testing—pilot test for effectiveness of the adaptation including implementation outcomes

expected to deliver the EBI and those targeted to receive it, the setting in which you are trying to implement, and the broader community, sub-national, national and even global settings. Multi-level analyses of contextual factors and mapping to relevant implementation strategies are particularly important within PHC systems and reflect the need to account for the interdependence between the individual provider, service delivery point (facility), community, subnational and national levels. For example, if you want to integrate the human papillomavirus (HPV) vaccine into PC, what are the attitudes of providers and targeted recipients? What is the infrastructure needed to stock and store the vaccine? What are the communities' attitudes toward the HPV vaccine? Will insurance and national policy support the costs and clinical standards?

As noted, one of the most common frameworks is the CFIR, which informs measurement in five domains (and a sixth one for low- and middle-income settings). The framework has a robust website that can help users understand how to measure these factors (www.CFIRGuide.org). In addition, work has been done to develop a tool to map from these factors to strategies, building from work to identify some best bets in approaches to address barriers (see later discussion). Other frameworks that may also be helpful include the socioecological model and PRISM.[9,11]

19.2.3 What Are Implementation Strategies?

Once you have identified your barriers and facilitators, you will need to map these to strategies that can help overcome barriers and leverage facilitators. For example, if the community does not know about or trust the HPV vaccine, then you might choose community engagement and education as a strategy. Researchers have developed a set of recommendations: Expert Recommendations for Implementation Change (ERIC). These are grouped into nine categories (see Box 19.2).[12] Often, more than one strategy is needed. For example, a strategy of only investing in resources or capacities alone is unlikely to achieve progress towards better PC outcomes. Instead, the interdependencies of primary health care (PHC) system components should be considered. For example, system resources such as the staff, supplies and space are managed through

BOX 19.2 NINE CATEGORIES OF STRATEGIES ADAPTED FROM EXPERT RECOMMENDATIONS FOR IMPLEMENTATION CHANGE (ERIC)[12]

1. Engage consumers
2. Develop stakeholder relationships
3. Use evaluative and iterative strategies
4. Utilise financial strategies
5. Change infrastructure
6. Support clinicians (or other providers)
7. Adapt and tailor to context
8. Provide interactive assistance
9. Train and educate stakeholders

TABLE 19.2 Selected Implementation Outcomes and Definitions

Implementation Outcome	Definition
Acceptability	Perception or option that an intervention is agreeable or satisfactory
Adoption	Uptake of an intervention by providers of the intervention
Appropriateness	The fit of an intervention to a particular context or setting
Cost	Resources (financial or otherwise) and effort needed to implement an intervention
Feasibility	The extent to which the intervention can be implemented
Fidelity	The match between how an intervention is intended to be delivered and how it is actually delivered
Reach/Penetration	The degree to which an intervention reaches the targeted population
Sustainability/Maintenance	The extent to which an intervention (or its effect) can be or is sustained over time. It can also be measured as the degree to which it becomes part of an organisation's everyday practice

Adapted in part from E Proctor, 2011. *Outcomes for implementation research: Conceptual distinctions, measurement challenges, and research agenda*[33]

system capacities, including monitoring, motivation and measurement of quality to achieve key PHC performance measures, including continuity, comprehensiveness, coordination, first-contact access and people-centredness.[13]

Once you choose your strategies, you need to define them. Imagine doing training, but each trainer does it differently (on different days, with different content, and different delivery processes and frequency). This would make it difficult to understand if and why training was effective (or not). Powell's guidance on defining strategies can help by guiding implementers to describe the key parts of a strategy (Table 19.2). However, even with all this work, you may need to adapt the strategy after you begin to put it into practice. This need is why it is important to monitor if strategies lead to the early changes you want (e.g., knowledge, attitudes, delivery) and, if not, how you need to change the strategies. There are very useful tools (FRAME-IS and LiST) that can help you track these changes and if they worked.[14]

19.2.4 Measuring Implementation Outcomes

In implementation research, you will want to know if your EBI is reaching the right people (reach or penetration), being delivered (adoption and feasibility) and being delivered correctly (fidelity), and that your strategies support maintenance of delivery over time (maintenance or sustainability). Definitions of some of the implementation outcomes are presented in Table 19.2. The two most common frameworks for guiding what to measure are RE-AIM (see also RE-AIM website) and Proctor's framework, which includes implementation outcomes as well as those related to health systems and clinical outcomes.[15,16] Understanding these outcomes is also

TABLE 19.3 Examples of Mapping from Barrier and Facilitator to Strategies and Outcomes

Barrier or Facilitator	Implementation Strategy	Mechanism	Implementation Outcome
Provider knowledge deficit	Education (provision of information)	Awareness-building, knowledge-acquisition	Feasibility, acceptability, appropriateness, adoption
Provider skill deficit	Training (teaching and practice with corrective feedback)	Skill acquisition, refinement, mastery	Fidelity to EBI
Turnover of staff	Train-the-trainer	Continuous on-site expertise available for consultation	Sustainability
Provider engagement	A clinical champion-led implementation team	Change the attitudes and motivation for Implementation	Feasibility, acceptability, appropriateness
Unstandardised clinical care options	Clinical guidelines	Clarity of clinical care	Fidelity

important to understand any drop in the expected population benefits. If there are problems with any of these outcomes, then the number of people, potentially the effectiveness at the individual level (if poor fidelity), and the population benefit will not be achieved. Implementation outcomes can also be measured for your strategies. For example, for training strategy: training the targeted providers (reach), training delivered correctly (fidelity), knowledge gained (effectiveness) and knowledge maintained over time (maintenance).

19.2.5 Putting It Together

Implementation science methods can help you map from a barrier or facilitator to a strategy, explain why you think it should work (mechanism) and the outcomes you expect to see. Some examples are shown in Table 19.3.

19.3 Using Implementation Research to Close Implementation Gaps to Improve Access and Quality of Primary Care Services

PHC system frameworks, such as the WHO/UNICEF Primary Health Care Measurement Framework and Indicators, can help navigate this complexity as they provide a theory of change for the critical inputs, processes and outputs that contribute to the delivery of PC services that drive better health outcomes.[17] These frameworks can help map the contextual factors that could be barriers or facilitators to any PC intervention. Additionally, tools to capture patient perspectives through the voice of the people being served, such as the People's Voice Survey and expansion of the use of patient-reported outcome measures, supplement more traditional technical quality measures with the lived experience of people accessing and using

PC and measuring outcomes that matter to them.[18] These frameworks and measurement resources provide ways to understand and measure contextual factors relevant to implementing EBIs into PHC.

One example where implementation research can help is in working to implement an integrated care model that centres on the individual rather than the disease. Barriers have included siloed funding, weak care delivery and supply chain systems. Integration as an overarching strategy can help break down traditional disease programme siloes, such as HIV, maternal and child health, and tuberculosis, at service delivery points to integrate more coordinated and comprehensive care (an important quality measure of PHC). For example, in Nigeria, implementation research was used to identify contextual factors and then choose and adapt strategies to guide the implementation of an integrated task-shifting strategy for integrating hypertension diagnosis and management into HIV clinics.[19]

Networks of care, also referred to as networks of practice in some countries, are being used to integrate PC services horizontally and vertically across service delivery points. These networks of care link community and PC service delivery points through data and patient management referral systems and protocols to guide where and how patients receive the care they need. For instance, the administration of a malaria test to a feverish child by a community health worker might require a referral to a local health clinic for more comprehensive management. If that child becomes more ill, they may be transferred to a PC centre or hospital for inpatient treatment.

Another example, from the Ghana Health Services, is a network of care model that links public and private community-based PC services, serving as "spokes," to Model Primary Health Centers, serving as referral "hubs", where acute inpatient and some specialist services are provided.[20]

Implementation research can support the rollout of networks of care by providing a structured approach to understand readiness challenges and identify suitable strategies to transition from the current model of care (see Table 19.4 for illustrative examples).

TABLE 19.4 How Implementation Research Can Support the Implementation of a Network of Care to Transform Vertical Services into Integrated People-Centred PC

Potential Barriers	Potential Strategies
Individual levels • Individual providers' lack of knowledge and skills • Poor quality of care (technical and experience)	• Guidelines and training • Supportive supervision • Engagement of community for accountability (e.g., community score cards)
Health systems • Inadequate human resources for health to delivery services • Cost of medications to patients • Availability of medication at service delivery points	• Task sharing • Change insurance policies and essential drug list • Strengthen integrated supply chain • Drug revolving fund • Engage stakeholders, including for advocacy
Networks of practice • Data and process to track individuals over time • Gaps in referral across health system levels	• Active empanelment • Linkage with CHWs for outreach and follow-up

Implementation success of networks of care can be measured by implementation outcomes both for the EBI and strategies. For example, for the EBI of basic emergency obstetric and newborn care (EmONC) delivery: appropriate women in care at the right level (reach), people receiving quality care at the appropriate level with dignity (adoption and acceptability), timely referral to higher levels of care (effectiveness) and reduced maternal and neonatal morbidity and mortality (effectiveness), and persistence of readiness to deliver EmONC (maintenance). Measuring outcomes of the strategies can help determine if they are being implemented. For example, for supportive supervision: supportive supervision occurring (reach), correctly (fidelity), and maintained over time. These implementation outcome measures can help us understand where strategies need to be adapted, added or stopped and provide generalisable insights to inform broader scale-up within Ghana and to other countries in the region interested in network of practice (NOP) implementation.

19.3.1 Using Implementation Research to Scale Solutions

Done well, implementation research can support the scale-up of EBI implementation by creating replicable learning on the process of planning, implementing, monitoring and scaling interventions to new settings. Particularly relevant for PC, implementation research underscores the importance of understanding the contextual factors and relevant strategies at multiple levels. Two projects to strengthen possible serious bacterial infection (PSBI) management amongst newborns when referral was not possible in Ethiopia and Kenya illustrate how implementation research can be used to address contextual similarities and differences through implementation strategies.[21]

During the COVID-19 pandemic (2020–2022), implementation research was used to understand contextual facilitators and barriers to improve the implementation of a possible serious bacterial infection (PSBI) treatment cascade in two projects in Ethiopia and Kenya. Within each country, the projects utilised determinant and evaluative frameworks (CIFR and RE-AIM, respectively) to identify barriers and facilitators and to develop strategies designed to address implementation challenges and measure targeted implementation outcomes, including reach, acceptability and fidelity to evidence-based PSBI treatment protocols when referral was not possible. Figure 19.1 shows how strategies targeted many of the determinants, providing an understanding of the mechanism by which they were thought to facilitate the targeted outcomes.

Some barriers and facilitators were common across both country projects, while some were unique to each. Understanding system and individual capacities at the national, local and provider levels informed the development of implementation strategies. Strategies were grouped into the WHO health system building blocks and organised according to the PSBI care cascade: identify and screen newborns for illness, diagnosis and treatment, correct treatment and adherence, follow-up and cure. Some strategies were developed to address barriers or leverage facilitators across multiple steps of the care cascade. For example, existing CHW cadres in both Ethiopia and Kenya could support the integration of PSBI management into existing primary care systems, and programme monitoring and data use infrastructure and procedures could support quality improvement efforts. Given weak surveillance across both

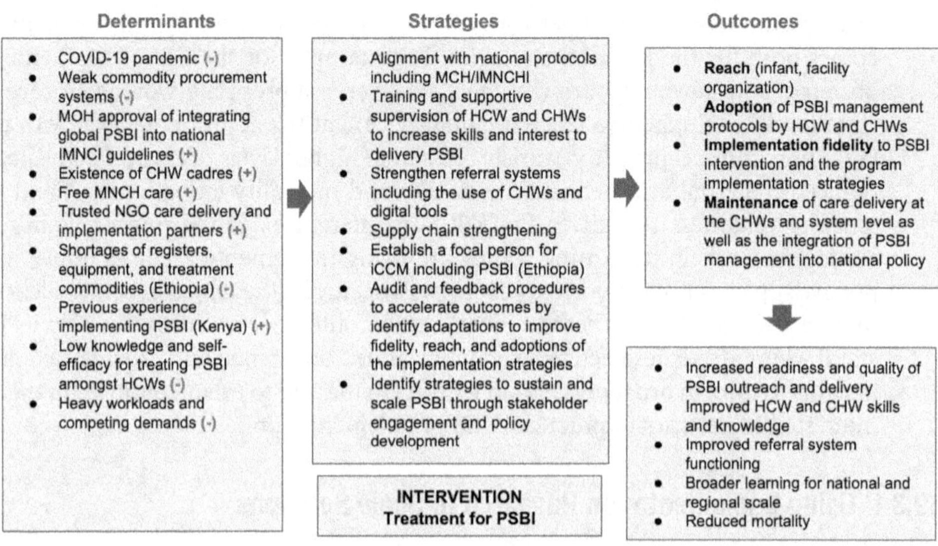

FIGURE 19.1 Implementation research logic model for projects in Ethiopia and Kenya. Possible serious bacterial illness (PSBI) access and delivery when referral is not possible

IMNCI: integrated management of maternal, newborn and child illness; HCW: healthcare worker; CHW: community health worker; MOH: Ministry of Health; MCH: maternal and child healthcare; NGO: non-governmental organisation; PSBI: possible serious bacterial infection; ICCM: integrated community case management. Adapted from Tiruneh et al[25] Reproduced with permission.

contexts, the projects developed specific strategies to improve the identification, screening and diagnosis of PSBI cases among newborns. This included the implementation of home visits to identify newborns with potential cases of sepsis for follow-up. Digital health data strategies were tailored to each context. In Kenya, digital data collection was used to support newborn identification and screening, and in Ethiopia it was used to support tracking of care (adherence) and follow-up.

Both projects identified challenges at multiple levels including the community (lack of belief in PSBI) and facility (availability of treatment medication, provider knowledge). These barriers were addressed by strategies at different levels, including community education, provider training, and better national commodity supply management, all informed by strong stakeholder engagement.

Another example of how implementation research supports the adaptation and implementation of EBIs across diverse settings is the spread of the WHO HEARTS technical package for cardiovascular disease management. In 2016, the WHO published the HEARTS technical package to improve cardiovascular care by implementing evidence-based, multi-level implementation strategies to improve hypertension treatment and control rates through health behaviours and pharmacotherapy at the PC level. The technical package is based on the Kaiser Permanente Northern California model of hypertension control and includes a number of strategies: (1) patient registration and empanelment (health system level), (2) standard treatment protocol (national policy level), (3) encouragement of fixed-dose combination therapy (health system level), (4) team-based care (health worker level) and (5) home blood pressure monitoring and health coaching (patient-level).[19]

Between 2017 and 2022, the WHO, the non-profit organisation Resolve to Save Lives, national governments and implementing partners designed, tested and scaled the HEARTS hypertension intervention in 32 low- and middle-income countries through the Global Heart Program, providing treatment to 12.2 million patients in 165,000 PC facilities.[22]

In Nigeria, where nearly one-third of non-communicable disease-related deaths are due to cardiovascular disease and the estimated prevalence of hypertension amongst adults ranges from 25% to 40%, the Global Hearts Program was implemented as part of the hypertension treatment in Nigeria in the Federal Capital Territory.[23] Understanding implementation barriers was critical, and started using the WHO Service Availability and Readiness Assessment (SARA) to measure facility readiness to diagnose, treat and manage hypertension and diabetes mellitus.[24] Additional qualitative assessment was done to understand provider and community knowledge, and attitudes towards hypertension care access and delivery in PC.[25] Using implementation research, the implementing strategies were designed or adapted with new ones, including supportive supervision to support task sharing and development of a drug revolving fund to address availability and cost of medications. To support sustainability and scale, advocacy at the national level was done to expand insurance coverage. The implementation was successful, with improvement in hypertension treatment, evidence of sustainability, and work underway to scale-up to additional states in the country.

19.3.2 How to Move Forward

There are a number of opportunities to better leverage implementation research to address gaps in PHC implementation and impact. There are important opportunities to learn from countries who have had better outcomes in PHC and PHC-delivered care to identify their implementation strategies adapted to their contexts.[26] Embedded implementation research can also help ensure that these methods can strengthen how programmes are planned, structured, financed and implemented.

For example, programme budgets should include support to integrate implementation research methods to strengthen adaptive learning and management and engage stakeholders in planning for sustainability and scale. To continue the important learning will also require continued building of robust capacity at country and regional levels where the work will be taking place. This work is especially important since local researchers often have the needed knowledge and perspective to identify and understand contextual factors and therefore are well suited to develop feasible, acceptable, effective implementation strategies.

19.4 Conclusion

PHC has the potential to save more lives, reduce suffering and serve as the core to deliver the EBIs needed to accelerate improvement in global health. Implementation science has the potential to help policymakers, implementers, clinicians and communities identify barriers that may prevent effective and equitable implementation of interventions proven to improve the health of individuals and communities. It is critical to continue to expand implementation research capacity building and work in universities, government institutions and for frontline providers to improve the effectiveness of healthcare and PHC systems throughout the world.

References

1. Kruk ME, Gage AD, Arsenault C, et al. High-quality health systems in the sustainable development goals era: Time for a revolution. *Lancet Glob Health.* 2018;6(11):e1196–e252. https://doi.org/10.1016/S2214-109X(18)30386-3
2. Jamison DT, Summers LH, Chang AY, et al. Glob health 2050: The path to halving premature death by mid-century. *Lancet.* 2024;404(10462):1561–614. https://doi.org/10.1016/S0140-6736(24)01439-9
3. Mash RNJ, Malan Z, Hirschhorn L. Understanding implementation research. *Afr J Prm Health Care Fam Med.* 2025;16(2):a4934. https://doi.org/10.4102/phcfm.v17i2.4934
4. Binagwaho A, Frisch MF, Udoh K, et al. Implementation research: An efficient and effective tool to accelerate universal health coverage. *Int J Health Policy Manag.* 2020;9(5):182–4. https://doi.org/10.15171/ijhpm.2019.125
5. National Institute of Health. PAR-19-274: Dissemination and implementation research in health (R01 clinical trial optional). 2019. [cited 1 Mar 2025; Available from: https://grants.nih.gov/grants/guide/pa-files/PAR-19-274.html]
6. Bauer MS, Damschroder L, Hagedorn H, et al. An introduction to implementation science for the non-specialist. *BMC Psychol.* 2015;3(1):32. https://doi.org/10.1186/s40359-015-0089-9
7. Peters DH, Adam T, Alonge O, et al. Implementation research: What it is and how to do it. *BMJ.* 2013;347:f6753. https://doi.org/10.1136/bmj.f6753
8. World Health Organization. Implementation research training materials. 2025. [cited 1 Mar 2025; Available from: https://tdr.who.int/home/our-work/strengthening-research-capacity/implementation-research-training-materials#:~:text=This%20provides%20an%20overview%20to,TDR%20supported%20regional%20training%20centres]
9. Feldstein AC, Glasgow RE. A practical, robust implementation and sustainability model (PRISM) for integrating research findings into practice. *Jt Comm J Qual Patient Saf.* 2008;34(4):228–43. https://doi.org/10.1016/s1553-7250(08)34030-6
10. Wingood GM, DiClemente RJ. The ADAPT-ITT model: A novel method of adapting evidence-based HIV Interventions. *J Acquir Immune Defic Syndr.* 2008;47(Suppl 1):S40–6. https://doi.org/10.1097/QAI.0b013e3181605df1
11. Lee BC, Bendixsen C, Liebman AK, et al. Using the socio-ecological model to frame agricultural safety and health interventions. *J Agromedicine.* 2017;22(4):298–303. https://doi.org/10.1080/1059924X.2017.1356780
12. Powell BJ, Waltz TJ, Chinman MJ, et al. A refined compilation of implementation strategies: Results from the Expert Recommendations for Implementing Change (ERIC) project. *Implement Sci.* 2015;10:21. https://doi.org/10.1186/s13012-015-0209-1.
13. Bitton A, Veillard JH, Basu L, et al. The 5S-5M-5C schematic: Transforming primary care inputs to outcomes in low-income and middle-income countries. *BMJ Glob Health.* 2018;3(Suppl 3):e001020. https://doi.org/10.1136/bmjgh-2018-001020
14. Miller CJ, Barnett ML, Baumann AA, et al. The FRAME-IS: A framework for documenting modifications to implementation strategies in healthcare. *Implement Sci.* 2021;16(1):36. https://doi.org/10.1186/s13012-021-01105-3
15. Glasgow RE, Harden SM, Gaglio B, et al. RE-AIM planning and evaluation framework: Adapting to new science and practice with a 20-year review. *Front Public Health.* 2019;7:64. https://doi.org/10.3389/fpubh.2019.00064

16. Proctor EK, Landsverk J, Aarons G, et al. Implementation research in mental health services: An emerging science with conceptual, methodological, and training challenges. *Adm Policy Ment Health*. 2009;36(1):24–34. https://doi.org/10.1007/s10488-008-0197-4
17. World Health Organization & United Nations Children's Fund. Primary health care measurement framework and indicators: Monitoring health systems through a primary health care lens. 2022. [Available from: https://www.who.int/publications/i/item/9789240044210]
18. Kruk ME, Lewis TP. Introduction to the Lancet global health's series on the people's voice survey on health system performance. *Lancet Glob Health*. 2024;12(1):e14–e15. https://doi.org/10.1016/S2214-109X(23)00512-0
19. Iwelunmor J, Ezechi O, Obiezu-Umeh C, et al. Factors influencing the integration of evidence-based task-strengthening strategies for hypertension control within HIV clinics in Nigeria. *Implement Sci Commun*. 2022;3(1):43. https://doi.org/10.1186/s43058-022-00289-z
20. Ghana Health Service. Implementation guidelines for networks of practice–2024. p. 75. [Available from: https://p4h.world/app/uploads/2024/07/NoP-Implementation-Guidelines-GHS-FINAL-24-Launched.x69485.pdf]
21. Tiruneh GT, Odwe G, Kamberos AH, et al. Optimizing integration of community-based management of possible serious bacterial infection (PSBI) in young infants into primary healthcare systems in Ethiopia and Kenya: Successes and challenges. *BMC Health Serv Res*. 2024;24(1):280. https://doi.org/10.1186/s12913-024-10679-9
22. Moran AE, Gupta R, Global hearts initiative C: Implementation of global hearts hypertension control programs in 32 low- and middle-income countries: JACC international. *J Am Coll Cardiol*. 2023;82(19):1868–84. https://doi.org/10.1016/j.jacc.2023.08.043
23. Baldridge AS, Orji IA, Shedul GL, et al. Enhancing hypertension education of community health extension workers in Nigeria's federal capital territory: The impact of the extension for community healthcare outcomes model on primary care, a quasi-experimental study. *BMC Prim Care*. 2024;25(1):334. https://doi.org/10.1186/s12875-024-02579-y
24. Orji IA, Baldridge AS, Omitiran K, et al. Capacity and site readiness for hypertension control program implementation in the Federal Capital Territory of Nigeria: A cross-sectional study. *BMC Health Serv Res*. 2021;21(1):322. https://doi.org/10.1186/s12913-021-06320-8
25. Okoli RCB, Shedul G, Hirschhorn LR, et al. Stakeholder perspectives to inform adaptation of a hypertension treatment program in primary healthcare centers in the Federal Capital Territory, Nigeria: A qualitative study. *Implement Sci Commun*. 2021;2(1):97. https://doi.org/10.1186/s43058-021-00197-8
26. Peterson SS. Embedded implementation research in programming at scale—the new normal to be! *BMC Pediatr*. 2024;23(Suppl 1):650. https://doi.org/10.1186/s12887-023-04470-8
27. Curran GM. Implementation science made too simple: A teaching tool. *Implement Sci Commun*. 2020;1:27. https://doi.org/10.1186/s43058-020-00001-z
28. CFIR Research Team-Center for Clinical Management Research. Consolidated Framework for Implementation Research (CFIR). 2025. [Available from: https://cfirguide.org/]
29. University of Denver Colorado. 4 steps to complete the iPRISM webtool. 2025. [cited 3 Apr 2025; Available from: https://prismtool.org/]
30. Bergstrom A, Ehrenberg A, Eldh AC, et al. The use of the PARIHS framework in implementation research and practice-a citation analysis of the literature. *Implement Sci*. 2020;15(1):68. https://doi.org/10.1186/s13012-020-01003-0
31. EPIS Framework. The EPIS implementation framework. [cited 1 Feb 2025; Available from: https://episframework.com/]
32. RE-AIM. [cited 1 Feb 2025; Available from: https://re-aim.org/]
33. Proctor E, Silmere H, Raghavan R, et al. Outcomes for implementation research: Conceptual distinctions, measurement challenges, and research agenda. *Adm Policy Ment Health*. 2011;38(2):65–76. https://doi.org/10.1007/s10488-010-0319-7
34. Damschroder LJ. Clarity out of chaos: Use of theory in implementation research. *Psychiatry Res*. 2020;283:112461. https://doi.org/10.1016/j.psychres.2019.06.036

CHAPTER

20

Patient-Centred Approaches to Primary Care Research

Patient and Public Involvement and Patient-Reported Measurement

Jose M Valderas and Candan Kendir

20.1 Introduction

Clinical practice, as well as health policy, has long recognised the merits of placing patients at the centre of the system and decision-making.[1,2] In research, the values of patients, alongside their first-hand experience and knowledge, provide unique information for identifying priorities, improving its quality and enhancing its relevance, actionability and impact. The vision for a shift from research 'on' or 'about' patients to doing it 'with' (or even 'by') patients has gradually emerged over the past years, albeit most of the progress has centred around establishing appropriate methods.[3]

Primary care provides extraordinary opportunities for anchoring patient-centred research approaches in clinical settings. It is the natural gateway for access to health services (first contact) for a broad range of health needs regardless of age, gender, condition (comprehensiveness) and, in particular, it has a focus on developing long-term relationships (continuity).[4] The adoption of patient-centred approaches in primary care research can therefore not just enhance research conduct and translation of findings to primary care itself, but it can also catalyse its extension to all other parts of the healthcare system.[5] Adoption of patient-centred approaches is, unfortunately, not part of standard practice in primary care research yet.

With the aim of accelerating the incorporation of patient-centred approaches in primary care research, this chapter reviews the concept, need and approaches to patient-centred research in the context of primary care. While doing that, it also provides actionable tools and empirical study examples for co-developing research with patient and public involvement and using patient-reported measurements for assessing their own health and healthcare delivery.

DOI: 10.1201/9781003652106-24

20.2 Understanding Patient-Centred Research

Patient-centred care is responsive to patients' values, needs and preferences.[1,6] A similar approach to research can ensure that research is aligned with the principles of the care it aims to inform. In patient-centred research, decision-making is thus guided by values, preferences, first-hand knowledge and experiences of people. It entails active, meaningful and collaborative participation of people across all stages of the research pathway, from identification of research questions and study design all the way to dissemination and implementation of findings.

Patient-centred approaches help identify priorities from people's perspectives, ensure relevance to their values and needs, and increase uptake and use of research findings in practice. They also serve as a means to enhance patient engagement in their own care, build trust between patient and researcher, address patients' preferences and promote better outcomes. Such approaches can also promote participation of patients in research and encourage ethical research practices that prioritise patient welfare.

A patient-centred approach to primary care research requires consideration of the core functions of primary care: first point of contact, coordinated, comprehensive and continuous.[4] It also ensures contextual relevance to primary care settings where diversity and social context are important. By combining user knowledge and experience with community needs and service realities, a patient-centred approach can produce results that are more likely to be used by and in primary care practices.

Patient-centredness in primary care research can be achieved through different approaches. In this chapter, we will detail two specific approaches to operationalise and ensure patient-centredness in primary care research of particular relevance. The first focuses on a generic approach to research in which patients participate in research as team members with varying degrees of roles and responsibilities. The second details a specific approach through which patients contribute to the assessment of interventions and delivery of primary care.

20.3 Implementing Patient and Public Involvement

Patient and public involvement (PPI) ideally starts early and takes place throughout the research pathway, from design to dissemination and implementation of findings. In such an approach, patients' insights can shape study objectives, design and methods to ensure appropriateness and applicability. Varying terms have been used in the literature to define such participation and the level of participation.[7] Those most used are PPI, patient engagement, participation or involvement, co-creation or co-development. In this chapter, we will adopt PPI to refer to the participation of people in primary care research with varying degrees of participation levels. The level of participation may vary from co-development, through shared decision-making, to informational activities focused on awareness-raising (Table 20.1).

TABLE 20.1 Framework for Different Levels of Patient and Public Involvement in Research

Level (From Most Engaged to Least Engaged)	Descriptor	Characteristic	Example Practices
Co-develop/Co-lead	Equity in governance, shared power	People with lived experience co-lead governance, strategy and dissemination. Decision-making is shared.	Patient-led research agendas, funded co-public involvement grants, co-leading work packages, participatory research
Involve/Collaborate	Structured contribution	Partners influence specific aspects (eg question setting) but within pre-defined roles.	Advisory panels, review panels
Consult	Occasional input	Feedback is sought but not integrated systematically. Decision-making remains researcher-led.	Surveys, focus groups, public consultations
Inform	Awareness raising	One-way information flow. People are *subjects* of outreach, not partners.	Factsheets, newsletters, websites, information leaflets

Several frameworks and guides have been developed to provide structural support for PPI in research.[3,8,9] Guidance from national institutions is also provided in some countries (Table 20.2). For example, the UK Standards for Public Involvement provide a framework for researchers, detailing good engagement practices with standards and putting the standards into practice. The Canadian Institutes of Health Research similarly provides a framework establishing key concepts, principles and areas for PPI. The Patient-Centered Outcomes Research Institute (PCORI) in the United States offers foundational expectations for meaningful engagement and provides templates, rubrics and tools to operationalise it. Some international organisations also support patient engagement in research by addressing key areas, such as the Professional Society for Health Economics and Outcomes Research (ISPOR)'s Patient-Centred Special Interest Group, which provides a common definition for patient engagement in research.[7]

PPI begins at the design stage of research and requires adequate support and resourcing. Financial support such as honoraria, travel reimbursement and compensation for time helps remove participation barriers. Equally important, non-financial support includes flexible scheduling, administrative support and accessible information. The research team should plan for these resources and include them in funding applications, staff planning and timelines.

Recruitment should include a broad and diverse group of PPI participants with relevant background and lived experiences. This means actively reaching out to people with varied experiences, including under-represented groups. Clear roles and responsibilities should be defined and shared early in the process to develop a common understanding and establish trust. Patient and civil society organisations can support identifying and reaching out to relevant participants. Once PPI are established, appropriate training should take place from basic research literacy to specific

TABLE 20.2 Leading PPI Initiatives in Different Countries

Country	National Framework	Mandated in Grants	Patient Governance Role	Support Structures
United Kingdom	NIHR INVOLVE	Yes	Strong (including ethics)	Extensive (Applied Research Collaborations, toolkits)
Canada	SPOR	Yes	Yes (co-leads in governance)	SUPPORT Units
Australia	NHMRC State-level	Growing	Yes (varies by state)	Consumer programmes
Netherlands	ZonMw Federatie	Often	Moderate to strong	Patient networks
United States	PCORI	Yes	Yes (patients on panels)	PCORI Engagement Team

NIHR: National Institute for Health and Care Research; SPOR: Strategy for Patient-Oriented Research; CIHR: Canadian Institutes of Health Research; NHMRC: The National Health and Medical Research Council; ZonMw: Netherlands Organisation for Health Research and Development; PCORI: Patient-Centred Outcomes Research Institute

research methods, depending on the research. In addition to research training, equipping researchers with communication as well as facilitation skills can foster reciprocal learning and meaningful engagement.

Some organisations provide publicly available courses to train researchers and partners on how to ensure meaningful PPI in health research. One example is the Canadian Institutes of Health Research's (CIHR) Institute of Musculoskeletal Health and Arthritis (IMHA), which developed a set of online, self-directed, free modules applicable to any research where PPI take place.

Research funders and journals increasingly require reporting on PPI, although this is usually addressed in a standard text with minimal detail. For more advanced and transparent reporting, tools such as the GRIPP2 reporting checklist offer structured templates detailing about the aims, methods, outcomes and reflections on PPI.[10] While improving advanced learning, such tools also encourage transparency and further develop respect and trust.

Central to all PPI is building a relationship of trust, respect and transparency. Using participatory techniques such as co-design workshops and storytelling enhance engagement and amplifies perspectives that otherwise might not be heard. Meaningful engagement, built on a relationship of trust, is iterative and relational. That's why primary care provides extraordinary opportunities to cultivate this relationship and support mutual growth. Recognition of contributions is also equally important to build a relationship of trust and be equitable. Such recognition could take the form of publication authorship, acknowledgement in presentations and opportunities to (co-)present the research.

Despite growing interest and support for PPI, several challenges exist.[5,11,12] Poor planning usually leads to quick, reactive and superficial engagement activities, limiting participation. Implementing PPI is resource intensive, requiring time, financial resources and flexibility. Even if these are planned in the initial research funding opportunity, sustainability is rarely established, with most funding opportunities being episodic and time-limited. Such episodic funding also hampers building and maintaining a relationship of trust over time, leading to inefficiencies with each research project starting from the beginning. In addition, communication issues due to unclear purposes, roles, structures, inadequate training (ie lack of experience) and inaccessible language create frustration and hamper meaningful PPI.

Effective and meaningful PPI requires thoughtful planning of support and resources, inclusive and diverse recruitment, appropriate training covering both research and communication skills, transparent reporting and a respectful relationship of trust. Aligning funding, legal frameworks, data systems and institutional support is crucial for the implementation and maintenance.

20.4 Implementing Patient-Centred Measurement

One particularly interesting approach to operationalising patient-centredness is through the routine use of patient-reported information about their health and healthcare. When systematically collected using standardised questionnaires, these data are referred to as patient-reported outcome measures (PROMs) and patient-reported experience measures (PREMs). As illustrated in Boxes 20.1 and 20.2,

BOX 20.1 SUCCESSFUL INTEGRATION OF PROMS AND PREMS

Heart Failure Pathway Pilot in Tuscany, Italy

A well-documented case of integrating both patient-reported outcome measures (PROMs) and patient-reported experience measures (PREMs) in a primary care context is the heart failure pathway pilot study conducted in Tuscany, Italy. This study specifically set out to collect and analyse both PROMs and PREMs along the care continuum, including primary care, to gain a comprehensive understanding of patient health outcomes and care experiences.

The study was conducted across the care pathway for heart failure patients, involving both primary care and hospital settings. Data collection points included after hospital discharge and during follow-up in the community, where primary care providers played a central role. Results were shared with general practitioners, nurses, cardiologists and health system managers, fostering a multidisciplinary approach to care improvement.

PROMs: The Kansas City Cardiomyopathy Questionnaire (KCCQ-12) (patient-perceived health outcomes related to heart failure).

PREMs: A tailored experience questionnaire was developed in collaboration with primary care professionals and cardiologists to capture patient experiences at different points along the care pathway.

Data from PREMs illuminated aspects of the care process that could explain variations in PROMs, helping teams identify and address discontinuities in care.

This Tuscany heart failure pathway pilot is a clear example of how PROMs and PREMs can be successfully integrated into primary care to inform clinical practice, support quality improvement and enhance care integration from the patient's perspective. The study demonstrates feasibility, value and actionable insights when both types of patient-reported measures are used together in routine primary care settings.[33,34]

BOX 20.2 THE OECD'S PATIENT-REPORTED INDICATOR SURVEYS (PARIS)

The OECD's patient-reported indicator surveys (PaRIS) initiative measures health outcomes and healthcare experiences that matter to people. PaRIS aims to fill a critical gap in primary healthcare, by asking about aspects such as physical functioning, psychological well-being, experiences of healthcare and self-management support. Participating countries collaborate in the development, standardisation and implementation of indicators.

Both patient and primary care practice questionnaires, created based on the PaRIS conceptual framework, were developed and piloted through extensive collaboration with patients, healthcare professionals, academics and policymakers to ensure relevance and comparability across countries. The survey captures health outcomes and experiences of primary and ambulatory care patients aged 45 and older who visited their primary care practice in the past six months.

A first iteration of the survey in 19 countries across three continents revealed significant variations in patient-reported outcomes and experiences across countries.[24] Although some countries excel in patient-centred care through self-management support, better care coordination and communication, others struggle with providing effective care to those living with chronic conditions. The data highlight the added value of collecting and using patient-reported measurements to identify areas where actions are needed and drive improvements in quality and efficiency.

PaRIS, designed as a series of systematic cross-sectional surveys conducted every five years, uses patient-reported measurements to assess the performance of healthcare systems in primary care. The next iteration is currently underway with an expansion to additional countries and optimisation of its delivery and performance.[35]

PROMs and PREMs are powerful tools for informing various aspects of care: they can guide shared decision-making in clinical encounters, support self-management, monitor and evaluate healthcare performance, and even inform value-based payment models.

PROMs capture how patients evaluate their symptoms, functioning and overall health status. In the classical Donabedian model, they are considered outcomes of care. PROMs can be generic—such as the Patient-Reported Outcomes Measurement Information System-10 (PROMIS-10), WHO-5 Well-Being Index, Medical Outcomes Study Short Form 36 (SF-36) or EuroQol (EQ-5D)—or specific to populations (eg KIDSCREEN, a health-related quality of life questionnaire for children and young people), diseases (eg Patient Health Questionnaire [PHQ] for depression) or concepts (eg Brief Pain Inventory).[13–19] Some PROMs allow a high degree of individualisation, such as the Schedule for the Evaluation of Individual Quality of Life (SEIQoL).[20] Generic measures are especially useful in primary care as they capture holistic outcomes aligned with whole-person care. Specific measures are better suited for research on particular conditions or patient subgroups. PREMs, in contrast, assess patients' experiences with the care they receive. In the context of primary care, PREMs often evaluate core functions such as accessibility, continuity, communication, coordination and patient-centredness—either directly or through indicators such as waiting times or satisfaction with information provided. Prominent examples include the General Practice Patient Survey (GPPS) in the UK and the OECD PaRIS Patient Questionnaire (PaRIS-PQ), both of which provide structured insights into patients' lived experiences in primary care settings.[21,22]

It is increasingly common to use PROMs and PREMs in tandem, either as part of integrated instruments—such as the Patient-Reported Experiences and Outcomes of Safety in Primary Care (PREOS-PC)—or through the coordinated use of separate tools.[23] The OECD's PaRIS initiative exemplifies how international organisations are using both PROMs and PREMs to benchmark healthcare system performance across countries and strengthen patient-centred care globally (Figure 20.1).[24]

Numerous resources and repositories support the identification and application of PROMs and PREMs. These include the Patient-Reported Outcome and Quality of Life Instruments Database (PROQOLID), which catalogues validated instruments across health conditions, and the International Consortium for Health Outcomes Measurement (ICHOM), which promotes standardised outcome sets.[25–27] Local experiences, such as institutional implementation and academic research in primary care settings, also contribute valuable evidence.

Choosing the right instrument requires careful evaluation of its psychometric properties:

- *Validity*: whether an instrument measures what it is intended to. This includes content validity (relevance of items), construct validity (alignment with theoretical expectations) and criterion validity (correlation with established measures).
- *Reliability*: consistency of results across time or observers. Test-retest reliability, internal consistency and inter-rater reliability are commonly assessed.
- *Sensitivity to change*: ability of a measure to detect meaningful changes over time—critical for evaluating treatment impact.

Several systems have been developed to support the evaluation of measurement tools. Evaluating the Measurement of Patient-Reported Outcomes (EMPRO) and Consensus-based Standards for the selection of health Measurement Instruments (COSMIN) provide structured criteria for appraising the quality and applicability of PROMs and PREMs.[28,29]

Instrument development typically begins with gathering content from relevant sources—patients, healthcare professionals and existing literature—followed by drafting items, piloting the questionnaire and performing psychometric evaluation. Interpretation of scores can be informed by established norms, minimally important differences or content-based thresholds.

To ensure transparency and quality in research involving PROMs and PREMs, reporting guidelines such as the CONSORT extension for PROs provide structured

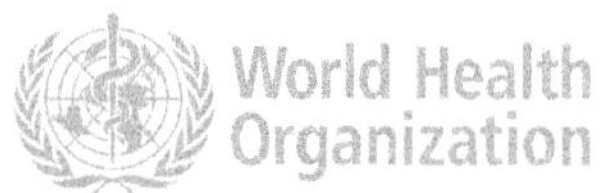

The World Health Organization-Five Well-Being Index (WHO-5)

Please indicate for each of the five statements which is closest to how you have been feeling over the last two weeks. Notice that higher numbers mean better well-being.

Example. If you have felt cheerful and in good spirits more than half of the time during the last two weeks, select number three.

		All of the time	Most of the time	More than half of the time	Less than half of the time	Some of the time	At no time
1	**I have felt cheerful and in good spirits**	5	4	3	2	1	0
2	**I have felt calm and relaxed**	5	4	3	2	1	0
3	**I have felt active and vigorous**	5	4	3	2	1	0
4	**I woke up feeling fresh and rested**	5	4	3	2	1	0
5	**My daily life has been filled with things that interest me**	5	4	3	2	1	0

FIGURE 20.1 Reproduction of WHO-5 Well-Being Index

recommendations for trial reporting. Other guidelines support observational studies and instrument development.

Despite the promise of PROMs and PREMs, several challenges remain. These include integrating them into routine workflows, ensuring representativeness in responses and building capacity for data collection and interpretation. Solutions include investments in data collection systems, ongoing training and capacity building, and international standardisation of instruments and domains. By embedding PROMs and PREMs into the fabric of healthcare systems, particularly in primary care, we can operationalise a more patient-centred, accountable and responsive model of care.

The future of patient-centred research in primary care focuses on both scaling and sustaining meaningful PPI and leveraging digital innovations for standardised measurement. Wider adoption of formal frameworks as mandatory practices with dedicated funding and training programmes is underway in numerous countries. Sustainability of PPI efforts through fostering long-term community partnerships and creating supportive funding opportunities are also likely developments. Mobile apps, wearables and AI-driven solutions will enable real-time collection, interpretation and feedback of PROMs/PREMs to patients and their healthcare professionals. Incorporating appropriate training in patient-centred research into undergraduate and postgraduate curricula, as well as continuing professional development, will enhance knowledge and encourage action based on the results. Although many of the most widely used tools are based on standard forms that were developed using Classical Test Theory, newer approaches to measurement have emerged. Methodological developments based on Item Response Theory (including Rasch Analysis) have allowed the development of robust banks of items with electronic administration. Computerised adaptive testing (CAT) allows a targeted administration that selects the most informative items based on the previous responses, thereby significantly shortening administration burden while retaining high levels of reliability.[30] The Patient-Reported Outcomes Measurement Information System (PROMIS) is one such system.[31] Adaptive approaches that extend CAT logic by incorporating item characteristics related to applicability, desirability and relevance can further personalise questionnaire content, thereby improving engagement and data quality.[32]

20.5 Conclusion

Incorporating patient-centred approaches into primary care research is both a necessary and transformative step towards ensuring that research is relevant, ethical and impactful. Through meaningful patient and public involvement and the systematic use of patient-reported measures, research can more effectively reflect real-world needs, values and experiences. These approaches enhance the quality and applicability of findings, foster trust and promote uptake in practice. As this chapter has outlined, tools, frameworks and strategies exist to support this transition. The challenge now lies in their sustained, thoughtful implementation to truly embed the patient voice at the heart of primary care research.

References

1. Mead N, Bower P. Patient-centredness: A conceptual framework and review of the empirical literature. *Soc Sci Med*. 2000;51(7):1087–1100.
2. Organisation for Economic Co-operation and Development (OECD). Health for the people, by the people: Building people-centred health systems. OECD Health Policy Studies. Paris: OECD Publishing; 2021. [cited 4 Jul 2025; Available from: https://doi.org/10.1787/c259e79a-en]
3. Kirwan JR, de Wit M, Frank L, et al. Emerging guidelines for patient engagement in research. *Value Health*. 2017;20(3):481–6.
4. World Health Organization, United Nations Children's Fund (UNICEF). A vision for primary health care in the 21st century: Towards universal health coverage and the Sustainable Development Goals. Geneva: WHO; 2018.
5. Béland S, Lambert M, Delahunty-Pike A, et al. Patient and researcher experiences of patient engagement in primary care health care research: A participatory qualitative study. *Health Expect*. 2022;25(5):2365–76.
6. Berntsen G. Person-centred care systems: From theory to practice [Internet]. Dublin: ISQua; 2022. [cited 4 Jul 2025; Available from: https://isqua.org/media/attachments/2022/10/03/person-centred-care-systems_-from-theory-to-practice.pdf]
7. Harrington RL, Hanna ML, Oehrlein EM, et al. Defining patient engagement in research: Results of a systematic review and analysis: Report of the ISPOR Patient-Centered Special Interest Group. *Value Health*. 2020;23(6):677–88.
8. Greenhalgh T, Hinton L, Finlay T, et al. Frameworks for supporting patient and public involvement in research: Systematic review and co-design pilot. *Health Expect*. 2019; 22(4):785–801.
9. Chudyk AM, Horrill T, Waldman C, et al. Scoping review of models and frameworks of patient engagement in health services research. *BMJ Open*. 2022;12(8):e063507.
10. Staniszewska S, Brett J, Simera I, et al. GRIPP2 reporting checklists: Tools to improve reporting of patient and public involvement in research. *BMJ*. 2017;358:j3453.
11. Gonzalez M, Ogourtsova T, Zerbo A, et al. Patient engagement in a national research network: Barriers, facilitators, and impacts. *Res Involv Engagem*. 2023;9(1).
12. Heckert A, Forsythe LP, Carman KL, et al. Researchers, patients, and other stakeholders' perspectives on challenges to and strategies for engagement. *Res Involv Engagem*. 2020;6(1).
13. Hays RD, Bjorner JB, Revicki DA, et al. Development of physical and mental health summary scores from the patient-reported outcomes measurement information system (PROMIS) global items. *Qual Life Res*. 2009;18(7):873–80. https://doi.org/10.1007/s11136-009-9496-9
14. Topp CW, Østergaard SD, Søndergaard S, et al. The WHO-5 well-being index: A systematic review of the literature. *Psychother Psychosom*. 2015;84(3):167–76. https://doi.org/10.1159/000376585
15. Ware JE Jr, Sherbourne CD. The MOS 36-item short-form health survey (SF-36): I. Conceptual framework and item selection. *Med Care*. 1992;30(6):473–83.
16. EuroQol Group. EuroQol: A new facility for the measurement of health-related quality of life. *Health Policy*. 1990;16(3):199–208. https://doi.org/10.1016/0168-8510(90)90421-9
17. Ravens-Sieberer U, Gosch A, Rajmil L, et al. KIDSCREEN-52 quality-of-life measure for children and adolescents. *Expert Rev Pharmacoecon Outcomes Res*. 2005;5(3):353–64. https://doi.org/10.1586/14737167.5.3.353
18. Kroenke K, Spitzer RL, Williams JB. The PHQ-9: Validity of a brief depression severity measure. *J Gen Intern Med*. 2001;16(9):606–13. https://doi.org/10.1046/j.1525-1497.2001.016009606.x
19. Cleeland CS, Ryan KM. Pain assessment: Global use of the brief pain inventory. *Ann Acad Med Singap*. 1994;23(2):129–38.

20. O'Boyle CA, McGee H, Hickey A, et al. Individual quality of life in patients undergoing hip replacement. *Lancet*. 1992;339(8801):1088–91. https://doi.org/10.1016/0140-6736(92)90673-q
21. NHS England. GP patient survey 2025 questionnaire [Internet]. London: NHS England; 2024. [cited 6 Jun 2024; Available from: https://gp-patient.co.uk/downloads/2025/qandletter/GPPS_2025_Questionnaire_PUBLIC.pdf]
22. Organisation for Economic Co-operation and Development (OECD). PaRIS patient questionnaire [Internet]. Paris: OECD. [cited 6 Jun 2024; Available from: https://www.oecd.org/content/dam/oecd/en/about/programmes/patient-reported-indicator-surveys/PaRIS%20patient%20questionnaire.pdf]
23. Ricci-Cabello I, Avery AJ, Reeves D, et al. Measuring patient safety in primary care: The development and validation of the 'Patient Reported Experiences and Outcomes of Safety in Primary Care' (PREOS-PC). *Ann Fam Med*. 2016;14(3):253–61.
24. OECD. Does healthcare deliver? Results from the Patient-Reported Indicator Surveys (PaRIS). OECD Health Policy Studies. Paris: OECD Publishing; 2025. [cited 4 Jul 2025; Available from: https://doi.org/10.1787/c8af05a5-en].
25. MAPi Trust. About PROQOLID. Lyon: MAPi Trust. [cited 6 Jun 2024; Available from: https://eprovide.mapi-trust.org/about/about-proqolid]
26. International Consortium for Health Outcomes Measurement (ICHOM). Home. Boston: ICHOM. [cited 6 Jun 2024; Available from: https://www.ichom.org]
27. Gangannagaripalli J, Albagli A, Myers SN, et al. A standard set of value-based patient-centered outcomes and measures of overall health in adults. *Patient*. 2022;15(3):341–51. https://doi.org/10.1007/s40271-021-00554-8
28. Valderas JM, Ferrer M, Mendívil J, et al. Development of EMPRO: A tool for the standardized assessment of patient-reported outcome measures. *Value Health*. 2008;11(4):700–8. https://doi.org/10.1111/j.1524-4733.2007.00309.x
29. Mokkink LB, Terwee CB, Patrick DL, et al. The COSMIN checklist for assessing the methodological quality of studies on measurement properties of health status measurement instruments: An international Delphi study. *Qual Life Res*. 2010;19(4):539–49. https://doi.org/10.1007/s11136-010-9606-8
30. Evans JP, Gibbons C, Toms AD, et al. Use of computerised adaptive testing to reduce the number of items in patient-reported hip and knee outcome scores: An analysis of the NHS England National Patient-Reported Outcome Measures programme. *BMJ Open*. 2022;12(7):e059415. https://doi.org/10.1136/bmjopen-2021-059415
31. Terwee CB, Ahmed S, Alhasani R, et al. Comparable real-world patient-reported outcomes data across health conditions, settings, and countries: The PROMIS International Collaboration. *NEJM Catalyst Innov Care Deliv*. 2024;5(9). https://doi.org/10.1056/CAT.24.0045
32. Porter I, Gonçalves-Bradley D, Ricci-Cabello I, et al. Framework and guidance for implementing patient-reported outcomes in clinical practice: Evidence, challenges and opportunities. *J Comp Eff Res*. 2016;5(5):507–19. https://doi.org/10.2217/cer-2015-0014
33. Pennucci F, De Rosis S, Passino C. Piloting a web-based systematic collection and reporting of patient-reported outcome measures and patient-reported experience measures in chronic heart failure. *BMJ Open*. 2020;10(10):e037754. https://doi.org/10.1136/bmjopen-2020-037754
34. De Rosis S, Ferrè F, Pennucci F. Including patient-reported measures in performance evaluation systems: Patient contribution in assessing and improving the healthcare systems. *Int J Health Plann Manage*. 2022;37(Suppl 1):144–65. https://doi.org/10.1002/hpm.3596
35. Bloemeke-Cammin J, Groene O, Ballester M, Guanais F, Groenewegen P, Kendir C, et al. International cross-cultural development and field testing of the primary care practice questionnaire for the PaRIS survey (PaRIS-PCPQ). *BMC Prim Care*. 2024;25(1):168. https://doi:10.1186/s12875-024-02375-8.

CHAPTER

21

Community Engagement and Co-Design

Siobhan Tu'akoi, Samuela Ofanoa and Felicity Goodyear-Smith

21.1 Introduction

Traditional models of research are typically top-down processes of scientific inquiry, starting with a hypothesis or theoretical framework and drawing conclusions based on evidence. This model typically prioritises the views of academics, scientists and experts to develop and test theories. As a result, community voices have historically not been prioritised, often being incorporated in implementation and dissemination phases later in the research process or left out altogether. However, there is increasing acknowledgement among research and academic sectors that there is significant value in ensuring that communities engage both in research and intervention development. For primary care research, the prioritisation of community partnership draws parallels to shared decision-making in patient-centred care, acknowledging the power of patients who are actively empowered in their own health management.[1] This chapter outlines community engagement and co-design principles, focusing on a case study with Pacific communities and primary care experts in *Aotearoa* New Zealand (NZ) and the value that this can have for intervention design, uptake and outcomes.

21.2 Communities Engaging in Research

Participatory action research approaches bring together community members, researchers and other stakeholders to co-create knowledge and push for social change.[2] Key considerations for participatory action research includes building relationships, forming working practices, establishing a common understanding of the issue, observing, gathering and generating materials, collaborative data analysis, and planning and taking action.[2] Under the umbrella of participatory methodologies, co-design is a specific method that aims to achieve the active participation and involvement of community members or 'end-users'.[3] By definition, co-design is a collaborative approach to solving problems and designing solutions that aims to be

DOI: 10.1201/9781003652106-25

better targeted and impactful due to the involvement of community stakeholders.[3] It centres on trusting relationships, shared decision-making, open communication and reciprocity, paving the way for lived experiences to be prioritised. The co-design process is intended to be an iterative, reciprocal journey of design, development and feedback among stakeholder groups, rather than a one-off or linear process. Research or interventions that are undertaken using co-design importantly prioritise the views and experiences of communities throughout the entire process, and in turn ensure the end product is better aligned for relevance and impact.[4]

Due to its foundation in community engagement, co-design approaches are increasingly used with vulnerable or underserved communities who experience significant health inequities because of social and systemic barriers. Although this has significant potential for engaging communities who have historically been excluded from research,[5] it must be carried out thoughtfully and with critical reflection. Moll and colleagues outline key factors for researchers to consider in this process, namely for co-design facilitators to understand their own worldviews and assumptions, the values and worldviews of the population they are working with, and the system in which the co-design will take place.[5] Understanding the cultural worldviews of the communities involved in the co-design is essential, as this can dictate the success of engagement. Till, Farao and colleagues outline methodological lessons from their community-based approaches in South Africa, acknowledging that, as a concept with Western origins, co-design must be undertaken in the context of local cultural norms and geographies.[6] Specific examples arising from their work include the need to balance cultural politeness and traditional gender roles while ensuring the active engagement of all participants. They also discuss inherent cultural hierarchies, power relations and differences between urban and rural sites that exist within these community settings.[6] Therefore, while co-design and participatory frameworks empower communities to engage in research, it is important that contextual factors and cultural dynamics are upheld.

21.3 Case Study with Pacific Communities in Aotearoa, New Zealand

Applying participatory methodologies, co-design methods and cultural frameworks, we present a case study example of how these principles have worked in practice for Pacific communities living in South Auckland, New Zealand (NZ). Pacific people are a diverse community who come from Pacific Island countries across Polynesia, Melanesia and Micronesia. In NZ, the largest populations of Pacific people identify with Samoan, Tongan, Cook Islands Māori and Niuean ancestry.[7] The cultures are distinct and diverse, but Pacific communities share common values of a holistic worldview centred around the importance of *vā*—relationships with people, the surrounding environment, time, space and the spiritual world of the non-living.[8] Family and collectivism are priorities, extending beyond the nuclear kinship to encompass the extended family, village, islands and ancestral linkages.[7] The concept of relationality extends beyond time and death, whereby Pacific elders, who are bestowed higher status and respect as knowledge-holders, are responsible for transferring history, cultural customs, traditions and protocols to the younger generations to maintain the connection between the past and present. Through these relationships, the values of respect, reciprocity, love, spirituality and service are maintained over time. In research with Pacific peoples, it is important to uphold these worldviews to create safe, empowering environments.

The case study we present here is a collaboration that comprises a partnership among academic researchers, Pacific community members and primary healthcare professionals, jointly known as the Pacific Research Collective. The research project was initially conceptualised after Rose Lamont, a Samoan patient from NZ, and her general practitioner travelled together to attend the North American Primary Care Research Group conference in 2016.[9] After attending a patient and clinician engagement workshop, Rose learned about research approaches that prioritised communities, clinicians and researchers working together to achieve equitable health outcomes. Understanding more about participatory research and patient-led interventions, she was empowered to establish her own community group upon returning to NZ. This became what is now known as the Pacific Peoples Health Advisory Group (PPHAG), comprising Pacific people living in South Auckland, aged 18 years and older, from a diverse range of social, educational and Pacific ethnic backgrounds.[9]

Concurrently, the primary health organisation of which the general practitioner was medical director formed a parallel group named the Pacific Practice-Based Research Network (PPBRN).[9] This consisted of primary healthcare professionals, such as doctors, practice nurses and managers, who worked in general practices with high numbers of enrolled Pacific patients.

The purpose of the community group PPHAG and the health professional network PPBRN was to come together and *talanga* (interactive talk with a purpose)[10] about health issues affecting Pacific people and what they might be able to do about it. To build their own research capacity and become upskilled in methods and methodologies, the groups sought out broader networks with academics and researchers at the University of Auckland. Experts in primary healthcare and Pacific health research were invited to run workshops with PPHAG and PPBRN. Workshops were focused on basic research concepts such as quantitative and qualitative approaches, how to ask research questions that are answerable and where findings may have direct impact on community health and well-being, and understanding different methodologies such as Western versus Pacific frameworks, thus building their skills and capabilities. These *talanga* sessions among community, health professionals and academics started to build on the lived experiences of Pacific people in South Auckland and the health inequities they faced. In a session on how to ask meaningful research questions, PPHAG and PPBRN drafted lists of specific health issues they felt were priorities for Pacific communities, and they then designed associated research questions. Eight key areas were workshopped into specific research questions with topics ranging from gout, rheumatic fever, skin infections, disability, elderly Pasifika, teenage pregnancy and mental health through to effective engagement with general practice.

After critical deliberations, the communities ranked the research questions by importance and selected gout and rheumatic fever as the two most in need of critical community-led intervention. In NZ, Pacific peoples experience significant inequities in both gout and rheumatic fever, with the highest rates of both health issues compared to other ethnic groups. Similarly, PPHAG and PPBRN outlined their personal experiences of struggling with these health issues, noting challenges in Pacific communities of both accessing primary healthcare services and understanding what the diseases are and how to treat them effectively.[11,12] To shape the strategic direction of research projects focused on both gout and rheumatic fever as the community had decided, an initial Health Activation grant was secured from the Health Research Council of NZ for a year. This grant provided funding for the groups to meet and continue their discussions with University of Auckland researchers, including capacity building of their own research skills and collaboratively developing longer-term grant applications. Two emerging Pacific researchers then came onboard to lead the parallel co-design research projects. Grants for each health issue were obtained in 2021 to investigate the burden of disease among Pacific people in Auckland general practices, explore what has been done before and co-design innovative, novel approaches for Pacific communities.[13,14] The design of these participatory research projects centred on bringing together diverse perspectives, prioritising the voices of the Pacific community groups who started this process.

The initial workshops with PPHAG and PPBRN on Pacific methodologies presented a range of both pan-Pacific and ethnic-specific models and frameworks to the groups. After discussions together, the groups selected the Samoan *fa'afaletui* model as an underlying framework to guide the research (Figure 21.1).[15,16] This model promotes the way of (*fa'a*) weaving together (*tui*) diverse perspectives or 'houses' (*fale*) to achieve consensus. The framework symbolises this using three levels: the top of the mountain (big-picture view), top of the tree (middle-stance lens) and person in the canoe closest to the school of fish (lived experience). Applied to the two research projects, the top of the mountain perspective refers to international and national data, obtained through literature reviews of previous interventions and national data. The top of the tree perspective refers to primary healthcare professionals (such as PPBRN members) who work in local communities with patients who are affected by gout and rheumatic fever. The person in the canoe sees the finer details and, in this case, represents the views of Pacific community members (PPHAG) and their families. The *fa'afaletui* model brings together diverse perspectives to achieve a consensus and thus upholds key Pacific values of relationships, respect, reciprocity and responsibility. PPHAG and PPBRN acknowledged that the *fa'afaletui* model emphasised these values and that maintaining these values throughout the entirety of each research project will ensure success.

Eight half-day co-design workshops were then undertaken with the PPHAG and PPBRN groups, adopting the *talanga* method of interactive talking with a purpose. In order to co-design interventions later down the track, the initial workshops aimed to empower the groups to understand and critically reflect on existing approaches. These involved presentations on what interventions had been developed nationally so far, enabling the community to brainstorm new and innovative approaches. Subsequent workshops focussed on co-designing specific interventions and selecting one to refine based on considerations of feasibility, cost, effectiveness and impact. This was a back-and-forth iterative process whereby the community were the key decision-makers at every step. While the project is ongoing, one example of a co-designed intervention in the gout project focuses on a multifaceted intervention aimed at improving awareness and understanding of gout in the

Top of the mountain
See the whole landscape (big picture)
Top of the tree
Middle-stance lens
Person in the canoe fishing
Closest to 'school of fish'.
Knows the small details

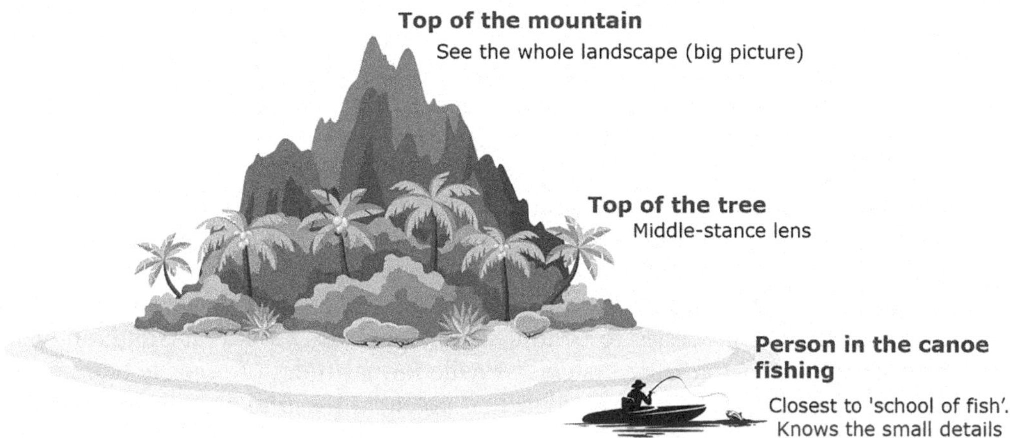

FIGURE 21.1 *Fa'afaletui*

Pacific community. This includes a short, engaging video resource co-created by the groups that simplifies complex gout concepts in a Pacific way and is intended to be delivered in primary care settings. Alongside the video, short, informative brochures were co-designed to be printed in seven different Pacific languages.

These approaches are currently being evaluated in a randomised trial using pre- and post-surveys to measure the effectiveness through potential changes in community knowledge (comparing those who view the video with controls who do not). Additionally, qualitative *talanga* interviews are being conducted with primary healthcare professionals external to the co-design partnership to explore the wider usefulness and feasibility in a clinical setting. While these studies are still in progress, health professionals in this study are anecdotally reporting existing gaps of gout educational material for Pacific people and are responding positively to the co-designed resources. Following the evaluation, these co-designed educational interventions will be rolled out in clinics across South Auckland.

21.4 Challenges for Co-Design in the Future

Despite the potential of co-design methods to improve the relevancy of interventions, there are inherent challenges in undertaking this type of research. In order to develop strong, trusting partnerships, significant time input is often needed to build trust and to enable safe, non-hierarchical environments.[4,5] Timelines for proposals, funding outputs and other necessary research milestones may not align with the time needed to facilitate deep and meaningful discussion with community groups. Equally, the time it takes to develop, pilot and evaluate interventions from a quality research perspective may not meet the expectations of community members who rightfully want to see real change. Timeline challenges are commonly acknowledged across co-design projects; getting the balance right hinges on having a foundation of strong relationships and understanding among all parties. The iterative feedback process can be a useful tool to mediate tensions, ensuring that all partners are regularly up-to-date and meaningfully involved in every step. Open and clear communication to community members on the challenges and opportunities of research processes is critical, and understanding and flexibility is equally needed from researchers on the realities of community-based projects that are never truly linear.

It is important that community members have sufficient research skills and understanding to be able to meaningfully contribute to a project. Research capacity-building though provision of training and support can help bridge these skill gaps and ensure that their input improves the research quality.

Challenges for co-design research also exist in other traditional research structures, such as the processes to obtain ethical approvals. Goodyear-Smith and colleagues outline that current systems provide formal codes of practice that aim to ensure "the methodology is rigorous; that potential harm to participants is minimised; that people know exactly what they are signing up to; and that the potential benefits of study outcomes outweigh possible risks of safety or confidentiality".[17] Intervention studies are viewed to involve greater risk and specific protocols, and documentation must be supplied at application and adhered to throughout the study.[17] By nature, the design and particulars of a co-designed intervention will generally not be known when ethical approvals are applied for, which clashes with the need to provide detailed and specific accounts of what will be carried out. There is a need for ethics committees to acknowledge the diversity in research projects and participatory methods, and their understanding that co-design, in its power-sharing approach, serves to reduce participant risk.[17] There is also an opportunity for stakeholders to work alongside committees to create specific protocols and rules for this type of research, to ensure that co-design projects can be carried out while ensuring that ethical integrity is maintained and participants are protected.

21.5 Value of Co-Design in Primary Healthcare

There is significant value in conducting co-design research in primary healthcare settings, firstly from a social justice and community empowerment perspective. Co-design explicitly involves power sharing among all collaborators and stakeholders in the partnership, acknowledging the unique and valuable knowledge brought forward by each party. Researchers come with technical knowledge of research methods; primary care professionals have significant health expertise; and communities have knowledge of contextual factors and lived experience.

Working together in a strong, reciprocal partnership where each voice is valued can have significant benefits for a rigorous research approach, interventions that are better designed for real impact and potential for higher community uptake and engagement.[4,18] As a result, there is significant potential for co-design and participatory methodologies to reduce research waste, that is, research that has limited relevance for clinicians, patients and other end-users.[4] Research to date into the effectiveness of co-designed interventions is generally positive, although methods often focus on qualitative approaches and short-term impacts.[4] To build the knowledge based on co-design research in health and the benefits of it for broader use across primary healthcare, it is important that strong evaluations are employed to investigate efficacy in the long-term.

21.6 Conclusion

Traditionally, health research has prioritised the views of academics and experts; however, communities hold significant knowledge and experiences that can help improve research methods, leading to better solutions. The case study presented in this chapter describes two community-initiated research projects, on gout and rheumatic fever respectively, that are grounded by the Samoan *fa'afaletui* model and co-design methodology. Key learnings from this process for other health research projects include the importance of upholding cultural values and worldviews, and empowering communities to be key decision-makers at every step of design and development. If health inequities and barriers in healthcare are to be overcome, then the meaningful engagement and participation of the communities affected by these disparities is critical.

References

1. Goodyear-Smith F. Use of codesign in primary care research: Real-life examples. *Fam Med Community Health*. 2021;9(Suppl 1):e001181.
2. Cornish F, Breton N, Moreno-Tabarez U, et al. Participatory action research. *Nat Rev Methods Primers*. 2023;3(1):34.
3. Vargas C, Whelan J, Brimblecombe J, et al. Co-creation, co-design and co-production for public health: A perspective on definitions and distinctions. *Public Health Res Pract*. 2022;32(2).
4. Slattery P, Saeri AK, Bragge P. Research co-design in health: A rapid overview of reviews. *Health Res Policy and Syst*. 2020;18:1–13.
5. Moll S, Wyndham-West M, Mulvale G, et al. Are you really doing 'codesign'? Critical reflections when working with vulnerable populations. *BMJ Open*. 2020;10(11):e038339.
6. Till S, Farao J, Coleman TL, Shandu LD, Khuzwayo N, Muthelo L, Mbombi MO, Motlhatlhedi M, Mabena G, Van Heerden A, Mothiba TM, Norris S, Verdezoto N, and Densmore M. 2022. Community-based Codesign across Geographic Locations and Cultures: Methodological Lessons from Co-design Workshops in South Africa. In *Participatory Design Conference* 2022: Volume 1 (PDC 2022 Vol. 1), August 19–September 1, 2022, Newcastle upon Tyne, United Kingdom. ACM, New York, NY, USA, 13 pages. https://doi.org/10.1145/3536169.3537786.
7. Ponton V. Utilizing Pacific methodologies as inclusive practice. *Sage Open*. 2018;8(3): 2158244018792962.
8. Teariki MA, Leau E. Understanding Pacific worldviews: Principles and connections for research. *Kōtuitui: NZ J Soc Sci*. 2024;19(2):132–51.
9. Lamont R, Fishman T, Sanders PF, et al. View from the canoe: Co-designing research Pacific style. *Ann Fam Med*. 2020;18(2):172–5.
10. Ofanoa M, Percival T, Huggard P, et al. Talanga: The Tongan way enquiry. *Sociol Stud*. 2015;5(4):334–40.
11. Ofanoa S, Ofanoa M, Tu'akoi S, et al. Pacific community's perceptions on how to improve uptake of urate-lowering therapy for Pacific gout patients. *Int J Equity Health*. 2025;24(1):91.
12. Tu'akoi S, Ofanoa M, Ofanoa S, et al. 'Not a short fix': A participatory approach to exploring challenges and opportunities for rheumatic fever prevention with Pacific people in South Auckland, New Zealand. *J Health Equity*. 2025;2(1):2444001.
13. Ofanoa M, Ofanoa SM, Heather M, et al. Design and implementation of a Pacific intervention to increase uptake of urate-lowering therapy for gout: A study protocol. *Int J Equity Health*. 2021;20(1):262.
14. Tu'akoi S, Ofanoa M, Ofanoa S, et al. Co-designing an intervention to prevent rheumatic fever in Pacific People in South Auckland: A study protocol. *Int J Equity Health*. 2022;21(1):101.

15. Goodyear-Smith F, 'Ofanoa M. Fa'afaletui: A Pacific research framework. *J Mix Methods Res*. 2022;16(1):34–46.
16. Tuia TT, Cobb D. Decolonizing Samoan fa'afaletui methodology: Taking a closer look. *AlterNative*. 2021;17(2):275–83.
17. Goodyear-Smith F, Jackson C, Greenhalgh T. Co-design and implementation research: Challenges and solutions for ethics committees. *BMC Med Ethics*. 2015;16:1–5.
18. O'Brien J, Fossey E, Palmer VJ. A scoping review of the use of co-design methods with culturally and linguistically diverse communities to improve or adapt mental health services. *Health Soc Care Community*. 2021;29(1):1–17.

CHAPTER

22

Thematic Analysis Approaches

A Multiplicity

Martina Kelly and Patricia Thille

22.1 Introduction

Thematic analysis (TA) is among the most widely used—and often misconstrued—approaches to qualitative analysis in health research. So why does this book, which emphasises future directions in primary care research, include a chapter about a familiar method? Although TA is widely used in qualitative health services research, too often the term is employed generically, limiting the quality of primary care research. In this chapter, we introduce readers to key concepts and terms associated with TA, which is not a singular data analysis method but rather one which encompasses a range of approaches, each rooted in different conceptual foundations. Our aim is to guide researchers in making informed decisions about the type of TA they select, ensuring coherence between research question and analysis to improve research quality.

By the end of this chapter, you will be able to:

- Differentiate among three approaches to thematic analysis.
- Recognise the conceptual foundations supporting each approach.
- Make a well-informed methodological choice when conducting a thematic analysis.

22.2 What Is Thematic Analysis?

Perhaps the two most common misunderstandings regarding TA are:

1. It is treated as a singular method, with one set of procedures.
2. It is a synonym for, or the only analysis method within, qualitative research.

The first problem occurs in manuscript after manuscript, which either lack a citation specific to the method or inappropriately cite the outdated 2006 manuscript by Braun and Clarke.[1] This makes reading and judging the quality of the research problematic.

DOI: 10.1201/9781003652106-26

The second problem is seen in a lack of justification for the choice of TA over a range of other qualitative analysis methods. Narrative, discourse and phenomenological methodologies each have their own qualitative analysis traditions, for example, that align with many of the research questions we pose in primary care health services research.

TA is best understood as a spectrum of methods,[2,3] which co-exist with other analysis methods in the long history of qualitative research. Different versions of TA explore and develop patterns (themes) from data in varied ways.[2,3] Each approach has its own strengths and limitations, methodological commitments and ways of attending to the researchers' underlying values.[2,3]

What TA approaches share, typically, is a coding process to support the analysis in some way. Researchers develop codes (see Table 22.1), segment the data into codes, and engage with all the data labelled under each code to progress toward themes, but the similarities end there; approaches to TA differ in how they understand what a theme is and the extent to which they describe, summarise or interpret data.[2,3]

In this chapter, we outline three approaches or 'schools' of TA, as Braun and Clarke (2019)[3] categorise them: coding reliability, codebook and reflexive TA (Figure 22.1). These types of TA differ in their philosophical and methodological

TABLE 22.1 Glossary of Key Terms in Thematic Analysis

Term	Explanation
Code	A label that is applied to chunks of data
Inductive coding	Coding is data-driven; researchers develop codes from raw data without using pre-determined categories from a theory or framework; a 'bottom-up' approach
Deductive coding	Coding is driven by theory or a conceptual framework; researchers start with a pre-defined set of codes and applies these codes to analyse data—a 'top-down' approach
Semantic meaning	Explicit or overt meaning
Latent meaning	Implicit or underlying meaning; involves researcher interpretation
Theme	Patterns in the data that shed new light on the phenomenon under investigation
Domain summary	A summary of what participants say in relation to a topic, often compiled based on semantic (explicit) meaning
Reflexivity	The process of maintaining awareness to researcher assumptions and how these shape interpretation
Paradigm	Beliefs that researchers share about how the chosen research topic can be understood and studied; two commonly described paradigms in health research are post-positivism and constructivism
Post-positivism	In post-positivism, researchers believe that the topic they are studying—the reality of that topic—exists in a singular form, but human experiences and values make it difficult to know in a pure way
Constructivism	In constructivism, researchers believe that they topic they are studying—the reality of that topic—exists in multiple forms, which depend on the individual and context, and how people continually 'construct' their knowledge based on their experiences over time

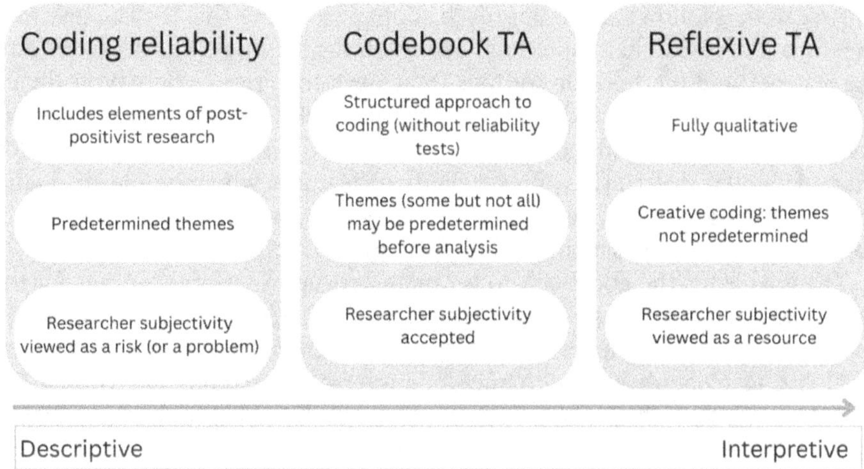

FIGURE 22.1 Three schools of thematic analysis (based on Braun and Clarke, 2019,[3] 2022[4])

commitments to coding and theme development. They may be conceptualised as a continuum from reliability to reflexive approaches.[3]

Before outlining key features of these approaches to TA, in Table 22.1 we define some terms commonly used when describing different approaches to TA.

22.3 How to Choose the Approach to Use When Conducting Thematic Analysis

To help readers determine what approach to TA might best align with a research question, we invite you to imagine the following scenario:

> *You are a family physician working in an inner-city group practice with an aging population. Recently, you introduced several new services to help seniors access care. You are curious to know if your efforts have been effective and how to further tailor accessible healthcare for this population. You decide to conduct some research. You approach your local Department of Family Medicine, and they offer you support, suggesting you analyse your data using 'thematic analysis'. However, they ask you to consider which approach would work best for you and your team. What are your options, and how do you decide?*

22.3.1 Coding Reliability Approaches

Coding reliability approaches to TA emphasise coding accuracy, in keeping with a post-positivist paradigm. This means that the researchers assume that there is a singular reality and a singular truth for the topic they study, and they attempt to surface it through research. Coding reliability approaches attempt to translate quantitative thinking into a qualitative method; some methodologists argue that coding reliability approaches are only 'partially qualitative'.[3]

Researchers following this approach adopt procedures that they believe minimise the impact of researcher values and beliefs on the findings. This includes establishing a structured method for coding. To achieve this, researchers typically create a codebook in a top-down, deductive way that relates to their research question. A codebook consists of a list of codes, each with a definition, often illustrated by an example, and a description of exclusions or features which would disqualify text from belonging to a particular code. Codebook codes may also directly match data collection tools, such as using the topic of interview questions as a code.[3]

The goal is for the codebook to be an agreed-upon set of meanings for multiple researchers to apply to the data. Multiple researchers often work independently to code the data, then compare accuracy; levels of agreement between raters are calculated, using Cohen's kappa to measure inter-coding reliability (Box 22.1). The assumption is that a high level of agreement (usually 0.80 or higher) signifies reliable coding. This approach to coding and theme development has been described as consensus coding, as it builds towards a singular, 'correct' analysis, consistent with post-positivism.[3] The emphasis is on following a rigid framework, following procedure to produce coding accuracy.

Researchers using coding reliability approaches typically conceptualise themes as analytic inputs—that is, themes are developed relatively early in data analysis, often after an initial phase of data familiarisation, which drives the data coding process.[3] Themes may also be described as analytic outputs, typically presented as descriptive domain summaries of the data, derived based on semantic meaning of the data—for example, barriers or facilitators to engaging in a health activity or achieving quality improvement. Using this approach, the focus is on summarising data in response to the questions asked, rather than on searching for or exploring implicit meaning that may be under the surface.

Scenario revisited: In your practice, there are two senior colleagues who have conducted research before and are familiar with quantitative research. They share their sense about what has worked (teleconsults and transport) and what has not (nutrition services) in the new services and are keen to describe these. You do interviews, focusing your questions around the specific services offered. While reading the interview transcripts, your senior colleagues suggest the team works deductively, focusing on the patients' comments about these services—ie, the services are themes that drive the data analysis. You and your co-researchers each highlight text that relates to these categories, adding code labels about each service and whether patients report a positive, neutral or negative impact. After reading two interviews each, the team meets again to compare coding and ensure that everyone

BOX 22.1 SAMPLE TEXT DESCRIBING A CODING RELIABILITY APPROACH TO TA

To achieve inter-rater reliability, two investigators worked independently to apply codes for each document in the dataset. Investigators met to compare coding and resolved discrepancies through discussion, redefining code descriptions as needed. Data were reanalysed until at least 80% agreement was reached.

is coding in a similar way, to eliminate any bias and produce reliable, objective results. They suggest that all the 'codes' will fit under the thematic headings, and they provide useful descriptive summaries (analytic outputs) of the newly introduced services.

22.3.2 Codebook Approaches

Codebook approaches to TA serve as a middle ground between post-positivist coding reliability and fully reflexive methods (Box 22.2). Although codebook approaches do not measure inter-rater reliability, they often adopt structured approaches to analysis, including developing structured coding frameworks or templates. Simultaneously, the coding approach retains some flexibility to recognise the role of inductive insights and researcher reflexivity. The purpose of the codebook is to label segments of data of interest. Using this approach, coding of data is primarily concerned with mapping and charting the data, proving helpful when managing the substantial amounts of data generated in some qualitative studies. Additionally, this method is well suited for teamwork, particularly multidisciplinary collaboration, which may involve researchers with varying levels of familiarity with qualitative research.

Popular approaches which adopt this approach to TA include template analysis[5,6] and the framework method.[7] The emphasis is on having a structured approach to coding, whilst remaining open to identifying new codes and new analytic insights.

Themes in codebook TA may be descriptive or interpretive, depending on the level of researcher reflexivity and study framing/research question.

Scenario revisited: Your clinic's new resident has some experience conducting qualitative research, and they offer to help you analyse the data. They agree with the senior partners that telehealth, transport and nutrition are important categories to consider, but when they read the interviews, they also note some additional categories come through, including the role of the pharmacist and social worker. The team decides to continue coding with the pre-arranged categories of telehealth, transport and nutrition, but also to keep an open mind for new categories, which the team agrees to discuss at subsequent meetings. As meetings continue, the team

BOX 22.2 SAMPLE TEXT DESCRIBING A CODEBOOK APPROACH TO TA, E.G., TEMPLATE ANALYSIS

The first template comprised a mix of tentative *a priori* codes identified as salient from existing literature and inductive codes derived from close reading of the data. These initial codes were considered tentative and provisional. Two members of the research team applied this initial template to code the next three interviews, whilst remaining open to identification of new codes. They met to discuss the template, add new codes, modify and re-organise codes, to refine the next iteration of the template. The list of codes was modified through successive readings of the data such that the template continued to develop until it represented the data as fully as possible.

realises that issues of transport are not as important as originally thought and could be better considered in relation to patient safety, and data under that category are reassigned. As you move to write up the analysis, you speak to both the deductive and inductive codes.

22.3.3 Reflexive Approaches

Reflexive thematic analysis (RTA), as the name suggests, considers researcher reflexivity as central to data analysis. Reflexivity is not a synonym for reflection, as is well covered in Chapter 8. RTA recognises that no single truth represents the topic and its reality; rather, there are multiple 'realities'—meaning is contextual and situated as per constructivism. Thus, RTA sits well with a constructivist paradigm and fits nicely with research questions that explore and interpret people's experiences or beliefs.

In RTA, coding is an open, generative, creative and iterative process, as the researcher draws on their own understandings of the data and the topic.[2,3] As researchers become more engaged with the data, they may evolve their codes, renaming or combining with other codes to become 'candidate themes', refined through returning to data and analytic writing. Reflexive researchers argue strongly that themes do not 'emerge'; instead, researchers actively create themes, by the data interacting with the researchers' interpretative frameworks, experiences and assumptions.[2,3] Said another way, RTA creates interpretive themes that cannot be derived in advance, but instead through a deep, interpretive process. Themes in RTA 'unite data that might otherwise appear disparate, or meaning that occurs in multiple and varied contexts; they (often) explain large portions of a dataset; they are often abstract entities or ideas, capturing implicit ideas "beneath the surface" of the data, but can also capture more explicit and concrete meaning'.[3]

22.4 Reflexive Openness

Due to the central role of the researcher in constructing themes, it is essential that researchers using RTA share their assumptions—and their best understanding of how they have impacted analysis—with the reader. This means more than a superficial reporting of researchers' own gender, ethnicity and disciplinary background(s). Reflexive openness requires researchers to situate their theoretical assumptions and share how these impacted analysis. Several practical strategies exist to help researchers demonstrate reflexivity. Perhaps the simplest and most common is maintaining a reflexive research diary, where the researcher documents their research journey, including initial thoughts and preconceptions about the study, and journals how these change throughout the research process. In Chapter 8, Crabtree and Miller[8] provide a useful set of exercises for individual and teams of researchers.

In RTA, themes are the output of interpretive processes that may include coding (Box 22.3). Themes in RTA far more often interpret latent meaning and are named to represent meaning-based patterns that are not immediately apparent but often possess narrative explanatory power of the data. The goal is to develop a coherent interpretation of the data that is grounded in the data, while recognising that different researchers could offer a different reflexive interpretation, thanks to their different background knowledge and beliefs.[3] Good themes convey a coherent, insightful story about the data concerning the research question, created through a reflexive process.[3]

Braun and Clarke are the key methodologists of RTA, sharing extensive guidance to support high-quality RTA. For an in-depth description of how to conduct RTA, we direct readers to Braun and Clarke, 2022.[4]

Scenario revisited: The team is joined by a senior researcher with extensive experience with qualitative research. Rather than focusing on 'what worked or not' in terms of service evaluation, the researcher suggests reframing the research question to focus on how older people experience the new services, keeping an open mind to whatever participants mention during the interviews. They suggest that before the team starts to read the transcripts, everyone should meet to discuss their interest in the project and their experience working with and caring for elderly patients. They open the meeting describing their experience caring for their elderly parents and their frustrations with accessing care. The researcher invites team members to express their ideas about the research and the services provided. They also suggest that perhaps an underpinning concept for the project may be about understanding how older people think about their health and aging, and what is important to them in relation to health services at this stage of life.

BOX 22.3 SAMPLE TEXT DESCRIBING RTA, BASED ON OUR PERSPECTIVES AS AUTHORS OF THIS CHAPTER

Martina is a family doctor, with more than 20 years of experience working in medical education. In her research, she draws on her experience caring for patients, as an Irish woman who moved to Canada. Her research practice is strongly influenced by her clinical work as a family doctor, which involves interpreting how patients subjectively experience symptoms. Much of her research is interpretive.

Patty is a hybrid scholar—a physiotherapist by first degree and medical sociologist by PhD. She has spent more than 20 years exploring the theory of methods. Most of her research is in the critical and/or constructionist paradigms, informed by sociological theories that draw attention to how systems of inequality manifest in practice or in meaning-making. As an educator in a Canadian graduate research programme, she teaches a range of paradigms and emphasises the importance of methodological coherence to create impactful research.

In writing this chapter, we drew on our experience as researchers and educators, working with graduate students, reflecting on some of the errors and assumptions made in our respective areas of scholarship. Martina, as a physician, recognised, for example, that reliability methods are widespread in qualitative research published in medical journals, perhaps because of the historical legacy of positivism, which values an assumption of objective truth. Patty is frustrated with atheoretical and un-reflexive qualitative research in health sciences and avoids TA, yet many graduate students in health fields gravitate to it. Both Martina and Patty acknowledge that RTA can seem abstract to physicians and physiotherapists alike, and reflexivity may feel uncomfortable when first engaging with this approach.

After reading the first two interview transcripts, the researchers meet to share what surprised or otherwise jumped out at them; for example, one interview participant talked about problems as a function of 'old age', giving this reason to explain why they don't make an appointment to see the doctor, despite having pain. One research team member recalls that this idea has been described in the wider literature but not in relation to family medicine clinic use.

For the next meeting, they suggest that all team members work inductively, that is, read the next two interviews, mark up words or phrases that seem of interest, and the team will meet again to discuss. When writing their manuscript, the researchers reflect on their interpretive process and address the way the interview guide, which was developed before the analysis method was chosen, shaped the findings.

22.5 How Do Theories and Conceptual Frameworks Fit with Different Thematic Analysis Approaches?

At times, a research study is guided by a theory or conceptual framework. For example, a quality improvement or implementation study about access may apply a conceptual framework to support interpretation, such as Levesque and colleagues' highly regarded patient-centred access model, which understands access on a continuum that results from a match between accessibility of services and patient resources.[9] TA approaches, across the different types, are flexible in this regard. Coding reliability and codebook approaches may integrate conceptual frameworks directly within their codebook. RTA, with a more constructivist leaning, can work with theories that share that orientation, such as narrative and phenomenological theories.

22.6 Reading and Evaluating Thematic Analysis

What makes for a good-quality TA is, in part, defined by the chosen TA approach. Coherence between the research question, the approach chosen and its execution improves the quality of TA.[3] If a theoretical or conceptual framework is used, it must be compatible with the paradigm of the research, described well and its use accounted for in the methods description. A good TA describes the analytic process in detail, such that a reader can understand how the final interpretation was constructed.[3]

Features of a weak or unconvincing TA may include the following:[3,10]

- *Too many or too few themes*: too many themes can signal poor analytic depth, while too many suggests a lack of analytic synthesis across different ideas in the data.
- *Too many theme levels*: for example, if a coding reliability or codebook TA has decided in advance to use 'facilitators' and 'barriers' as their primary codes, and then adds sub-codes and sub-sub-codes, the manuscript becomes more of a list than a meaningful engagement with data.

- *Confusion between codes and themes*: while coding reliability approaches may pre-determine themes and use them as codes, within more fully qualitative approaches, pre-determination is not acceptable.
- Mismatch between data extracts (e.g. quotations from the data) and analytic claims
- Too few or too many data extracts
- Overlap between themes

22.7 Practice Points

- There is rarely an 'ideal' way to approach a research question. What matters is coherence: your choice of method should align with the research question(s), paradigmatic/theoretical assumptions, data collection and analysis methods choices.
- When working in a team, consider an upfront discussion of different team members' approaches to, and perspectives on, thematic analysis.
- Identify, describe and cite your approach, ensuring that your analysis citation corresponds with your method.
- Justify your choice of approach.
- Outline the steps you took to develop your analysis, including strategies for enhancing reflexivity. For tips, see Crabtree and Miller (2023)[8] and Chapter 8.
- Ensure your use of terminology is appropriate. For example, if using RTA, themes do not 'emerge' from nowhere like buried treasure.

References

1. Braun V, Clarke V. Using thematic analysis in psychology. *Qual Res Psychol.* 2006; 3(2):77–101.
2. Braun V, Clarke V. Can I use TA? Should I use TA? Should I *not* use TA? Comparing reflexive thematic analysis and other pattern-based qualitative analytic approaches. *Couns Psychother Res.* 2021;21(1):37–47.
3. Braun V, Clarke V, Hayfield N, Terry G. Thematic analysis. In: Liamputtong P, ed. Handbook of research methods in health social sciences. Singapore: Springer Singapore; 2019. p. 843–60. [cited 28 Mar 2025; Available from: http://link.springer.com/10.1007/978-981-10-5251-4_103]
4. Braun V, Clarke V. Thematic analysis: A practical guide. Los Angeles: SAGE; 2022. 376 p. [Available from: https://study.sagepub.com/thematicanalysis]
5. Brooks J, McCluskey S, Turley E, King N. The utility of template analysis in qualitative psychology research. *Qual Res Psychol.* 2015 Apr 3;12(2):202–22.
6. King N. Doing template analysis. In: Symon G, Cassell C, eds. Qualitative organizational research: Core methods and current challenges. SAGE; 2012. p. 426–50.
7. Gale NK, Heath G, Cameron E, Rashid S, Redwood S. Using the framework method for the analysis of qualitative data in multi-disciplinary health research. *BMC Med Res Methodol.* 2013 Sep 18;13(1):117.

8. Crabtree BF, Miller WL. Doing qualitative research (3rd edition). Thousand Oaks: SAGE; 2023.
9. Levesque JF, Harris MF, Russell G. Patient-centred access to health care: Conceptualising access at the interface of health systems and populations. *Int J Equity Health*. 2013;12(1):18.
10. Finlay L. Qualitative research: The 'good', the 'bad' and the 'ugly'. *Eur J Qual Res Psychother.* 2024;14. [Available from: https://ejqrp.org/index.php/ejqrp/article/view/294]

Further Reading

Braun V, Clarke V, Hayfield N, Terry G. Thematic analysis 48. In: Liamputtong P, ed. Handbook of research methods in health social sciences. Springer; 2019. p. 843–60. https://doi.org/10.1007/978-981-10-5251-4_103

CHAPTER

23

Embedding Economic Reasoning in Primary Care Research

Toward Value-Driven and Equitable Health Systems

Akim Tafadzwa Lukwa and Plaxcedes Chiwire

23.1 Introduction

23.1.1 Defining Primary Health Care, Primary Care and Health Economics

Health systems globally are under increasing strain from rising multimorbidity, population ageing and fiscal pressures,[1,2] particularly in low- and middle-income countries (LMICs), where limited resources, workforce shortages and structural inequities constrain service delivery.[3,4] In this context, primary health care (PHC) and its clinical subsystem, primary care (PC), are central to achieving equitable, efficient and sustainable health systems. According to the World Health Organization (WHO),[5] PHC is a whole-of-society approach built around three interrelated components:

1. Integrated health services that prioritise primary care and essential public health functions
2. Multisectoral policy and action to address the broader social, economic and environmental determinants of health
3. Empowered people and communities who are engaged in their own health and the health systems that serve them.

In contrast, Primary care refers to the patient-facing clinical platform and community-based services that operationalise PHC at the individual and household levels.[6] Primary care embodies integrated, person-centred care and is key to realising universal health coverage (UHC). Despite this centrality, economic reasoning remains

DOI: 10.1201/9781003652106-27

peripheral to the design, financing and evaluation of PC systems. Decisions about what to fund, how to pay and which technologies to adopt often lack a systematic assessment of value or affordability. Health economics (HE) provides the analytical framework for addressing these questions, helping health systems allocate scarce resources to maximise health gains, ensure financial protection and sustain service delivery over time.[7,8]

This chapter focuses on three interrelated domains of health economics that are foundational to embedding economic reasoning within PC research and policy.

1. *Economic evaluation and analysis*: Cost-effectiveness analysis (CEA), cost-utility analysis (CUA) and cost-benefit analysis (CBA) assess whether interventions offer good value for money (see Box 23.1).
2. *Healthcare financing and systems*: Examining how health services are funded, how risks are pooled and how strategic purchasing mechanisms can improve efficiency and equity.
3. *Health technology assessment (HTA)*: Systematically evaluating the costs and consequences of new drugs, diagnostics and digital tools before adoption. Integrating these domains into PC research transforms it from documenting what works to assessing what is worth doing, anchoring value creation in the pursuit of efficiency, equity and sustainability.

BOX 23.1 DISTINGUISHING TYPES OF FULL ECONOMIC EVALUATION

The core types of full economic evaluation in healthcare are defined by how they measure and value the consequences (outcomes) of interventions.

- *Cost-Effectiveness Analysis (CEA)* measures consequences in natural clinical units (e.g., life years gained, cases prevented). It results in a cost-effectiveness ratio (e.g., cost per life year gained) and is used to compare interventions with a common, specific health goal.
- *Cost-Utility Analysis (CUA)* is a specific form of CEA where consequences are measured in quality-adjusted life years (QALYs) or disability-adjusted life years (DALYs). This allows for comparisons across different disease areas and health programs by combining mortality and morbidity into a single "utility"-based metric. CUA is often considered the gold standard for informing broad health policy and resource allocation.
- *Cost-Benefit Analysis (CBA)* values all consequences in monetary units. By comparing costs and benefits both measured in currency, it determines whether the benefits of an intervention outweigh its costs, providing a direct answer for economic efficiency that is useful for decisions beyond healthcare (e.g., environmental or public health regulation).

23.2 Conceptual Linkages Between Primary Care and Health Economics

23.2.1 Integrating Health Economics Within the Primary Care System

The relationship between PC and HE can be understood as a dynamic interplay between system performance and resource optimisation. PC provides the structural and service-delivery foundation of a health system, while HE offers the analytical tools to evaluate, prioritise and sustain those functions under resource constraints. In essence, PC defines the 'what' and 'how' of service delivery, whereas HE describes the 'why' and 'with what consequence' in economic and societal terms. Within this interface, health economics informs PC through three complementary functions:

1. Measurement of value, quantifying costs and outcomes across interventions, facilities and population groups.
2. Resource allocation and incentive design guiding how financial and non-financial resources are distributed across levels of care to maximise efficiency and equity; and
3. Policy translation providing decision rules and evidence to align PC financing, technology adoption and service delivery with system-wide sustainability goals.

Conversely, PC provides the empirical and institutional context that makes economic analysis meaningful. Data generated in PC (e.g., service utilisation, outcomes, costs) allows economists to assess the performance and efficiency of real-world delivery models. This bidirectional relationship ensures that economic reasoning is not external to PC but embedded within its continuous quality improvement and accountability processes.

Embedding health economics within PC also supports adaptive policy design. Economic evaluation evidence guides the inclusion of high-value interventions in essential benefit packages, financing analysis informs capitation, pay-for-performance, and strategic purchasing models, and HTA frameworks ensure that new technologies strengthen rather than fragment PC. Together, these mechanisms translate economic evidence into learning systems that improve performance, reduce waste and sustain equitable coverage.

In summary, HE operationalises the principles of value, efficiency and equity that underpin PC, ensuring that limited resources generate the greatest possible health and societal benefit. This integration forms the conceptual foundation for the framework presented in Figure 23.1.

23.2.2 The Health Economics Lens on Primary Care Systems

The conceptual framework (Figure 23.1) positions PC within the broader health system, linking core system functions to service delivery, outputs and eventual health outcomes. At the top level, the six WHO health system building blocks, leadership and governance, financing, health information systems, workforce, medicines and supplies, and infrastructure, form the structural foundation on which PC

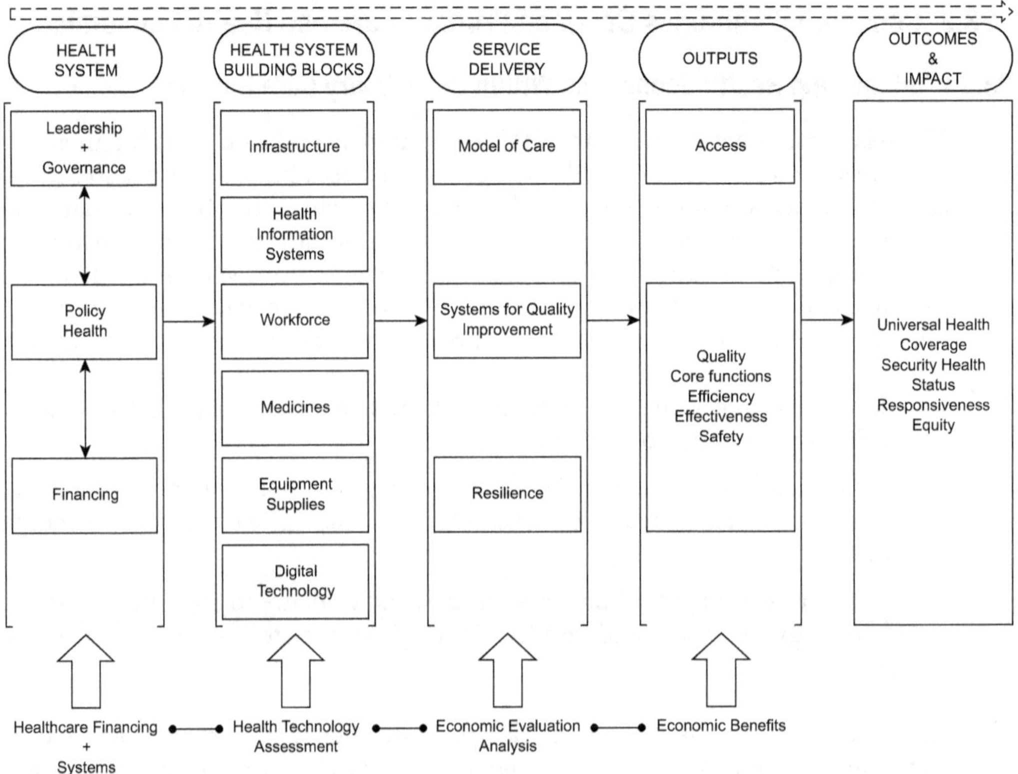

FIGURE 23.1 Conceptual framework linking primary care and health economics

Source: Adapted from (Lukwa et al., 2025; World Health Organisation and United Nations Children's Fund, 2021)

is organised and delivered.[9] These building blocks shape the model of care, service quality and resilience that together underpin effective PC delivery. Beneath these system functions, three health-economics domains serve as decision-support mechanisms that guide PC in achieving efficiency, equity and improved outcomes.

23.2.3 Interpreting the Conceptual Framework

The conceptual framework in Figure 23.1 presents a horizontal pathway that shows how PC performance emerges from the interaction among health system structures, service delivery processes and economic decision-making. It begins with the core health system functions, leadership and governance, health policy and financing, which create the strategic and regulatory environment within which primary care is organised. These functions determine how priorities are set, how resources are mobilised and how institutions shape the delivery of PC services.

The next section of the framework highlights the health system building blocks. These include the workforce, infrastructure, health information systems, medicines, equipment and supplies, and digital technologies,[9] which together form the operational foundation for PC. Their availability, distribution and quality influence the extent to which services can be delivered effectively and equitably. Strong building blocks support a reliable platform for patient care, while weaknesses in any component can constrain PC performance.

Moving along the pathway, the service delivery domain captures how these inputs are translated into actual care. This includes the model of care, systems for quality improvement and patient safety as well as resilience. These elements determine what services are provided, how they are organised and where they are provided. They determine whether PC functions as a trusted first point of contact and can adapt to shocks, such as epidemics or resource shortages.

The framework then links service delivery to immediate system outputs, including access and availability of care as well as the quality of that care in terms of core PC functions (first contact accessibility, continuity, coordination, comprehensiveness, people-centredness), efficiency, effectiveness, and safety. These outputs serve as measurable indicators of the system's performance. Improvements in these areas signal that primary care is functioning as intended, while persistent weaknesses point to areas requiring policy or managerial intervention.

Finally, the pathway connects these outputs to broader outcomes and impacts, such as improved population health, enhanced health security, increased system responsiveness, and progress toward UHC and better equity. These outcomes represent the long-term societal value of strong primary care and reflect both health and social gains.

Beneath this main pathway, the three health economics domains—economic evaluation, healthcare financing and health technology assessment (HTA)—function as analytical engines that support decision-making throughout the system. They guide how resources are allocated, which technologies are adopted, and how purchasing arrangements are structured. By informing these decisions, the economics domains reinforce efficiency, equity and sustainability across all components of the framework and ultimately generate wider economic benefits. The continuous interactions across the pathway illustrate how evidence from health economics strengthens primary care performance, and how strong PC in turn contributes to a more resilient and sustainable health system.

23.3 Operationalising the Three Health-Economics Domains in PC Research

23.3.1 Domain 1: Economic Evaluation

23.3.1.1 Economic Evaluation for PC: From Questions to Decisions

An economic evaluation in primary care begins by defining the decision problem. This should be clearly structured using the PICO framework: Population, Intervention, Comparator and Outcome,[10] and supported by a specified time horizon, setting, and an explicit analytical perspective (eg provider, patient or societal). The choice of perspective is central because it determines which costs and effects are included. For example, a patient perspective may capture direct out-of-pocket expenses, travel costs, lost income and time spent providing informal caregiving.

In contrast, the societal perspective is broader and accounts for all costs and consequences to society, such as productivity losses from illness or premature mortality, the value of unpaid caregiver labour, costs to employers and broader social impacts like reduced economic output.[7,8] The aforementioned capture the full economic consequences of health interventions; the patient and, especially, the societal perspectives are often the most policy-salient in primary care settings.

Measuring costs requires a 'stacked' approach tailored to PC. This involves a facility layer using step-down costing to allocate overheads (management, utilities, capital) to specific cost centres such as clinics or community health worker platforms;[11] a service layer employing Activity-Based Costing (ABC) to quantify resources (staff time, diagnostics, consumables) used per visit or episode to price distinct service lines;[12,13] and a patient-contact layer utilising Time-Driven ABC (TD-ABC), which leverages time and flow data to capture actual person-level costs, a method critical for evaluating re-designed workflows, task-sharing or digital tools.[7]

In practice, a mixed costing approach is recommended using top-down methods for overheads and bottom-up methods for high-cost or variable activities while documenting price sources, reporting the base year for costs and applying Purchasing Power Parity (PPP) conversions where cross-country comparability is important.[14–17]

23.3.1.2 Within Clinical Trials versus Model-Based Approaches

When decision-makers need rapid, budget-relevant signals rooted in programme accounts, it is helpful to embed CEA or CUA within clinical trials that typically have a six to 24-month follow-up (eg blood pressure control, viral suppression). For example, adding lab-equipped health posts in rural Rwanda produced measurable increases in utilisation and reductions in mortality within two years and yielded a favourable cost per DALY averted.[18]

Shift to model-based CEA or CUA when effects extend beyond follow-up, events are rare but consequential, or options imply system re-design. The Bridging Income Generation with Group Integrated Care (BIGPIC) trial used a Markov model to project cardiovascular events and disability-adjusted life years (DALYs) over 20 years for integrated group care.[19] For diagnostics, decision-analytic models are essential because pathways diverge post-test. South Africa's Xpert MTB/RIF adoption combined real-world costing with a decision model to estimate downstream outcomes and value.[17]

23.3.1.3 Uncertainty, Reporting and Translation to Policy

Handling uncertainty is critical for the credibility of any economic evaluation and for informing decisions under constrained resources.[20,21] To this end, a multi-faceted analytical approach is required. Deterministic sensitivity analysis should be employed to test the individual influence of key model parameters, such as drug costs or intervention efficacy, on the results.[22,23]

For assessing joint parameter uncertainty, probabilistic sensitivity analysis is the preferred method, in which all parameters are varied simultaneously according to their predefined probability distributions.[24,25] The output of this analysis is best presented as Cost-Effectiveness Acceptability Curves (CEACs), which illustrate the probability of an intervention being cost-effective across a range of willingness-to-pay thresholds. Where significant decision uncertainty remains, the Expected Value of Perfect Information (EVPI) can be calculated to quantify the potential value of acquiring additional evidence through future research.

Transparent, standardised reporting is the foundation on which evidence is translated into policy. All evaluations must adhere to the Consolidated Health Economic Evaluation Reporting Standards (CHEERS) 2022 guidelines.[26,27] This ensures a complete and transparent account of the model's structure, data sources, price years, currency conversions and methods for characterising uncertainty.

Finally, translating technical results into actionable intelligence for decision-makers is a non-negotiable final step. The presentation of an Incremental Cost-Effectiveness Ratio (ICER) should always be accompanied by a Budget Impact Analysis (BIA) to assess the financial consequences of adoption within a specific health system context. Furthermore, a policy brief must be developed to distil the evidence. This brief should clearly state the recommended decision, summarise the findings on value for money and affordability, highlight any material distributional effects across population subgroups and outline the key operational requirements for successful implementation. This integrated approach ensures that economic evidence moves beyond an academic exercise to directly support efficient, equitable and sustainable resource allocation.

23.3.2 Domain 2: Healthcare Financing and Systems for PHC

Financing determines which resources reach the primary care front line and how reliably they do so. Three core functions shape this process: revenue raising, risk pooling and strategic purchasing.[28] Revenue raising refers to how funds are collected, while risk pooling determines how financial risks are shared across members of a population to protect individuals from high out-of-pocket costs. Strategic purchasing then governs how these pooled resources are allocated to providers to improve access, quality and efficiency.

Figure 23.2 does not illustrate risk pooling directly but instead shows the three dimensions of progress toward UHC: extending population coverage ('who is covered?'), expanding the range of services included ('which services are covered?'),

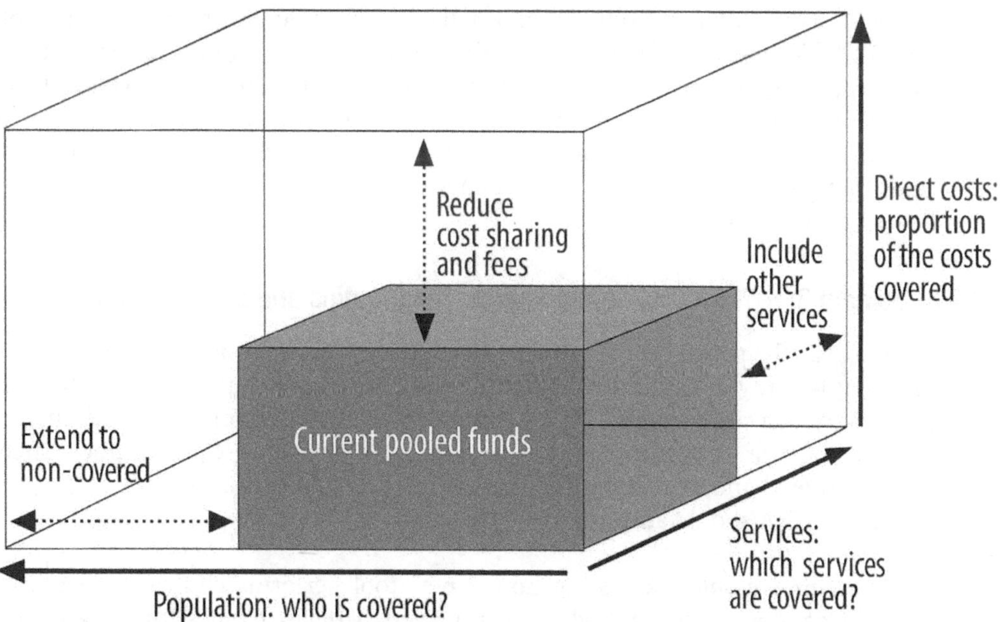

FIGURE 23.2 The WHO Universal Health Coverage (UHC) Cube

Source: Adapted from the *World Health Organisation Bulletin* (Evans and Etienne, 2010)

and increasing financial protection by reducing direct payments ('what proportion of costs are covered?'). These dimensions are directly influenced by how effectively countries raise revenue, pool risks and purchase services, making financing a central determinant of primary care's contribution to UHC.

Purchasing choices, particularly purchaser-provider payment methods, form the 'behavioural operating system' of PC:

- Capitation and blended capitation models (capitation combined with fee-for-service and quality incentives) can strengthen continuity of care and support the prevention of avoidable illness, complications and unnecessary hospital use when they are risk-adjusted and paired with strong accountability mechanisms.[29,30]
- Pay-for-performance or Results-Based Financing (RBF) can improve selected service-delivery outputs but requires strong verification systems and must demonstrate value for money. In Malawi, maternal–newborn RBF improved key process measures such as timely management of obstetric complications and adherence to evidence-based practices when incentives were tied to clearly defined indicators and independently verified, contributing to gains in effective coverage,[31] and aligning with broader evidence that P4P can enhance process quality in LMICs.[32] Comparative analyses further highlight that programme design features rather than geography drive performance, including indicator choice, incentive size and verification mechanisms.[33]

Equity and financial protection are foundational objectives of PC, and financing reforms must be explicitly designed to reduce catastrophic out-of-pocket expenditures. This can be assessed through distributional cost-effectiveness analysis (DCEA) when interventions differentially benefit poorer or more vulnerable groups.[34,35] To ensure that signals of value for money are actionable for commissioners, PC studies must report not only the Incremental Cost-Effectiveness Ratio (ICER) and Budget Impact Analysis (BIA) but also critical operational details of the financing model, including the specific payment mechanism, the purchasing rules that govern it (eg gatekeeping, panel size, quality bonuses) and the precise flow of funds to PC teams.

23.3.3 Domain 3: HTA for PHC Technologies, Diagnostics and Digital Tools

HTA acts as the gatekeeper for primary care technologies by assessing whether an intervention provides additional value at the first point of contact and at what system cost.[36,37] In primary care, HTA compares a new technology with the current standard of care to determine both its clinical performance (e.g., accuracy, effectiveness, safety) and its economic value (e.g., cost-effectiveness, resource use).

For PC, HTA should address:

- *Comparative value*: assessing how a new tool performs clinically relative to existing alternatives and whether it delivers better outcomes for a reasonable additional cost.

- *Budget impact and affordability*: estimating the financial implications of adopting the technology across PC facilities.
- *Delivery fit*: evaluating whether the technology can be implemented effectively, considering training needs, maintenance requirements, supply chains, interoperability with existing digital systems, and workflow compatibility.
- *De-implementation*: identifying technologies that offer low or no value and should be phased out.

The evaluation of diagnostics and digital health technologies within PC necessitates the use of decision-analytic modelling, as patient trajectories and thus downstream clinical outcomes and costs diverge significantly following a test result or a triage algorithm. This is exemplified by the model-based assessment of South Africa's Xpert MTB/RIF rollout, which captured the long-term value of improved tuberculosis diagnosis.[17] Similarly, for technologies such as digital blood pressure monitoring, lifetime models demonstrate how modest initial investments can yield substantial long-term value by preventing costly cardiovascular events, as evidenced by PC in the United Kingdom.[38] However, an equity lens is critical in this domain. Health Technology Assessment (HTA) for PC must proactively examine targeting rules; identify access barriers related to connectivity, language or disability; and assess the distributional impacts of technologies that shift the locus of care from hospitals to communities.

23.4 Cross-Cutting Methods, Data and Translation for PC Decisions

23.4.1 Learning-System Data for Economic Decisions

Credible economic decisions in PC are contingent upon integrated data systems.[39] Moving beyond siloed information requires a deliberate 'data plumbing' strategy that connects routine health information systems (HIS) with dedicated costing cells and patient outcome tracking.[40] The operational anchor for this is a versioned, regularly updated unit-cost library, directly linked to PC performance dashboards.

This creates a dynamic, auditable resource aligned with the WHO PHC Measurement Framework, enabling managers to move beyond activity tracking to assess the efficiency and resource intensity of care delivery.[41] Although ICERs from decision-analytic models remain the gold standard for allocative efficiency, understanding the complex, system-wide behaviour of PC requires complementary modelling approaches. System dynamics and agent-based models are increasingly used to capture patient heterogeneity, care-seeking behaviour and feedback loops inherent to multimorbidity and service integration,[42] making them ideal for examining emergent effects such as clinic congestion, optimal outreach coverage and referral bottlenecks.

23.4.2 Equity, Sustainability and Place

Economic evaluations must transcend a narrow focus on aggregate efficiency to address who benefits from PC investments. Distributional Cost-Effectiveness Analysis adds an explicit equity lens, estimating how costs and health gains are distributed across socioeconomic groups and quantifying equity-efficiency trade-offs.[34,35] This methodology is crucial for appraising policies such as community outreach, community health worker (CHW) models and pro-poor targeting, ensuring the pursuit of value for money does not inadvertently exacerbate health disparities.

Concurrently, the economic rationale for PC must be reframed in line with the imperatives of planetary health and system resilience. Given that the global healthcare sector contributes significantly to carbon emissions,[43] evaluations should report the co-benefits of climate-smart investments. This includes quantifying how transitions to clean energy for clinics, telehealth substitutions and electrification of fleet vehicles for outreach not only reduce the environmental footprint but also bolster PC continuity and resilience against climate shocks.[44]

23.4.3 From Analysis to Action: Decision Products

To ensure economic evidence informs practice, every evaluation must be translated into a 'minimum translation pack' tailored for decision-makers. This pack should comprise three core elements: (1) a CHEERS 2022-compliant short report to ensure technical transparency and reproducibility; (2) a Budget Impact Analysis (BIA) to assess affordability over a three- to five-year horizon; and (3) a policy brief that outlines concrete rollout scenarios, specifying implications for district teams, outreach coverage and staffing. This final product distils technical findings into actionable intelligence for scale-up.

23.4.4 PC Value Pack: What to Hand to a District Manager

A district manager should be provided with a one-page summary containing the ICER range and its interpretation against local opportunity-cost thresholds; a Cost-Effectiveness Acceptability Curve (CEAC) to visualise decision uncertainty; a three- to five-year BIA; clear staffing and supply chain implications; and equity notes on the distributional impacts across population subgroups.

23.5 Building Capacity and Institutionalising Economic Reasoning in PC

Embedding health economics within PC requires a deliberate, multi-level implementation strategy. We propose a crisp, four-pillar plan to systematise economic reasoning and move from ad-hoc analysis to institutional routine.

23.5.1 Human Capital

The first pillar, human capital, focuses on building a workforce that is fluent in economic principles. This involves mainstreaming health economics into PC curricula and offering targeted short courses and mentorship for researchers, clinicians and managers. The objective is to foster the routine application of reporting standards like CHEERS and the interpretation of findings against context-specific, opportunity-cost thresholds that reflect real budget constraints.

23.5.2 Institutional Infrastructure

The second pillar, institutional infrastructure, refers not to physical buildings but to the organisational systems, structures and processes that enable routine, high-quality economic analysis. This includes establishing dedicated costing units or 'cells' within health departments, supported by standard operating procedures, digital tools and staff capacity for producing and updating price books and versioned unit-cost libraries. These units should be integrated with National Health Accounts (NHA) and PC performance dashboards so that economic data consistently feed into planning, budgeting and monitoring cycles.

23.5.3 Collaborative Methods Cores

The third pillar, collaborative methods cores, promotes interdisciplinary rigour from start to finish. By embedding economists, epidemiologists and implementation scientists within PC research teams from the protocol design stage through to BIA and implementation, studies are co-designed to be more decision-relevant, scalable and methodologically robust.

23.5.4 Global Partnerships

The fourth pillar, global partnerships, leverages collective intelligence to accelerate progress. Formal alliances between global bodies like the World Organization of Family Doctors (WONCA) and the International Health Economics Association (iHEA) can broker south–south training and mentorship exchanges. At the same time, a commitment to open repositories for unit costs and PC-adapted HTA reference cases will improve methodological consistency and comparability across health systems.

23.6 Conclusion: A Practical Agenda for PC Value Creation

To translate the potential of health economics into tangible improvements in primary care, we propose a focused three-point agenda aligned with the three core domains. First, embed routine Domain-1 integration by ensuring that every major PC clinical trial or service re-design clearly states its analytical perspective, addresses uncertainty through deterministic and probabilistic sensitivity analysis, and reports ICERs alongside a BIA. Crucially, all findings should be mapped to the established goals of high-quality primary care, including access, continuity, person-centredness, coordination and comprehensiveness.

Second, pursue financing alignment (Domain-2) by requiring studies to explicitly describe and evaluate the payment rules, incentive structures and purchasing mechanisms that determine whether interventions are scalable and sustainable. Where feasible, this should incorporate Distributional CEA (DCEA) to illuminate effects on equity and financial protection.

Finally, install HTA at the front door (Domain-3) by adopting a PC-appropriate HTA reference case for diagnostics and digital tools, and by proactively planning for the de-implementation of low-value practices to reallocate resources efficiently. In short, value for money in primary care should be routine, auditable and decision-ready.

References

1. Khan HTA, Addo KM, Findlay H. Public health challenges and responses to the growing ageing populations. *Public Health Challenges*. 2024 Sep 21;3(3).
2. Colombo F, García-Goñi M, Schwierz C. Addressing multimorbidity to improve healthcare and economic sustainability. *J Comorb*. 2016 Jan 17;6(1):21–7.
3. Kumbhar ST, Bhatia M, Patel V. Health-care systems around the world: Diversity, challenges, and innovations. *Arch Med Health Sci*. 2025;13(1):95–9.
4. Mash R, Hirschhorn LR, Kakar IS, John R, Sharma M, Praveen D. Global lessons on delivery of primary healthcare services for people with non-communicable diseases: Convergent mixed methods. *Fam Med Community Health*. 2024;12(3):e002553.
5. World Health Organization. Building the economic case for primary health care: A scoping review; 2018.
6. World Health Organization. Strengthening primary health care as a key element towards achieving universal health coverage. In: Strengthening primary health care as a key element towards achieving universal health coverage; 2023.
7. Drummond M et al., Sculpher M, Claxton K, Stoddart G. Methods for the economic evaluation of health care programmes. Oxford:Oxford University Press; 2015.
8. Sanders GD, Neumann PJ, Basu A, Brock DW, Feeny D, Krahn M, et al. Recommendations for conduct, methodological practices, and reporting of cost-effectiveness analyses: Second panel on cost-effectiveness in health and medicine. *JAMA*. 2016;316(10):1093–103.
9. Manyazewal T. Using the World Health Organization health system building blocks through survey of healthcare professionals to determine the performance of public healthcare facilities. *Arch Public Health*. 2017;75:1–8.
10. Kloda LA, Boruff JT, Soares Cavalcante A. A comparison of patient, intervention, comparison, outcome (PICO) to a new, alternative clinical question framework for search skills, search results, and self-efficacy: A randomized controlled trial. *J Med Libr Assoc*. 2020 Apr 1;108(2).
11. Sanders GD, Neumann PJ, Basu A, Brock DW, Feeny D, Krahn M, et al. Recommendations for conduct, methodological practices, and reporting of cost-effectiveness analyses. *JAMA*. 2016 Sep 13;316(10):1093.
12. Anton CE. The activity based costing method applied to the analysis of the clients' profitability. *Series V—Econ Sci*. 2022 Jun 20;43–50.
13. Rajabi A, Dabiri A. Applying activity based costing (ABC) method to calculate cost price in hospital and remedy services. *Iran J Public Health*. 2012;41(4):100.
14. Špacírová Z, Epstein D, García-Mochón L, Rovira J, Olry de Labry Lima A, Espín J. A general framework for classifying costing methods for economic evaluation of health care. *Eur J Health Econ*. 2020 Jun 20;21(4):529–42.
15. Tatari P, Rezayatmand R, Nilchian F. Costs in dental care: A scoping review of methodologies and trends. *BMC Oral Health*. 2025 Oct 8;25(1):1571.
16. Laurence YV, Griffiths UK, Vassall A. Costs to health services and the patient of treating tuberculosis: A systematic literature review. *Pharmacoeconomics*. 2015;33(9):939–55.
17. Vassall A, Siapka M, Foster N, Cunnama L, Ramma L, Fielding K, et al. Cost-effectiveness of Xpert MTB/RIF for tuberculosis diagnosis in South Africa: A real-world cost analysis and economic evaluation. *Lancet Glob Health*. 2017;5(7):e710–9.

18. Shepard DS, Halasa-Rappel YA, Zeng W, Rowlands KR, Musange SF. Cost-effectiveness of expanding access to primary health care in rural rwanda by adding laboratory-equipped health posts: A prospective, controlled study. *Am J Trop Med Hyg.* 2023 May 3;108(5): 1042–51.
19. Chay J, Su RJ, Kamano JH, Andama B, Bloomfield GS, Delong AK, et al. Cost-effectiveness of group medical visits and microfinance interventions versus usual care to manage hypertension in Kenya: A secondary modelling analysis of data from the Bridging Income Generation with Group Integrated Care (BIGPIC) trial. *Lancet Glob Health.* 2024;12(8): e1331–42.
20. Petersohn S, Grimm SE, Ramaekers BLT, ten Cate-Hoek AJ, Joore MA. Exploring the feasibility of comprehensive uncertainty assessment in health economic modeling: A case study. *Value in Health.* 2021 Jul;24(7):983–94.
21. Limwattananon S. Handling uncertainty of the economic evaluation result: Sensitivity analysis. *J Med Assoc Thailand.* 2011;91(6):59.
22. Bae S, Lee J, Bae EY. How sensitive is sensitivity analysis? Evaluation of pharmacoeconomic submissions in Korea. *Front Pharmacol.* 2022 May 16;13.
23. Vreman RA, Geenen JW, Knies S, Mantel-Teeuwisse AK, Leufkens HGM, Goettsch WG. The application and implications of novel deterministic sensitivity analysis methods. *Pharmacoeconomics.* 2021 Jan 14;39(1):1–17.
24. Claxton K, Sculpher M, McCabe C, Briggs A, Akehurst R, Buxton M, et al. Probabilistic sensitivity analysis for NICE technology assessment: Not an optional extra. *Health Econ.* 2005 Apr;14(4):339–47.
25. Hatswell AJ, Bullement A, Briggs A, Paulden M, Stevenson MD. Probabilistic sensitivity analysis in cost-effectiveness models: Determining model convergence in cohort models. *Pharmacoeconomics.* 2018 Dec 27;36(12):1421–6.
26. Willke RJ, Pizzi LT. CHEERS to updated guidelines for reporting health economic evaluations! *Value in Health.* 2022;25(1):1–2.
27. Fayanju OM, Haukoos JS, Tseng JF. CHEERS reporting guidelines for economic evaluations. *JAMA Surg.* 2021;156(7):677–8.
28. Hanson K, Brikci N, Erlangga D, Alebachew A, De Allegri M, Balabanova D, et al. The Lancet Global Health Commission on financing primary health care: putting people at the centre. *Lancet Glob Health.* 2022 May;10(5):e715–72.
29. Glazier RH, Klein-Geltink J, Kopp A, Sibley LM. Capitation and enhanced fee-for-service models for primary care reform: A population-based evaluation. *Cmaj.* 2009;180(11): E72–81.
30. Vu T, Anderson KK, Devlin RA, Somé NH, Sarma S. Physician remuneration schemes, psychiatric hospitalizations and follow-up care: Evidence from blended fee-for-service and capitation models. *Soc Sci Med.* 2021;268:113465.
31. Chinkhumba J, De Allegri M, Brenner S, Muula A, Robberstad B. The cost-effectiveness of using results-based financing to reduce maternal and perinatal mortality in Malawi. *BMJ Glob Health.* 2020;5(5):e002260.
32. Das A, Gopalan SS, Chandramohan D. Effect of pay for performance to improve quality of maternal and child care in low-and middle-income countries: A systematic review. *BMC Public Health.* 2016;16(1):321.
33. Jamili S, Yousefi M, Pour HE, Houshmand E, Taghipour A, Tabatabaee SS, et al. Comparison of pay-for-performance (P4P) programs in primary care of selected countries: A comparative study. *BMC Health Serv Res.* 2023;23(1):865.
34. Asaria M, Griffin S, Cookson R. Distributional cost-effectiveness analysis: A tutorial. *Medical Decision Making.* 2016;36(1):8–19.
35. Cookson R, Griffin S, Norheim OF, Culyer AJ, Chalkidou K. Distributional cost-effectiveness analysis comes of age. *Value in Health.* 2021;24(1):118–20.

36. O'Rourke B, Oortwijn W, Schuller T. Announcing the new definition of health technology assessment. *Value in Health*. 2020;23(6):824–5.
37. O'Rourke B, Oortwijn W, Schuller T. The new definition of health technology assessment: A milestone in international collaboration. *Int J Technol Assess Health Care*. 2020 Jun 13;36(3):187–90.
38. Monahan M, Jowett S, Nickless A, Franssen M, Grant S, Greenfield S, et al. Cost-effectiveness of telemonitoring and self-monitoring of blood pressure for antihypertensive titration in primary care (TASMINH4). *Hypertension*. 2019;73(6):1231–9.
39. Clarke L, Anderson M, Anderson R, Klausen MB, Forman R, Kerns J, et al. Economic aspects of delivering primary care services: An evidence synthesis to inform policy and research priorities. *Milbank Q*. 2021 Dec 2;99(4):974–1023.
40. Choi T, Wallace SW, Wang Y. Big data analytics in operations management. *Prod Oper Manag*. 2018 Oct 1;27(10):1868–83.
41. PHCPI. Measuring primary health care performance | PHCPI [Internet]. PHCPI. 2018. [cited 29 Apr 2025; Available from: https://improvingphc.org/measuring-primary-health-care-performance]
42. Cassidy R, Singh NS, Schiratti PR, Semwanga A, Binyaruka P, Sachingongu N, et al. Mathematical modelling for health systems research: A systematic review of system dynamics and agent-based models. *BMC Health Serv Res*. 2019 Dec 19;19(1):845.
43. Or Z, Seppänen AV. The role of the health sector in tackling climate change: A narrative review. *Health Policy (New York)*. 2024 May;143:105053.
44. Martins FP, Paschoalotto MAC, Closs J, Bukowski M, Veras MM. The double burden: Climate change challenges for health systems. *Environ Health Insights*. 2024 Jan 20;18.

SECTION

5

Future Directions and Conclusions

CHAPTER

24

Capacity Building in Primary Care Research

Margarida Gil Conde and Paulo Jorge Nicola

24.1 Research Capacity Building

Research capacity building (RCB) is a structured process for developing the skills, resources and networks needed to conduct high-quality, sustainable research in primary health care (PHC). RCB is essential in family medicine, where evidence-based practice is critical to improving patient care, chronic disease management and health systems efficiency.[1–3]

Developing a strong research foundation in academic and non-academic family medicine has been a longstanding challenge, as research output falls behind other medical disciplines.[1–2] A key reason for this gap is the diverse and complex nature of PHC. Given this complexity, a 'one size fits all' approach to RCB is insufficient. Instead, multiple strategies are required to address the varying needs of researchers, institutions and healthcare systems.[2,4,5]

RCB operates on three levels:

Individual level: Enhancing and maintaining the research skills and competencies of PHC providers through training, mentorship and involvement in research projects.

Institutional level: Developing necessary infrastructure, securing funding and offering organisational support to sustain research activities.

Systemic level: Creating policies, networks and collaborations that strengthen research capacities.

RCB ensures that PHC professionals contribute to knowledge generation, influencing health policy and practice to improve patient outcomes.[5] To apply RCB principles effectively, two key approaches can be utilised:

1. *Top-down approach*: This involves institutional and policy-driven strategies such as providing protected research time, securing funding, recognising

DOI: 10.1201/9781003652106-29

research in career development, developing infrastructure and establishing research networks.

2. *Bottom-up approach*: This focuses on grassroots efforts, including training and mentorship programmes, networking opportunities, strategic communication and knowledge transfer mechanisms.

By consistently integrating both approaches and adopting long-term strategies, a supportive environment can be created, enabling PHC professionals to engage in impactful research, bridging the gap between research, policy and practice.

24.2 Strategies for a Top-Down Approach to RCB

24.2.1 Protected Time for Research, Career Development and Funding Support

Ensuring funding and protected research time is essential for RCB in PHC. Government and institutional support enable high-quality studies, training and infrastructure development, allowing researchers to strengthen networks, access specialised services and sustain impactful projects.[5,6] Protected research time helps reduce clinical workload, allowing PHC professionals to engage in research without compromising patient care. Structured institutional policies, career incentives and financial mechanisms such as grants and fellowships further encourage research involvement.[5–7]

Technological advancements, including artificial intelligence (AI), can support research by assisting with grant writing, data analysis and project management. However, AI should complement, not replace, dedicated funding and protected research time.[8]

Sustainable funding and institutional policies fostering research are particularly vital in low- and middle-income countries, where limited resources hinder research opportunities. A well-supported research environment drives innovation, improves patient care and informs health policy.[9,10] Examples include:

1. In the United Kingdom (UK), the Best Research for Best Health initiative provides protected time through funding mechanisms allowing general practitioners (GPs) to research.[4]
2. Australia's Primary Health Care Research, Evaluation and Development (PHCRED) Strategy provided funding to universities for training programmes, increasing PHC research capacity.[10]

Building a strong research infrastructure in PHC requires strategic investment in resources, personnel and technology. Leadership is essential for fostering research growth by supporting talent, identifying local strengths and gaps, and facilitating partnerships across communities, health systems and institutions.[5,11,12]

Essential infrastructure investments include research-optimised electronic medical records (EMRs) for high-quality data access, as well as financial and administrative structures such as grants management and auditing to sustain research efforts. Recruiting and retaining skilled researchers requires dedicated funding, mentorship and career development opportunities.[2,13]

Emerging technologies, including AI, can enhance research efficiency by assisting with data analysis, automating administrative tasks and improving patient recruitment. Although AI should complement traditional methods, it has the potential to streamline workflows and scale research initiatives.[8]

Integrating research into clinical practice includes promoting practice-based research networks (PBRNs), supporting data collection and engaging patients in study design. Flexible recruitment strategies and minimising disruptions to clinical workflows improve participation and feasibility. Prioritising infrastructure development alongside technological advancements can make PHC research more efficient, impactful and accessible, particularly in low- and middle-income countries[13–15] An example is Canada's Primary Care Research Institute facilitated access to big data for researchers, improving evidence generation.[2]

24.2.2 Network Implementation and Support

Building and supporting research networks in PHC requires a tailored approach that addresses the diverse needs of clinician-researchers. Strong leadership is crucial to allocating resources and fostering a research-friendly environment. Without this support, other capacity-building efforts may struggle to succeed.[16]

Institutions should assess their specific context before implementing research strategies. Smaller departments may prioritise collaborations, whereas larger ones can focus on structured infrastructure and dedicated research time. Multilevel networks integrating hospital care, long-term care and public health can improve research. Including stakeholders such as community agents, patient associations and local healthcare providers strengthens research relevance, quality and impact.[10,11,16]

By aligning support structures with the specific needs of clinician-researchers, institutions can create sustainable networks that encourage active participation, collaboration and the successful integration of research into PHC practice.[15] For example, the UK's National Institute for Health Research (NIHR) funded PBRNs to encourage collaborative primary care research.[15]

24.2.3 Developing Research Blueprints

Developing national strategies for RCB in PHC ensures a structured and context-specific approach to advancing research. These strategies should define clear research agendas aligned with local healthcare needs. Key components include targeted training programmes, the development of PBRNs and the transparent dissemination of findings to stakeholders.[10,16,17]

Research focusing on improving lower-quality care, increasing access and assessing innovations in real-world settings can add significant value. These strategies enhance the quality and impact of PHC research and strengthen its role in shaping healthcare policies and improving patient outcomes.[17,18] Canada has a blueprint for primary care research, which emphasises strategic priority setting and knowledge translation.[2]

24.3 Strategies for a Bottom-Up Approach to RCB

A bottom-up approach focuses on empowering individuals and institutions through training, mentorship and knowledge-sharing.

24.3.1 Training and Mentorship Programmes

Training and mentorship programmes are essential for RCB in PHC, particularly in low- and middle-income countries. By connecting junior researchers with experienced mentors, these programmes develop research skills and foster professional growth. Effective mentorship relies on mutual respect, clear communication and shared goals, ensuring meaningful engagement.[19]

Training in study design, data analysis, project management and knowledge translation equips researchers to address local health challenges. Mentorship provides personalised guidance, helping researchers navigate complex issues and disseminate findings effectively.[13]

Sustained integration of structured training and mentorship programmes will be key to developing a skilled research workforce in PHC. Strengthening these relationships ensures that future health leaders are prepared to tackle global health challenges.[12,20,21] One example is the TUTOR-PHC programme in Canada, which fosters transdisciplinary mentorship, improving research outputs among early-career researchers.[22]

24.3.2 Networking and Collaboration

Collaborations are vital to RCB in PHC. Partnerships among clinician-teachers, full-time researchers and PBRNs enable the integration of academic research with clinical practice. PBRNs, which unite PHC practices with researchers, allow practices to engage in relevant research that improves patient care and enhances the quality of PHC.[21]

Successful collaborations depend on dedicated and sustained support, including research staff, regular updates and effective communication. Interdisciplinary partnerships, driven by leadership committed to research, help address complex health challenges in PHC. These teams, composed of motivated individuals, benefit from mentorship and resources, ensuring that research aligns with clinical needs and is applied to improve care.[23–25] As collaborations continue to grow, they will drive impactful research and enhance the quality of PHC.[19,24] The Victorian PBRN in Australia connects academic researchers with PHC practitioners to enhance research relevance and implementation.[21]

24.3.3 Strategic Communication Interventions

Strategic communication is a strategy for engaging healthcare professionals in RCB. Grounded in theories such as social learning and diffusion of innovation, it leverages oral, written and digital channels to share information and drive positive changes in attitudes and practices. Effective communication interventions use these channels to sustain engagement with research and development (R&D) over time.

Research seminars, bulletins and digital platforms create a continuous flow of information, fostering an innovative mindset and long-term commitment to research. By integrating strategic communication, PHC can embed research into its identity and standards of excellence. Targeted strategies and ongoing follow-up help shape positive staff attitudes toward R&D, strengthening collaboration and supporting long-term RCB for improved patient outcomes.[26] For example, a strategic communication programme in Sweden successfully increased PHC professionals' engagement in research.[26]

24.4 Knowledge Transfer and Exchange (KTE)

KTE is useful for closing the gap between research and clinical practice. Family physicians should focus on identifying knowledge gaps and setting research priorities aligned with clinical needs. By involving patients and stakeholders, KTE ensures that research findings are relevant and actionable in practice.[17,18]

Engaging family physicians in RCB activities enables their active participation in research that directly influences patient care. This ongoing exchange of knowledge ensures that research is not only informative but also applicable in real-world clinical settings, ultimately enhancing healthcare outcomes.[2] An example is the CBPHC Signature Initiative in Canada, which facilitates knowledge translation through cross-jurisdictional research teams.[27]

24.5 Promoting Research Among Young General Practitioners

Encouraging young GPs to engage in research is vital for sustaining a research culture in PHC. Strategies include the following:

1 Incorporating Research in Medical Training

Research methodology can be integrated into family medicine residency programmes, such as in Canada's Family Medicine Forum emphasises research training in GP education.[28]

2 Supporting Small-Scale Research Projects

Micro-research initiatives can be encouraged, where trainees work on small, manageable projects, such as in the 6for6 programme in Canada, which offers structured research training for rural family physicians.[20]

3 Creating Research Career Pathways

Fellowships, grants and career progression opportunities can be provided for research-active GPs; for example, the UK's Designated Research Teams initiative funds early-career researchers to develop their research skills.[4]

4 Fostering International Collaboration

Young GPs can be connected with international research networks, such as the AfriWon Renaissance programme within WONCA, which provides mentorship and networking opportunities for young PHC researchers in Africa.[19]

24.6 Future Directions

Future strategies for RCB in PHC should focus on sustainability, equity and adaptability. Local research diversity is a strength, especially when implementation is monitored, best practices are identified and lessons are widely shared. Academic institutions, scientific societies and public agencies play a crucial role in evaluating current strategies and fostering capacity development at individual, institutional and systemic levels.

Despite its unique challenges, PHC research capacity benefits from collaboration with academic centres, research institutes, contract research organisations, public health bodies and hospital-based research units. Coordinated efforts across these entities can enhance the impact of RCB initiatives.

Further studies are needed to assess the influence of policies, organisational models and evolving clinical practice on PHC research capacity. Balancing top-down support with bottom-up initiatives will be key to driving meaningful healthcare improvements and shaping evidence-based policies globally.

References

1. Gil Conde M, Costa I, Silvério Serra S, Ramos RC, Ribeiro C, Broeiro-Goncalves P, et al. Strategies for research capacity building by family physicians in primary healthcare: A scoping review protocol. *BMJ Open*. 2024;14(2).
2. Fortin M, Pereira J, Hutchison B, Ramsden VR, Menear M, Snelgrove D. Nurturing a culture of curiosity in family medicine and primary care: The section of researchers' blueprint 2 (2018–2023). *Can Fam Physician*. 2021;167(5):333.
3. Wangler J, Jansky M. Primary care involvement in clinical research—prerequisites, motivators, and barriers: Results from a study series. *Arch Public Health*. 2024 Dec 1;82(1).
4. Cooke J, Nancarrow S, Dyas J, Williams M. An evaluation of the "Designated Research Team" approach to building research capacity in primary care. *BMC Fam Pract*. 2008;9.
5. Morgado MB, Rodrigues V, Carmona Ramos R, Rente A, Nicola P, Gil Conde M. Strategies for the promotion of primary health care research in Portugal: A qualitative study. *Acta Med Port*. 2024 Feb 1;37(2):110–8.
6. Huas C, Petek D, Diaz E, Mu-Noz-Perez MA, Torzsa P, Collins C. Strategies to improve research capacity across European general practice: The views of members of EGPRN and WONCA Europe. https://doi.org/10.1080/13814788.2018.1546282
7. Collins C, EGPRN Strategy Authorship Group. The EGPRN research strategy for general practice in Europe. *Eur J Gen Pract*. 2022 Dec;28(1):136–141. https://doi.org/10.1080/13814788.2022.2080815

8. Bajwa J, Munir U, Nori A, Williams B. Artificial intelligence in healthcare: Transforming the practice of medicine. *Future Healthc J.* 2021 Jul;8(2):e188.
9. Westfall JM, Wittenberg HR, Liaw W. Time to invest in primary care research—commentary on findings from an independent congressionally mandated study. *J Gen Intern Med.* 2021;36(7):2117–20.
10. Brown LJ, McIntyre EL. The contribution of primary health care research, evaluation and development-supported research to primary health care policy and practice. *Aust J Prim Health.* 2014;20(1):47–55.
11. Kuzel A, James P. Research development stories from 7 departments of family medicine: 7 lessons for all departments. *Ann Fam Med.* 2011;9(4):373–4.
12. Girard A, Dugas M, Lépine J, Carnovale V, Jalbert L, Turmel A, et al. Strategies to engage family physicians in primary care research: A systematic review. *J Eval Clin Pract.* 2023 Feb 1;29(1):233–49.
13. Ponka D, Coffman M, Fraser-Barclay KE, Fortier RDW, Howe A, Kidd M, et al. Fostering global primary care research: A capacity-building approach. *BMJ Glob Health.* 2020 Jul 5;5(7).
14. Van Royen P, Beyer M, Chevallier P, Eilat-Tsanani S, Lionis C, Peremans L, et al. Series: The research agenda for general practice/family medicine and primary health care in Europe. Part 6: Reaction on commentaries—how to continue with the Research Agenda? *Eur J Gen Pract.* 2011 Mar;17(1):58–61.
15. Ryan BL, Thorpe C, Zwarenstein M, Wickett J, Talukdar N, Boisvert L, et al. Building research culture and capacity in academic family medicine departments. *Can Fam Physician.* 2019;65(1):E38–44.
16. Bonfim D, Belotti L, de Almeida LY, Eshriqui I, Velasco SRM, Monteiro CN, et al. Challenges and strategies for conducting research in primary health care practice: An integrative review. *BMC Health Serv Res.* 2023 Dec 1;23(1).
17. Diaz E, Petek D, Tatsioni A, Eliat-tsanani S, Lingner H, Assenova R, et al. Research strategies for General Practice in Europe. EGPRN. Oct 2021.
18. Collins C. The EGPRN research strategy for general practice in Europe. *Eur J Gen Pract.* 2022;28(1):136–41.
19. McGuire CM, Fatusin BB, Kodicherla H, Yakubu K, Ameh P, Van Waes A, et al. Implementation of online research training and mentorship for sub-saharan African family physicians. *Ann Glob Health* 2021;87(1):13.
20. McCarthy P, Bethune C, Fitzgerald S, Graham W, Asghari S, Heeley T, et al. Curriculum development of 6for6: Longitudinal research skills program for rural and remote family physicians. *Can Fam Physician.* 2016 Feb 1;62(2):e89.
21. Soós M, Temple-Smith M, Gunn J, Johnston-Ata'ata K, Pirotta M. Establishing the Victorian primary care practice based research network. *Aust Fam Physician.* 2010;39.
22. Nicholson K, Ganann R, Bookey-Bassett S, Garland Baird L, Garnett A, Marshall Z, et al. Capacity building and mentorship among pan-Canadian early career researchers in community-based primary health care. *Prim Health Care Res Dev.* 2020;21.
23. Elliott-Rudder M. Researcher networking drives change: An autoenthnographic narrative analysis from medical graduate to primary health researcher. *Aust J Prim Health.* 2010;16(1):108–15.
24. Rortveit G. Research networks in primary care: An answer to the call for better clinical research. *Scand J Prim Health Care.* 2014 Sep 1;32(3):107–9.
25. Foy R, Eccles M. Structured career pathways in academic primary care. *Fam Pract.* 2008 Feb;25(1):63–7.
26. Morténius H. Creating an interest in research and development as a means of reducing the gap between theory and practice in primary care: An interventional study based on strategic communication. *Int J Environ Res Public Health.* 2014 Aug 26;11(9):8689–708.

27. Wong ST, Langton JM, Katz A, Fortin M, Godwin M, Green M, et al. Promoting cross-jurisdictional primary health care research: Developing a set of common indicators across 12 community-based primary health care teams in Canada. *Prim Health Care Res Dev.* 2018;20:e7.
28. Archibald D, Hogg W, Lemelin J, Dahrouge S, St. Jean M, Boucher F. Building capacity for medical education research in family medicine: The Program for Innovation in Medical Education (PIME). *Health Res Policy Syst.* 2017 Oct 23;15(1).

CHAPTER

25

Charting the Path Ahead for Primary Care Research

Mehmet Akman, Bob Mash and Felicity Goodyear-Smith

Primary care research is entering an era defined by complexity, rapid technological change and global interdependence. The chapters in this book collectively underscore that the future of primary care can no longer be shaped by incremental adjustments to traditional models. Primary care is now expected to respond to multimorbidity, persistent inequities, rapid digital change and environmental threats, while remaining anchored in person-centred, continuous care. What is required is bold, systemic transformation grounded in evidence, equity and innovation.

Across very different topics presented in this book, the authors meet on a shared point: the future of primary care research will be shaped as much by how we produce evidence as by what we study. Better questions, stronger methods, richer partnerships and clearer routes from findings to action are all needed if research is to support primary care systems that are effective, equitable and sustainable.

25.1 Emerging Methodologies: Expanding the Research Toolkit

The methodological landscape described in this book reflects an important shift. Primary care is a setting where people live with multiple conditions, where care is delivered by teams, and where outcomes are shaped by context and time. As a result, the field is moving away from method-as-identity and towards method as-fit: selecting designs that match the question, the setting and the decisions that need to be made.

Two particularly exciting developments illustrate the creative directions primary care research is taking. The first is platform trials. Traditional randomised controlled trials often struggle to address the complexity of primary care. Platform trials offer a flexible, adaptive design that allows multiple interventions to be tested simultaneously under a single protocol. This approach accelerates evidence generation, reduces costs and reflects real-world diversity, making it ideal for chronic disease management and implementation research.

DOI: 10.1201/9781003652106-30

Secondly, beyond numbers and charts, arts-based research methods, such as narrative inquiry, photovoice and creative expression, bring the human experience of health and illness to the forefront. These approaches deepen understanding of patient perspectives, foster engagement with marginalised communities and generate insights that complement traditional methodologies. They remind us that healthcare is not only a science but also a profoundly human endeavour.

Additionally, routinely collected data, such as electronic health records, registries and linked datasets, are now central to much of this work. Used well, they can support population-level surveillance, target inequities and enable learning over time. Used poorly, they can generate false certainty. This book therefore emphasises the careful definition of exposures and outcomes, attention to missingness and bias, transparent analytic choices, and interpretability for clinicians, policymakers and communities.

25.2 Key Themes for the Future

25.2.1 The Person and Community at the Centre

There are several critical and key actions for the next decade. Firstly, we must embrace complexity and tailor to context. Health systems are dynamic, and primary care operates at the intersection of biological, social and environmental determinants. Research must move beyond reductionist approaches to embrace complexity science, mixed methods and longitudinal designs that reflect real-world conditions. A consistent thread throughout the book is the need to treat people not as 'cases' but as partners living within families, communities and wider social conditions. Research that privileges what matters to patients (function, participation, quality of life, treatment burden and meaningful outcomes) will be more aligned with primary care's core purpose than research that is focused narrowly on disease-specific endpoints. This emphasis also requires a stronger commitment to equity. Studies that ignore social determinants risk reproducing the very disparities primary care is asked to reduce. Future work should routinely consider deprivation, migration, gender, racism, disability and rurality, and should include methods that support meaningful engagement with communities, including co-design and community-based participatory approaches where appropriate.

This approach means treating equity as a core outcome—measuring who benefits, who is left behind, and why. Health equity is not a peripheral concern; it is central to the legitimacy and impact of primary care research. It is essential that we build research capacity in low- and middle-income countries, address systemic racism and co-design interventions with communities.

25.2.2 Services as Systems and Resilience as a Capability

Primary care rarely operates as a single intervention delivered in isolation. It is a system of access points, relationships, information flows and decisions made under uncertainty. The chapters point towards system-aware research, such as realist evaluation, complexity-informed approaches and modelling to understand how services function across settings and over time.

Resilience emerges as a practical capability rather than a slogan: the ability of teams and organisations to adapt, learn and maintain quality when faced with shocks and long-term pressures. Research that measures and explains resilience through workforce dynamics, continuity, teamwork, coordination and learning routines can help decision-makers move from short-term fixes to sustained system strengthening.

25.2.3 Digital Tools, Big Data and AI

Digital tools, artificial intelligence and big data environments are now integral to primary care research, from telehealth and remote monitoring to decision support and data linkage. They provide an opportunity for a more timely measurement, better reach to underserved groups, and a closer connection between care processes and outcomes, yielding more precision and efficiency.

However, we must harness technology responsibly. These tools must be deployed ethically, transparently and inclusively to avoid widening disparities. Responsible innovation frameworks and participatory approaches will be essential. New technologies should be evaluated with the same seriousness as for any clinical or service intervention: clear theories of change, attention to unintended consequences, careful assessment of bias and fairness, and transparent reporting. Where AI is used, its role should be to support clinical judgement and patient choice, not to replace them. Governance, privacy and accountability are conditions for legitimacy rather than an option.

25.2.4 Genomics, Health Economics and Planetary Health as Mainstream Concerns

The scope of primary care research is widening. Genomics and precision approaches will increasingly influence risk assessment and treatment decisions, but they must be studied in ways that fit primary care's ethical and practical realities, including consent, communication, uncertainty and equity of access. Health economics is equally central. With constrained resources, primary care needs evidence not only of effectiveness but also of value, opportunity costs and distributional impact. Finally, planetary health is no longer peripheral: climate-related events, air quality, heat stress and ecological change affect morbidity patterns and service demand.

Climate change and environmental degradation are reshaping health risks. Primary care research must integrate planetary health principles, developing models that are resilient, sustainable and responsive to ecological realities.

25.2.5 Transdisciplinary and Interprofessional Collaboration

The challenges ahead cannot be solved within disciplinary silos. Many of the book's strongest examples involve collaboration across professional and disciplinary boundaries: family doctors, nurses, pharmacists, allied health professionals, public health practitioners, social scientists, economists and data specialists working together. Partnerships across primary care teams, population health, medicine, social sciences, engineering and the arts, alongside patients and communities, will generate richer insights and more impactful solutions.

The barriers are also familiar: differences in language and epistemology, misaligned incentives, unequal authority and limited time. Future research programmes will need deliberate structures for collaboration, shared governance, clarity on roles, fair recognition of contributions and investment in team development, so that 'interprofessional' becomes a working practice rather than a label.

25.2.6 Capacity Building and Advocacy for Primary Care Research as a Community Asset

The future of primary care research demands courage: to question entrenched paradigms, to innovate responsibly and to prioritise relevance over convenience. It calls for investment in infrastructure, capacity building and global collaboration. Above all, it requires a commitment to research that serves people, not just systems, by addressing the determinants of health and amplifying the voices of those most affected. Approaching primary care research as a community asset will strengthen care for whole populations, enable fair allocation of resources and support health systems under pressure. Realising this public value depends on sustained capacity building: protected time for clinicians and teams, stable infrastructure in academic and service settings, mentorship pathways and funding mechanisms that recognise the long time-horizons of system change.

Capacity is not only technical; it is also institutional and political. Primary care research often remains under-funded relative to its system importance, and it is frequently assessed using criteria designed for hospital-based or laboratory science. Strong advocacy is needed to persuade universities, funders and governments that rigorous primary care research delivers measurable benefits in access, continuity, quality, equity and cost, and that long-term investment is therefore justified.

25.3 Final Remarks

High-quality primary care research depends on methodological integrity and transparent reporting. This means defining concepts and outcomes clearly. It also means addressing bias, confounding and missing data openly. Evidence should also be built for implementation and improvement. Working with service leaders, frontline teams and communities helps keep questions practical and outcomes meaningful. Embedding evaluation in quality improvement cycles and using mixed methods to understand context can speed translation into better care. Implementation is therefore part of good research design, not a separate final step.

Taken together, the chapters in this book argue for a confident, pragmatic and values-driven future for primary care research. Welcoming methodological innovation is crucial, but it must also protect the qualities that make primary care distinctive: its commitment to relationships, context, continuity and whole-person care. As we look forward, this book offers not only a roadmap for primary care research but also an invitation: to reimagine primary care research as a driver of health equity, resilience and human flourishing in an uncertain world.

Index

Note: Page numbers in *italics* indicate a figure and page numbers in **bold** indicate a table on the corresponding page.

Q

For Product Safety Concerns and Information please contact our EU representative GPSR@taylorandfrancis.com
Taylor & Francis Verlag GmbH, Kaufingerstraße 24, 80331 München, Germany

www.ingramcontent.com/pod-product-compliance
Lightning Source LLC
LaVergne TN
LVHW081316110826
845149LV00006B/1517

* 9 7 8 1 0 4 1 0 9 8 5 0 8 *